主编 陈月明

精繪中華本草

百〇八歲叟馬識途

科学出版社
北京

内 容 简 介

生物科学绘画是以客观还原生物本身的形态、生境等为主要描绘对象的一种艺术表现形式。由于其描绘对象的真实性，需要绘画者以科学性为准绳，以艺术性为追求，从科学的视角审视自然界万物生灵，通过恰当的表现形式精准地表现在画纸上，达到科学性与艺术性的有机结合。

陈月明教授在近60年的生物科学画创作中，经过不断的探索和创新，形成了在客观表现本体形态的同时、融合我国传统绘画技法的富有中国特色的艺术风格。

本书精选收录了陈月明教授自1975年至2022年以多种绘画技法创作的129幅具有代表性的药用植物科学画，并对这些药用植物的基源、形态特征、生境分布、采收加工、性味功能、主治用法、化学成分等内容配以中、英文介绍，以方便读者参考。

本书集专业性、艺术性、科普性为一体，值得广大中医药工作者、生物科学绘画从业者及博物学爱好者品读和收藏。

图书在版编目（CIP）数据

精绘中华本草 / 陈月明主编. — 北京：科学出版社，2023.1
ISBN 978-7-03-073834-9

Ⅰ.①精… Ⅱ.①陈… Ⅲ.①本草—中国—图集 Ⅳ.①R281.3-64

中国版本图书馆CIP数据核字(2022)第220740号

责任编辑：刘　亚 / 责任校对：申晓焕
责任印制：赵　博 / 装帧设计：李荣刚　刘文建　李　德

科学出版社 出版
北京东黄城根北街16号
邮政编码：100717
http://www.sciencep.com

北京市金木堂数码科技有限公司 印刷

科学出版社发行　各地新华书店经销

*

2023年1月第　一　版　　开本：889 × 1194　1/16
2024年5月第二次印刷　　印张：19 1/2
字数：365 000

定价：298.00元

（如有印装质量问题，我社负责调换）

主编简介

陈月明(1933年—)，浙江新昌人。就职于中国医学科学院药用植物研究所。中国植物学会植物科学画专业委员会委员。1955年绍兴师范肄业，后曾进修于首都师范大学美术系，并师从中国科学院文联副主席、美协主席中国科学院植物研究所冯晋庸先生。从事药用植物科学画50多年，先后参加《江西中草药》《常用中草药》的绘图工作。在《全国中草药汇编》和《中药志》中任编委（以上两书均于1978年获全国科学大会奖）。在《原色中国本草图鉴》1至8册中任编委。并参加《中国药用植物栽培学》及农业出版社出版的《农业大全》的绘图，参加世界卫生组织主编的《世界常用药用植物指南》等著作的绘图与编辑工作。主编《中华本草彩色图典》（英文精华版）。

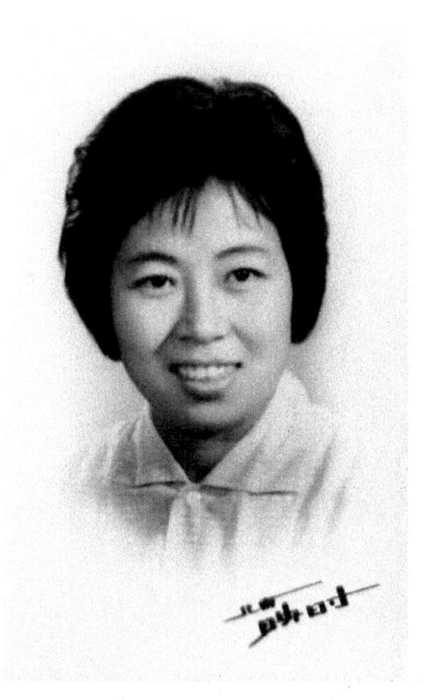

摄于1956年

1991年应美国加州世界生命研究所所长布鲁斯先生的邀请赴美，为该所完成 *Chinese Adaptogenic Nutritional Therapy for Radiation Sickness in Preparation* 和 *Chinese Materia Medica in Preparation* 两书的绘图工作。

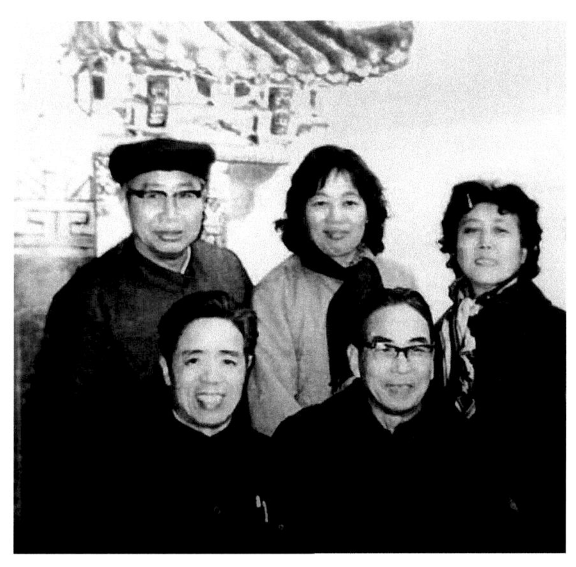

陈月明（后排中）与导师冯晋庸先生（后排左一）1984年摄于昆明

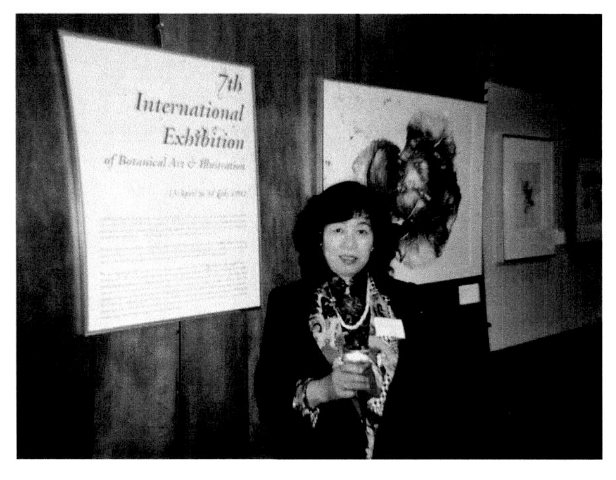

摄于 1992 年

1992 年 4 月参加在美国匹兹堡大学举办的第七届国际植物画展，作品《毛瓣绿绒蒿》被该大学收藏。同年 8 月美国加州圣贝纳迪诺市（San Bernardino, California）政府在该市的市政厅为其个人举办药用植物科学画画展，展出期的一切费用均由该市的市政府承担。当时在美国政府限制中草药使用的情况下，在美国却为中国的一位植物科学画画家举办“药用植物科学画画展”，这在美国是前所未有的。我国卫生部前部长钱信忠亲笔题词“妙笔生花”致贺。同年 9 月又被邀请参加美国洛杉矶师范学院画展，该市市长亲自在市长办公室为其颁授荣誉市民证书。

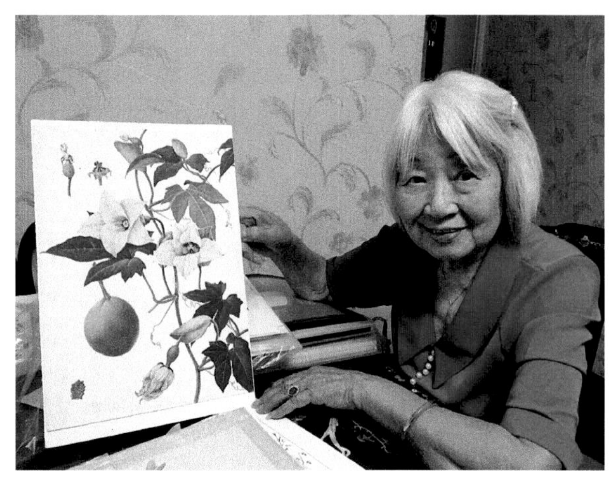

摄于 2019 年

1997 年应邀参加韩国顺天大学举办的画展，作品《朝鲜白头翁》被顺天大学校长收藏。在澳大利亚悉尼召开的第十三届植物画展中，作品《白头翁》获奖。《番红花》等多幅作品被外国友人收藏。她的植物科学画作品在国内外画展上多次获得最佳作品或优秀作品奖。

INTRODUCTION TO THE EDITOR IN CHIEF

Chen Yueming (1933—) was born in Xinchang County, Zhejiang Province. Professional plant scientific illustrator of the Institute of Medicinal Plant Development, Chinese Academy of Medical Sciences. Member of Botanical Scientific Illustration Committee of the Botanical Society of China. After studying in Shaoxing Normal School in1955, Professor Chen engaged in advanced studies in the School of Art, Capital Normal University and was taught by Mr. Feng Jinyong, the senior engineer of the Institute of Botany, Chinese Academy of Sciences, who was also the Vice chairman of the Federation of Literary and Art Circles, as well as the Chairman of the Art association, Chinese Academy of Sciences. Professor Chen was engaged in the field of medicinal plant scientific illustration for more than 50 years, participated in the illustration work in *Chinese Herbal Medicine in Jiangxi Province, Commonly Used Chinese Herbal Medicine*, worked as editorial board member of *Glossary of Chinese Herbal Medicine, Chinese Materia Medica* (Both of these books won the 1978 National Science and Technology Conference Award). Editorial board member of *Illustrated Atlas of Chinese Materia Medica, Volume 1-8*. She also participated in the illustration work of *Cultivation of Chinese Medicinal Plants*, and *Complete Book of Agriculture* published by Agriculture Press. Participated in the illustration and editing work of *Guide to Commonly Used Medicinal Plants in the World* edited by the World Health Organization. She is the Editor in Chief of *A Concise Illustrated Atlas of Chinese Materia Medica (English edition)*.

In 1991, she completed the illustration works of two books of *Chinese Adaptogenic Nutritional Therapy for Radiation Sickness in Preparation* and *Chinese Materia in Preparation* in the United States at the invitation of Bruce, Director of the World Life Institute in California, the United States.

In April 1992, she participated in the 7th International Botanical Illustration Exhibition held in the University of Pittsburgh, the United States, and the work of *Meconopsis torquata* was collected by the host University of Pittsburgh. In August 1992, she held an personal exhibition of her scientific illustrations of medicinal plants at the invitation of the government of San Bernardino, California. The exhibition was held in the municipal government of San Bernardino, and all expenses for the exhibition period were covered by the municipal government. At that time, Chinese herbal medicine was not allowed to treat patients under the strict control of the American government. However, it was unprecedented to hold an "exhibition of scientific illustrations of medicinal plants" in America for a Chinese painter of plant scientific illustration. Mr. Qian Xinzhong, former minister of the Ministry of Health of China, wrote a congratulatory inscription "Miao Bi Sheng Hua" (a Chinese idiom, meaning the wonderful painting that shows the soul of flower). In September 1992, she participated in the exhibition of paintings at the Normal College of Los Angeles, and was awarded the certificate of Honorary Citizen presented by the mayor of the city personally in the mayor's office.

In 1997, she participated in the exhibition of paintings held by Suncheon University, Korea, and the work "*Pulsatilla koreana*" was collected by the president of Suncheon University. At the 13th International Botanical Illustration Exhibition held in Sydney, Australia, her work "*Pulsatilla chinensis*" won the prize. Many of her works such as "*Crocus sativus*" were collected by international friends.Her plant scientific illustrations have won best or outstanding awards both domestically and internationally.

编辑委员会

顾　问

肖培根

主　编

陈月明

副主编

彭　勇　赵鑫磊

主　审

赵中振

编　委

（按汉语拼音音序排序）

陈月明　何春年　彭　勇　齐加力［美国］　荣念赫

宋沅燮［韩国］　谭　芳　谭晓蕾　赵鑫磊

主编单位

中国医学科学院
北京协和医学院
药用植物研究所

SCIENTIFIC ILLUSTRATIONS OF CHINESE MEDICINAL PLANTS

Editorial Committee

Consultant

Xiao Peigen

Editor in Chief

Chen Yueming

Associate Editors

Peng Yong, Zhao Xinlei

Chief Reviewer

Zhao Zhongzhen

Editorial Committee Members(Sorted according to Chinese pinyin)

Chen Yueming He Chunnian Peng Yong Elizabeth R Qi (USA) Rong Nianhe Song Won-Seob (Korea) Tan Fang Tan Xiaolei Zhao Xinlei

Edited by

The Institute of Medicinal Plant Development(IMPLAD),

Chinese Academy of Medical Sciences(CAMC) & Peking Union Medical College(PUMC)

序　一

在植物学和中药学研究领域，植物科学画是非常重要的基础研究资料，其意义是科学且精准地反映植物的形态特征，植物采集家们在野外采集回来压制干燥的腊叶标本失去了生活状态下的鲜艳颜色和立体质感，这些标本经过植物科学画家的整体构思，融合科学和美学、技术和艺术，在画纸上还原了植物的鲜活状态，换而言之，植物科学画就是新鲜植物的标准画像。

日前，陈月明教授带着即将付梓的《精绘中华本草》一书的样书和植物科学画作的原稿到我家交流，经陈教授系统地介绍，我了解到此书的构思和创作历程，为了追求科学性和艺术美，陈教授从采集标本到亲自栽培，不断观察，数易其稿，我对鲐背之年依然从事植物科学画创作的陈教授表示由衷敬佩。书中精选出 129 幅绘制精美的药用植物科学画作，并从植物形态、药用价值、功效应用、化学成分等方面给出了简要的介绍，这使我更为感叹我国植物区系实在是太丰富、太复杂了，药用植物的宝贵价值值得深入挖掘。在翻看样书时，让我震撼的是书中绘制的药用植物栩栩如生，有些植物还绘制有生境，翻看这些带有生境的画作原稿时，更为之惊艳，仿佛身临其境，这些植物就在眼前一般触手可及。

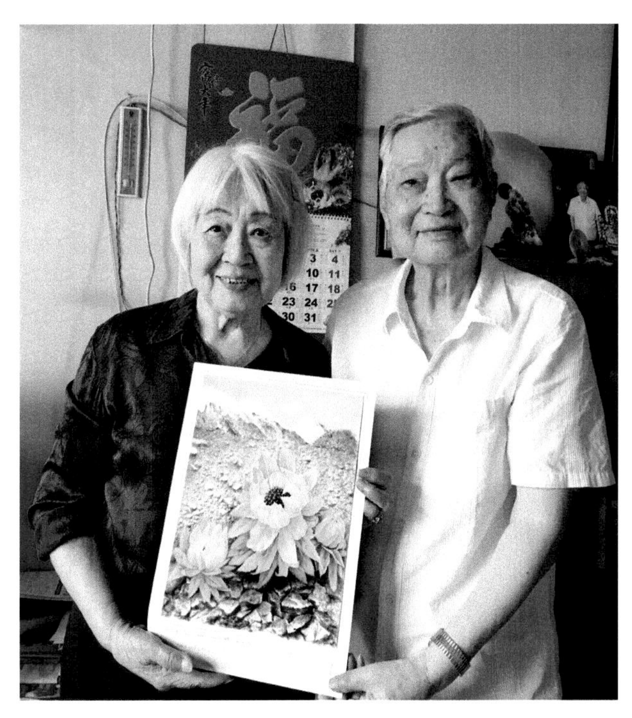

陈月明教授与王文采院士的合影

时光荏苒，陈月明教授与我相识已有半个世纪之久，多年前，

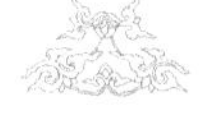

我到中国医学科学院药用植物研究所标本馆鉴定标本，彼时，即经常见到陈教授对着标本或是新鲜的植物埋头绘制植物科学画，陈教授丰富的野外考察写生经历和不断摸索创作的过程为植物科学画提供了丰富的素材，通过对中国传统绘画和西方现代科学绘画技法的融合和创新，也已形成了独树一帜的艺术风格。

端看这些画作时，我不禁想到中国近代植物学研究已有百年历史，取得了很大的成就，《中国高等植物图鉴》《中国植物志》等著作都离不开植物科学画家的辛勤劳动，植物科学绘画为中国的植物科学研究和国民经济发展，做出了巨大的贡献。遗憾的是，在《中国植物志》全书出版后，植物分类学的研究已有没落趋势，随之植物科学绘画的发展也陷入低谷，近些年，博物学逐渐兴起，植物科学画又有所发展，在科普和艺术领域焕发了新的生机，中国有大批优秀的植物科学画作品，有关部门应当有计划地收集、整理、保存和展示，这对于宣传科学文化有重要意义。

陈月明教授领衔的药学专家团队编著的《精绘中华本草》科学性与艺术性兼备，我对此书的完成表示衷心祝贺，希望它早日问世，供国内外药学家、植物学家和大众参考应用。

中国科学院　院士

中国科学院植物研究所　研究员　王文采

2021 年 6 月 15 日

本书即将付梓之际，惊悉王文采院士驾鹤西去，深感震惊与悲痛。回忆起自 20 世纪 60 年代认识王先生之始，半个多世纪以来，我一直得到他的指导与帮助。在本书编研期间，也数次得到王先生的鼓励与教诲，尤其他在病中依然关心本书的进展并亲题序言。而今天人永隔，回忆起王先生的音容笑貌，历历在目，我无比痛心遗憾。谨以此书，向最敬爱的王文采先生表示我的怀念与敬意，我也谨记王先生的教诲，愿将我的余生贡献给我国药用植物科学画事业的发展。先生之风，山高水长，深切缅怀王文采先生！先生千古！（陈月明于 2022 年 11 月 16 日）

Preface 1

In the research field of Botany and Chinese Materia Medica, the botanical scientific illustration is one of the most important basic research materials, which is of great significance to reflect the morphological characteristics of plants scientifically and accurately. The plants collected from the field have been pressed to dried herbariums, which had lost the vibrant color and three-dimensional texture in their living state. Through the overall conception as well as the convergence of science and aesthetics, technology and art by those botanical scientific illustrators, the herbariums have been restored to their vivid state of the plant on the drawing paper. In other words, the botanical scientific illustration is the standard portrait of the fresh plant.

A few days ago, Professor Chen Yueming brought a sample book of the upcoming *Scientific Illustrations of Chinese Medicinal Plants* and the original manuscripts of botanical scientific illustration to my house. After the systematic introduction from Professor Chen, I learned about the conception and creation journey of this book. In order to pursue scientific and artistic beauty, Professor Chen continued observing from collecting to cultivating the specimens by herself, and recreating the drafts many times. I would express my sincere admiration to Professor Chen who is still engaged in botanical scientific illustration in her old age. The book selects 129 beautifully drawn scientific illustrations of medicinal plants, and gives a brief introduction from the aspects of plant form, medicinal value, efficacy application, chemical constituents, etc., which makes me even more amazed that the Chinese Flora is that rich and complicated, and the precious value of medicinal plants is of that great worth. When looking at the sample book, I was shocked that the medicinal plants drawn in the book were that lifelike, and some plants were also painted togetherly with their habitats, which makes the plants generally within reach.

Time flies, Professor Chen and I have known each other for half a century. Many years ago, I went to The Institute of Medicinal Plant Development (IMPLAD) to identify the specimens (IMD). At that time, I often saw Professor Chen immersing herself in drawing botanical scientific illustrations in front of the specimens or fresh plants. Professor Chen's rich fieldwork, sketching experience and constant exploration and creation have provided rich materials for botanical scientific illustration. Through her integration and innovation of traditional Chinese painting and western modern scientific painting techniques, Professor Chen has formed her unique artistic style.

When looking at these paintings, I can't help thinking that modern Chinese botany research has had a history of a hundred years and has made great achievements. Books such as *Iconographia Cormophytorum Sinicorum* and *Flora Reipublicae Popularis Sinicae* are all inseparable from the hard work of experts on botanical scientific illustration. Botanical scientific illustration have made great contributions to China's plant scientific research and national economic development. Regrettably, after the publication of *Flora Reipublicae Popularis Sinicae*, the study of plant taxonomy has tended to decline, and the development of botanical scientific illustration has also hit a low point. In recent years, with the gradual rise of natural history and the development of botanical scientific illustration, botanical scientific illustration has gained new vitality in the field of popular science and art. China has a large number of excellent works of botanical scientific illustration, and relevant departments should collect, organize, preserve and display them in a planned way, which is of great significance for the promotion of scientific culture.

Scientific Illustrations of Chinese Medicinal Plants edited by a team of pharmaceutical experts led by Professor Chen is of both scientific and artistic value. I would like to express my heartfelt congratulations on the completion of this book for the reference of domestic and foreign pharmacists, botanists and the public.

Wen-Tsai Wang

Academician, Chinese Academy of Sciences

Professor, Institute of Botany, Chinese Academy of Sciences

June 15, 2021

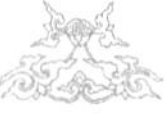

序　二

《精绘中华本草》，顾名思义，即将中国本草用绘画这种艺术形式精细完美地呈现在读者面前。植物科学画对艺术性和科学性都有较高的要求，而这方面的人才稀缺。

我与陈月明教授共事多年，20 世纪 60 年代，国家开展了轰轰烈烈的中药资源普查。应国家之需，陈教授做了大量的绘图工作。1983 年，陈教授在我力邀之下调入新成立的中国医学科学院药用植物研究所（原名为药用植物资源开发研究所），专职从事植物科学画的工作。在我进行乌头属 *Aconitum* 药用植物亲缘学的研究过程中，陈教授绘制的北乌头 *Aconitum kusnezoffii*、工布乌头 *Aconitum kongboense* 等精美的植物科学画为我的研究增色添彩。陈教授所绘制的多幅画作也被世界卫生组织和美国匹兹堡大学等知名机构收藏。

陈教授绘画功底深厚，虚心好学，勤于实践。年轻时深入山林旷野，反复观察植物形态，采集标本，掌握第一手资料；年迈仍不辍耕耘，委托年轻的团队在野外采集标本，拍摄照片，为新作品的诞生提供色彩的考量与科学上的支持，对画作的科学性一丝不苟。我了解到，她为了绘制提取青蒿素的原植物黄花蒿 *Artemisia annua*，托人采到幼苗，种植在家中的花盆里，精心呵护，仔细观察，从幼苗展叶到开花结果，记录每时每刻的变化，这样的科学精神和对绘画精益求精的态度令人钦佩。几十年来，陈

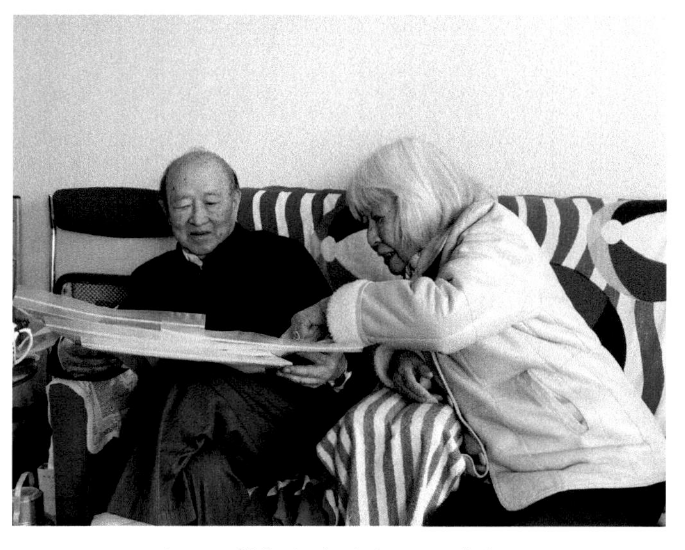

陈月明教授与肖培根院士的合影

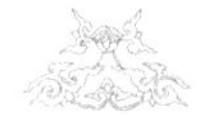

教授为教学与科研创作了大量科学性和艺术性兼俱的药用植物科学画，成为该领域不可多得的人才。

我曾力主陈教授将毕生作品编辑出版，呈现于社会，服务于中医药科学。不久前陈教授带着样稿和出版计划来我家交流征求意见，我甚感欣慰。陈教授带领团队即将出版的《精绘中华本草》将植物科学绘画的技艺和现代科学研究很好地结合，对继承和弘扬中医药事业有重要意义，为中医药的现代化和国际化添砖加瓦，实为可喜可贺之事！书中精美的植物科学画必将成为海内外读者手中极具观赏和收藏价值的珍本。此外，如此精美的植物科学画作品不仅会在植物科学画界和中医药研究者中产生重要影响，更会在大众科普和中小学中医药科普教育中做出更大的贡献。希望未来陈教授及其团队砥砺前行，精诚合作，以此书为蓝本，系统布局，再创辉煌。

祝愿《精绘中华本草》早日问世，祝贺陈月明教授再登科学和艺术的高峰。

欣为之序。

中国工程院　院士

中国医学科学院药用植物研究所　名誉所长

2019 年 11 月 28 日

Preface 2

Scientific Illustrations of Chinese Medicinal Plants presents illustrations of the Chinese materia medica with great artistic detail and scientific accuracy. People with such high degrees of understanding in both the arts and sciences are rare.

I have worked with Professor Chen Yueming for many years. In response to the public need in the 1960s, a comprehensive national survey of Chinese materia medica resources was carried out, and, as a result, Professor Chen completed an extensive amount of painted works. In 1983, I invited Professor Chen to transfer to the newly established Institute of Medicinal Plant Development in the Chinese Academy of Medical Sciences and specialize in scientific botanical illustrations. During my research on the pharmacophylogeny of *Aconitum*, Professor Chen's exquisite scientific botanical illustrations of *Aconitum kusnezoffii* and *Aconitum kongboense* notably enhanced my study. A number of Professor Chen's works have been collected by well-known institutions, such as the World Health Organization and the University of Pittsburgh.

Professor Chen has extraordinary painting skills paired with an openness to learn and diligence in practice. In her youth, she always trekked deep into the mountains and wilderness to continuously observe plants, collect specimens, and compile first-hand information. Even to this day, she continues to create new works, entrusting a younger team to collect specimens and provide photos in the field to capture accurate color schemes and scientific evidence. She is meticulous about the scientific nature of her paintings. I learned that to draw *Artemisia annua*, the original plant which artemisinin is extracted from, she asked people to collect seedlings and then planted them in her own home. She carefully tended to and observed the planted seedlings, fastidiously recording the changes from sprouting to flowering to fruit bearing. Her scientific spirit and pursuit

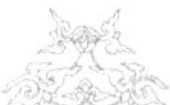

of artistic excellence are admirable. For decades, Professor Chen has created countless scientific and artistic paintings of medicinal plants for teaching and research purposes. She is a rare talent in this field.

I once urged Professor Chen to publish her life's works and present them to society to serve traditional Chinese medicine research. Not long ago, Professor Chen came to my home with a manuscript and publication plan, asking for comments and opinions. The forthcoming *Scientific Illustrations of Chinese Medicinal Plants*, led by Professor Chen, combines the techniques of scientific botanical illustration with modern scientific research. This collection is of great significance in preserving and advancing traditional Chinese medicine as well as contributing to modernization and globalization. To this feat, I extend my heartfelt congratulations! This book of exquisite scientific botanical illustrations is bound to become a coveted edition with high collection value for readers domestically and abroad. In addition, such exquisite scientific botanical illustrations will not only have an important impact on the field of scientific botanical illustration and traditional Chinese medicine but also make a greater contribution to the promotion and learning of traditional Chinese medicine in the Chinese public as well as in primary and secondary school education. I hope that Professor Chen and her team will continue to advance and collaborate sincerely in the future. Based on this book, may they create a systematic layout to achieve even more profound results.

I wish for this masterpiece, *Scientific Illustrations of Chinese Medicinal Plants*, to quickly publish and be available to the world. Congratulations to Professor Chen Yueming for reaching the pinnacle of the sciences and arts yet again.

It has been my great pleasure to pen this preface.

Xiao Peigen

Academician, Chinese Academy of Engineering

Honorary Director, Institute of Medicinal Plant Development,

Chinese Academy of Medical Sciences

November 28, 2019

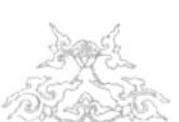

序　三

2019 年我在北京第一次见到陈月明教授和她主编的《中华本草彩色图典》一书。因与药用植物研究所的彭勇教授建立的良好友谊，我很荣幸地被陈教授夫妇邀请共进午餐。这段经历令我印象极为深刻，陈教授所散发出的美丽、博识和温柔的气息，都完整体现在她精绘的植物科学画中。她的著作和气质都深深吸引了我。《中华本草彩色图典》一书，将精美的插图与植物学知识和临床学知识相结合，很好地呈现出了 352 种药用本草的特性。

鉴于我并不在中国居住，我发现国外的中医专家能够获得高质量的培训，并成为优秀的中医临床医生。但通常情况下，中医专家在指导患者使用中药方剂和中成药时，对药用植物的相关信息缺乏深入了解。正是由于国外中医专家使用的这种务实办法，使我发现中医专家乃至于患者正努力地了解他们使用的药用植物的形态特征、药用部位等信息。由此可见，陈教授一书有其广泛需求和受众。

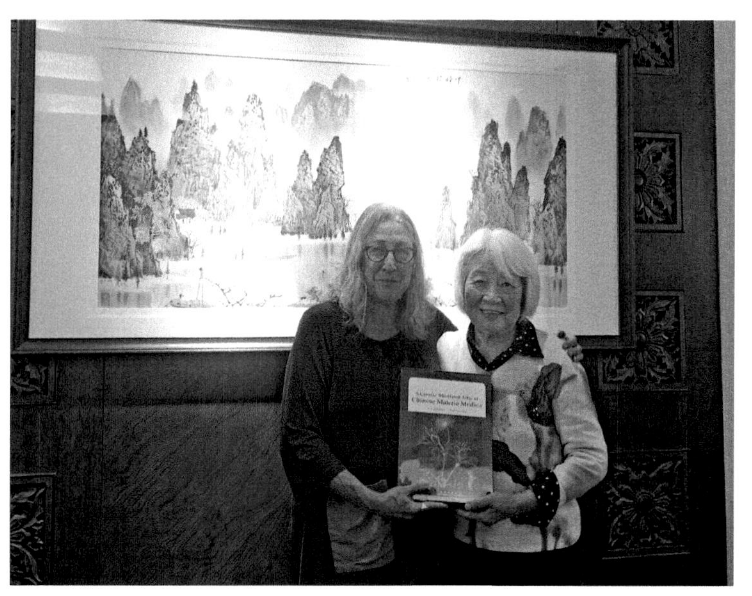

陈月明教授与巴西的 Elaine Elisabetsky 教授的合影

因此，我很高兴《精绘中华本草》一书的发行。在上一本著作中我学习到大量的药用植物学知识，但毫无疑问我将从这本新的著作中收获更多。我坚信，随着中医药在越来越多国家的医疗保健政策中变得更加突出，这本新书应

当在世界范围内推广。因此，我祝贺并感谢陈教授所取得的最新成果。我将继续贡献自己的力量，让她的书为科学界和临床界所知晓。

正如陈月明教授本人所走过的道路一样，我预见了一条美丽、实用、具有启发性的中华本草科学图典道路。我真的很荣幸有机会在此表达我对她及她所做工作的由衷钦佩。

传统药物学家

巴西南大河联邦大学生物化学系教授

2022 年 11 月 10 日，圣保罗

Preface 3

I first saw Dr. Chen Yueming's *A Concise Illustrated Atlas of Chinese Materia Medica at* the same time I met Prof. Chen herself, at Beijing in 2019. I was lucky enough to be invited for a lunch with her and her husband, a result of my good fortune to be friends with Professor Peng Yong from the Institute of Medicinal Plant Development (IMPLAD). It was one of the most remarkable meals I ever had, as I was mesmerized by her book as much as by herself. Dr. Chen exudes beauty, savvy, and gentleness. These qualities are expressed in her magnificent botanical illustrations. Her *A Concise Illustrated Atlas of Chinese Materia Medica* book combines the magnificent illustrations with well-organized information on botanical and clinical properties for 352 medicinal species .

As I do not live in China, I can observe that non-Chinese TCM experts can find good quality training and become fine TCM clinicians. But, more often than not, TCM experts have very little information of medicinal species that form the Chinese Materia Medica, as they instruct their patients to acquire the formulas and/or branded CM. While this is a pragmatic approach to TCM outside China, I find it of utmost importance that TCM expert - and even patients - learn about the plants they are using, how they look like, which part is used, etc. There is, therefore, a need and a niche for Prof. Chen botanical illustration books .

I am therefore delighted that *Scientific Illustrations of Chinese Medicinal Plants* has been launched, as I have already learned a great deal with the previous book and there is no doubt I will learn more with the new one. I truly believe the new book should be made available worldwide as TCM itself becomes more and more prominent in the pallet policies adopted for health care in more and more countries. Hence, I congratulate and

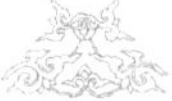

thank Dr. Chen for her newest achievement. I will continue my own efforts to make her books known to the scientific and clinical communities.

I foresee a beautiful, useful, and illuminating path for *Scientific Illustrations of Chinese Medicinal*, such as is the path of Dr. Chen Yueming herself. I am truly honored to have the opportunity to express my profound admiration for her and her work in these few words .

Professor, Ethnopharmacologist

Biochemistry Department, Universidade Federal do Rio Grande do Sul

São Paulo, November 10, 2022

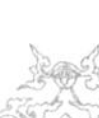

前　言

生物科学绘画是以客观还原生物本身的形态、生境等为主要描绘对象的一种艺术表现形式，一般用于生物分类学、古生物学、生态学等基础学科领域。生物科学绘画在创作过程中，不同于一般的绘画形式，不仅要求从业者具有较高的绘画基本功，还需具备一定的生物学知识素养。绘画者常常在实际创作中，面对着的是毫无生气的生物标本，仅仅利用肉眼和借助放大镜的观察，需要在画纸上复原出生物在生活史中的身姿，为科学研究提供生物的“标准肖像”。生物科学绘画由于其描绘对象的真实性，需要绘画者从科学的视角审视自然界万物生灵，通过恰当的表现形式精准地表现在画纸上，其重要意义主要表现在两方面：一是以科学性为准绳，需要准确地描绘生物的真实面貌；二是以艺术性为追求，跃然纸上，栩栩如生。科学绘画要达到科学性与艺术性的有机结合，常常离不开科学绘画工作者与科研人员的同心协力，因此，科学绘画更是理性与感性的完美融合。

真正意义上的生物科学绘画诞生于欧洲。文艺复兴时期，生物科学绘画就已达到极高的水平，而我国的科学绘画起步甚晚。20 世纪初，静生生物调查所的专职画师冯澄如先生（1896—1968 年）开启了我国生物科学绘画的先河，也被誉为我国生物科学绘画的奠基人。新中国成立后，随着我国科学事业的繁荣发展，生物科学绘画作为最基础的研究资料也受到前所未有的重视，培养了一批具有较高水平的从业者，也迎来了生物科学绘画的辉煌时刻。随着摄影技术的发展以及基础学科的定位，生物科学绘画人才逐渐凋零，近年来，博物学的兴起，为生物科学绘画又带来了新的生机。

本书主编陈月明教授自 20 世纪 60 年代开始，一直致力于药用植物科学绘画工作。1967 年在“五七”干校，被借调至江西省卫生厅协助绘画，参加《江

西中草药》一书的绘图工作。在那里认识了我国著名生物科学画大家冯晋庸老前辈，并一直得到冯先生的指导。在近六十年的创作中，陈教授经过不断的探索和创新，形成了在客观表现本体形态的同时，融合了我国传统绘画技法的富有中国特色的艺术风格，成为我国生物科学绘画事业中承前启后的代表人物之一。

1995 年陈月明教授退休后，中国工程院院士肖培根先生向陈月明教授建议，希望她能出版一本药用植物科学绘画的专著，一方面对自己钻研一生的本草科学画事业作一个系统总结，另一方面为我国药用植物研究提供重要的参考资料。有鉴于此，陈月明教授组织了我国一批中青年药用植物专家成立了编委会，开始了本书的编研工作。2019 年，陈月明教授时年八十有六，本书也完成了初步的编研工作，相关画作原稿送请中国科学院院士王文采先生和中国工程院院士肖培根先生指教，两位院士对陈月明教授的作品评价极高，表示祝贺并希望尽快出版为社会各界所用，但陈月明教授在追求艺术的道路上孜孜不倦，不断攀登艺术的高峰，创作了更多的药用植物科学绘画。编委会成员也受到极大鼓舞，不断充实完善内容，2022 年底终成此作。

本书收录了陈月明教授自 1975 年至 2022 年创作的药用植物科学绘画 129 幅，均是作者亲临实地写生创作。介绍中的内容主要参考了《中国药典》（2020 版）、《中华本草》、《中国植物志》、《原色中国本草图鉴》（日文版）、《中药志》、《全国中草药汇编》、《嘉卉》、*Flora of China*、*A Concise Illustrated Atlas of Chinese Materia Medica* 等专著；全书目录编排首先采用入药部位进行归类，每一类入药部位下采用物种的科名、属名的中文名，种名的学名分别进行排序，书后列有物种中文名、拉丁名、药材名的索引，供查阅检索。

本书从反映我国药用植物应用复杂性的角度出发，选择了常用大宗中药收录甘草、蒙古黄芪、宁夏枸杞等；民族民间药收录塔黄、沙棘等；海外本草收录西洋参、番红花等。从反映我国药用植物生境多样性的角度出发，选择了水生植物莲；沙生植物肉苁蓉等。从珍稀濒危药用植物资源保护的角度出发，选择了霍山石斛、冬虫夏草等。除此之外，还收录了我国高原山地极富特色的药用植物，如天山雪莲、唐古红景天、红花绿绒蒿及 2015 年获得诺贝尔生理学或医学奖的我国药学家屠呦呦研究员所研究的药用植物——黄花蒿。

本书集专业性、艺术性、科普性为一体，值得广大中医药工作者、生物科学绘画从业者、博物学爱好者品读和收藏。徜徉其中，相信大家会沉醉于植物科学绘画的艺术之美，也感叹于我国药用植物的魅力，成为大家民族自信、文

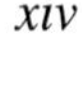

化自信的精神力量。希望通过本书的出版，推动我国生物科学绘画事业的传承和发展。

本书成稿之后，幸得时年 108 岁的著名书法家马识途先生挥毫题签；中国科学院王文采院士、中国工程院肖培根院士、前国际传统药物学会主席 Elaine Elisabetsky 教授及中国营养保健食品协会边振甲会长题序题词祝贺；著名本草学家赵中振教授担任主审；科学出版社大力支持本书出版。编委会向为本书的编研和出版提供指导和帮助的社会各界专家、学者、同仁表示深深的感谢。

我们反复斟酌了图文，力求科学严谨，但限于水平有限，难免存在疏漏错误之处，敬请广大读者提出宝贵意见。文中所涉及的功效用法、具体用药应在医师的指导下使用。

编委会

2022 年 12 月

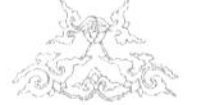

Foreword

Biological scientific illustration is a form of artistic expression that mainly objectively describes the form and habitat of biology itself. It is generally used in biological taxonomy, paleontology, ecology and other basic disciplines. Different from the general form of painting, during the creation process of biological scientific illustration, practitioners are not only required to possess a higher basic painting skills, but also need to have a certain biological knowledge accomplishment. In the actual creation, practitioners often face the lifeless biological specimens, only with their naked eye and with the help of a magnifying glass, they need to restore the body in the life history, to provide the "standard portrait" of biology for scientific research. Because of the authenticity of the object, the biological scientific illustration requires the illustrators to look at all the creatures in nature from the scientific perspective, then accurately represented on the drawing paper by the right form of expression, its significance is mainly reflected in two aspects: one is the scientific criterion, which need to accurately describe the true appearance; the second is the pursuit of artistry, which demand to be vivid as lifelike. In order to achieve the organic combination of science and artistry, scientific illustration is often inseparable from the concerted efforts of scientific illustrators and researchers. Therefore, scientific illustration is the perfect integration of sense and sensibility.

The real sense of biological scientific illustration was born in Europe. During the Renaissance period, biological scientific illustration has reached a very high level, while scientific illustration in China had a very late start. At the beginning of the 20th century, Mr. Feng Chengru (1896-1968), a full-time illustrator of Jingsheng Biological Survey Institute, opened the precedent of biological scientific illustration in China. He

was also known as the founder of biological scientific illustration in China. After the founding of the People's Republic of China in 1949, with the prosperity and development of scientific and technological undertakings in China, biological scientific illustration as the most basic research material has been attached with unprecedented importance, cultivated a number of high-level practitioners, and ushered in the brilliant moment of biological scientific illustration. With the development of photography technology and the positioning of basic disciplines, the talents of biological scientific illustration have gradually withered. In recent years, due to the rise of natural history, it has brought new vitality to the biological scientific illustration.

Professor Chen Yueming, the chief editor of this book, has been committed to the scientific illustration of medicinal plants since the 1960s. In 1967, in the Wuqi Cadre School, she was temporarily transferred to the Jiangxi Provincial Health Department to assist in illustration and undertaken the drawing work of the book *Chinese Herbal Medicine in Jiangxi Province*. During that time, she got to know Mr. Feng Jinyong, a famous biological scientific illustrator in China, and had been guided by Mr. Feng. In nearly 60 years of creation, after constant exploration and innovation, Professor Chen formed an artistic style with the combination of objective performance of noumenon form and a blend of rich Chinese artistic style of meticulous painting of flowers and birds as well as Chinese landscape painting techniques, which became one of the representatives in the scientific illustration in China serving as a link between past and future.

After Professor Chen's retirement in 1995, Mr. Xiao Peigen, academician, Chinese Academy of Engineering encouraged Professor Chen to publish her medicinal plant scientific illustration monograph. On the one hand, it will be a system summary to her lifetime career of Chinese materia medica scientific illustration, on the other hand, it will serve as the important reference for medicinal plant research. In view of this, Professor Chen organized a group of young and middle-aged medicinal plant experts in China to set up the editorial board, and began the compilation and research work of this book. In 2019, professor Chen was eighty six years old, the book also completed the preliminary research work, related manuscript was sent to Mr. Wang Wentsai, academician, Chinese Academy of Sciences and Mr. Xiao Peigen, academician, Chinese Academy of Engineering for advice. Two academicians gave extremely high evaluation

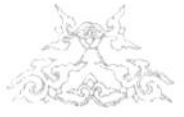

to professor Chen's works, congratulated and hoped the monograph can be published as soon as possible for the society. Professor Chen then constantly climbed the peak of art in the pursuit of art road, created more and more medicinal plant scientific illustration, making all members of the editorial board feel very touched and inspired, which made the volume of the monograph constantly added, all the way to the end of 2022.

The book includes 129 medicinal plant scientific illustrations of professor Chen from 1975 to 2022, all of which were personnally sketched from nature by the author, The main reference of the content of the book include *Chinese Pharmacopoeia(2020 edition), Chinese Materia Medica, Flora Reipublicae Popularis Sinicae, Illustrated Atlas of Chinese Materia Medica (Japanese edition), Chinese Medicinal Herbal, National Assembly of Chinese Herbal Medicine, Infinite Blooming, Flora of China, A Concise Illustrated Atlas of Chinese Materia Medica*, etc. The whole catalogue is firstly classified by medicinal parts. The Chinese name of the family and genus of the species and the scientific name of the species were respectively sorted under each medicinal part. The index of the Chinese names, scientific names and medicinal materials of the species are listed at the back of the book for reference and retrieval.

From the perspective of reflecting the complexity of the application of medicinal plants in China, this book selected *Glycyrrhiza uralensis*, *Astragalus membranaceus* var. *mongholicus*, *Lycium barbarum* and other commonly used Chinese medicine. Ethnic folk medicine included *Rheum nobile*, *Hippophae rhamnoides*, etc. Overseas medicine included *Panax quinquefolius*, *Crocus sativus* and so on. From the perspective of reflecting the diversity of medicinal plant habitat, the aquatic *Nelumbo nucifera* and the psammophyte *Cistanche deserticola* were selected. *Dendrobium huoshanense* and *Cordyceps sinensis* were selected from the perspective of the conservation of rare and endangered medicinal plant resources. In addition, the collection also includes highly featured medicinal plants in the mountainous areas of the Chinese plateau, such as *Saussurea involucrata*, *Rhodiola tangutica*, *Meconopsis punicea*, and *Artemisia annua*, a medicinal plant researched by Ms. Tu Youyou, the Chinese pharmacologist who was awarded the Nobel Prize in Medicine in 2015.

This book is a professional, artistic and popular science collection, and it is worth reading and collecting by the majority of traditional Chinese medicine workers,

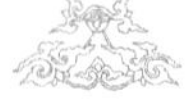

biological scientific illustration practitioners, and natural history lovers. Wandering in it, we believe that you will not only be immersed in the artistic beauty of plant scientific illustration, but also sigh at the charm of medicinal plants in China, which will eventually become the spiritual power of national confidence and cultural confidence. It is hoped that through the publication of this book, it will promote the inheritance and development of biological scientific illustration in China.

After the manuscript was about to be finished, Mr. Ma Shitu, a famous calligrapher who is already 108 years old, wrote the title of the book with best wishes. Mr. Wang Wentsai, academician of Chinese Academy of Sciences, Mr. Xiao Peigen, academician of Chinese Academy of Engineering, Professor Elaine Elisabetsky, former President of International Society for Ethnopharmacology and Mr. Bian Zhenjia, President of China Nutrition and Health Food Association wrote the prefaces and the inscriptions for congratulation; Professor Zhao Zhongzhen, a famous herbologist worked as the Chief Reviewer; Science Press also strongly supported the publication of this book. The editorial board would like to express its deep gratitude to the experts, scholars and colleagues who have provided guidance and help in the compilation, research and publication of this book.

We repeatedly consider the illustrations and texts, and strive to be scientific and rigorous, however, due to our limited level, it is inevitable that there might be mistakes and omissions. Please put forward your valuable suggestions. The indications of specific drugs mentioned in the book should be used under the guidance of doctors.

Editorial board

December, 2022

陳月明女士畫展開幕之喜

妙筆生花

錢信忠敬賀

一九九二年八月一日

卫生部前部长钱信忠先生的贺词

《精绘中华本草》
一部精美植物学著作
一部中医药科研教学教材
一部高级科普知识读本

边振甲
2022,12 北京

中国营养保健食品协会边振甲会长的题词

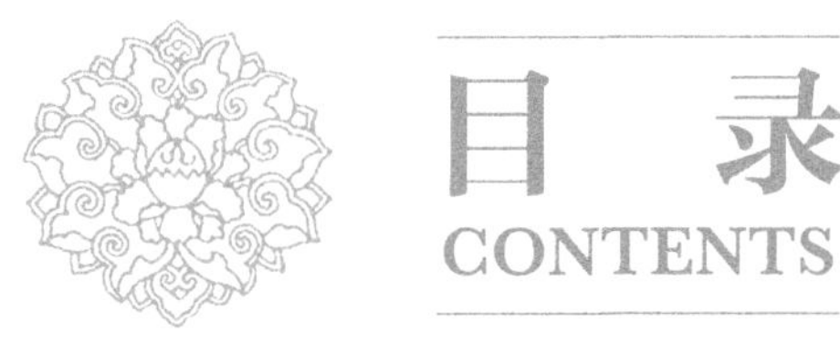

目录 CONTENTS

根及根茎类 | Roots and rhizomes

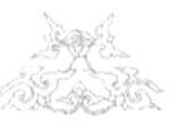

茎木类 | Stems and woods

皮类 | Tree barks and root barks

叶类 | Leaves

花类 | Flowers

果实种子类 | Fruits and seeds

全草类 | Whole Herbs

菌物类 | Fungus

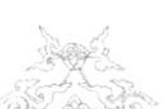

精绘中华本草

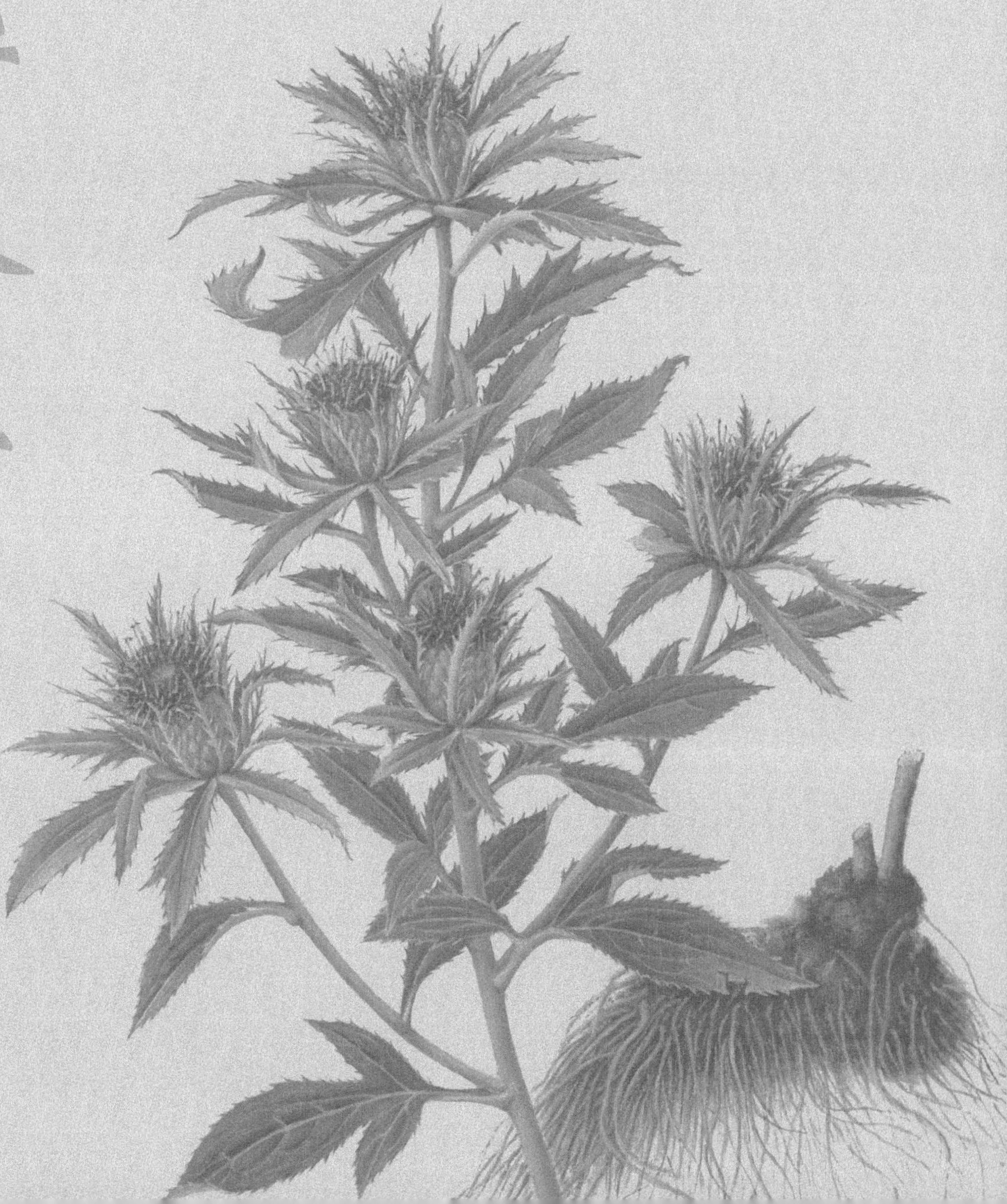

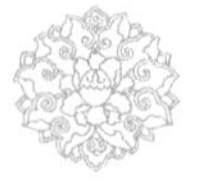

菘蓝

Songlan

Isatis indigotica

基　　源 十字花科 Brassicaceae 菘蓝属 *Isatis* 植物菘蓝 *Isatis indigotica* Fort. 的干燥根。药材名为“板蓝根”。

形态特征 二年生草本。茎直立，绿色，顶部多分枝，植株光滑无毛，带白粉霜。基生叶莲座状，长圆形，全缘或稍具波状齿，具柄；茎生叶长椭圆形。花瓣黄白色。短角果近长圆形，扁平，无毛，边缘有翅。种子长圆形，淡褐色。

生境分布 我国华北与华东地区常见栽培。

采收加工 秋季采挖，除去泥沙，晒干。

性味功能 寒，苦。清热解毒，凉血消斑。

主治用法 主要用于温病高热，神昏，发斑发疹，痄腮，喉痹，丹毒，痈肿。

化学成分 主要含有吲哚类成分，如靛蓝、靛玉红等；生物碱类，如告依春、表告依春等；有机酸类，如苯甲酸、水杨酸、丁香酸等；另外还含有氨基酸类、甾醇类化合物、腺苷、多糖、板蓝根甲素、芥子苷类、喹唑酮类等。

备　　注 菘蓝的叶为大青叶，叶经过加工可制成青黛，均具有清热解毒，凉血消斑等功用。

Source It is the dried root of *Isatis indigotica* Fort. (Brassicaceae). The medicinal material is called “Banlangen”.

Distribution *I. indigotica* is commonly cultivated in northern and eastern China.

Indications It is commonly used in warm diseases with high fever, loss of consciousness, macular and papular eruption, mumps, pharyngitis, erysipelas, and swollen welling-abscess.

Chemical Constituents It contains indoles such as indigo and indirubin, alkaloids such as goitrine and epigoitrin, organic acids such as benzoic acid, salicylic acid, and syringic acid. In addition, it also contains amino acids, sterols, adenosine, polysaccharides, isatan A, glucosinolate, quinazolone, etc.

Note The leaves of *I. indigotica* are called Folium Isatidis, which can be processed into Indigo Naturalis. Both can clear heat and resolve toxins, as well as cool blood and remove ecchymosis.

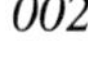

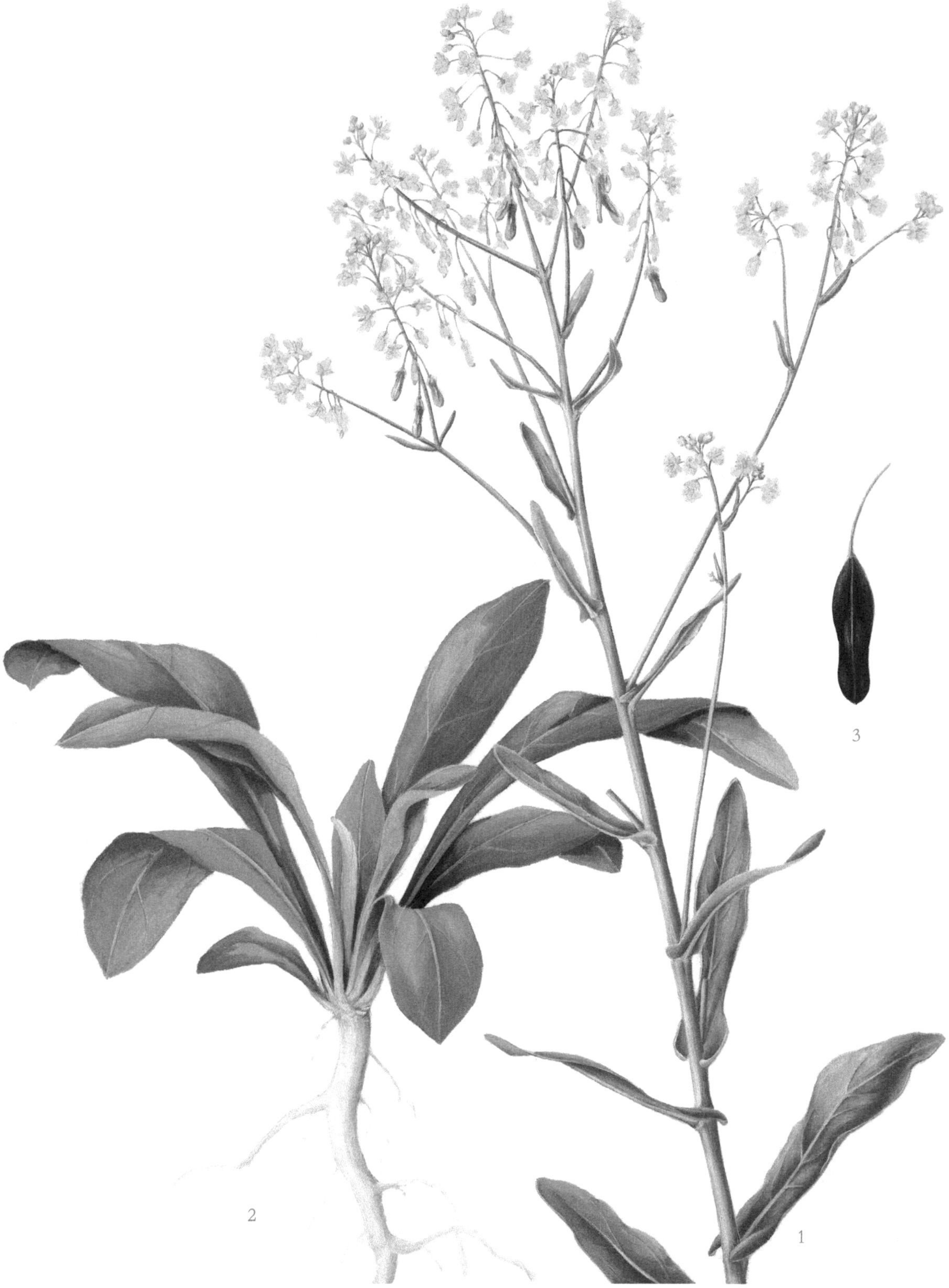

1

2

3

1. 花枝（flowering stem） 2. 基生叶及根（basal leaf and root） 3. 果实（fruit）

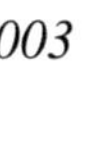

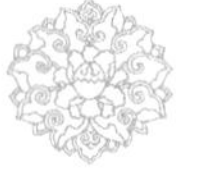

南五味子

Nanwuweizi

Kadsura longipedunculata

基　　源　木兰科 Magnoliaceae 南五味子属 *Kadsura* 植物南五味子 *Kadsura longipedunculata* Finet et Gagnep. 的干燥根。药材名为“红木香”。

形态特征　藤本。叶长圆状披针形、倒卵状披针形或卵状长圆形，先端渐尖或尖，基部狭楔形或宽楔形，边有疏齿，侧脉每边 5-7 条；上面具淡褐色透明腺点。花单生于叶腋，雌雄异株；雄花　花被片白色或淡黄色，8-17 片；雌花　花被片与雄花相似，雌蕊群椭圆体形或球形。聚合果球形，小浆果倒卵圆形，外果皮薄革质，干时显出种子。种子 2-3，肾形或肾状椭圆体形。

生境分布　分布于长江流域以南各地。生于海拔 200-1200 m 的山坡、阔叶林中的溪涧旁。

采收加工　立冬前后采挖，去净残茎、细根及泥土，晒干。

性味功能　温，辛、苦。理气止痛，祛风通络，活血消肿。

主治用法　主要用于胃痛，腹痛，风湿痹痛，痛经，月经不调，产后腹痛，咽喉肿痛，痔疮，无名肿毒，跌打损伤。

化学成分　根中含有木脂素类和三萜类成分，木脂素有右旋安五脂素、五内酯 B、五内酯 E、长南酸、内消旋二氢愈创木脂酸、五味子素、华中五味子醇 B、戈米辛、翼梗五味子酚、华中五味子酯 B 等；茎中含有苯甲酰日本南五味子木脂素 A、异戊酰日本南五味子木脂素 A、当归酰日本南五味子木脂素 A、日本南五味子木脂素 A、南五味子内酯、南五味子二内酯等。

Source　It is the dried root of *Kadsura longipedunculata* Finet et Gagnep. (Magnoliaceae). The medicinal material is called “Hongmuxiang”.

Distribution　*K. longipedunculata* is distributed in the south of the Yangtze River Basin, grown on mountain slopes, in valleys and beside streams of broad-leaf forests at an altitude of 200–1200 m.

Indications　It is mainly used to treat stomach pain, abdominal pain, wind–dampness impediment pain, dysmenorrhea, irregular menstruation, postpartum abdominal pain, sore throat, hemorrhoids, innominate toxin swelling, and traumatic injury.

Chemical Constituents　The root contains lignans and triterpenes as ingredients. The former includes (+)-anwulignan, schisanlactone B, schisanlactone E, changnanic acid, meso-dihydroguaiaretic acid, schisandrin, and schisandrol B, gomisin, schisanhenol, and schisantherin B. The stem includes benzoylbinankadsurin A, A, angeloylbinankadsurin A, binankadsurin A, kadsulactone, kadsudilactone, etc.

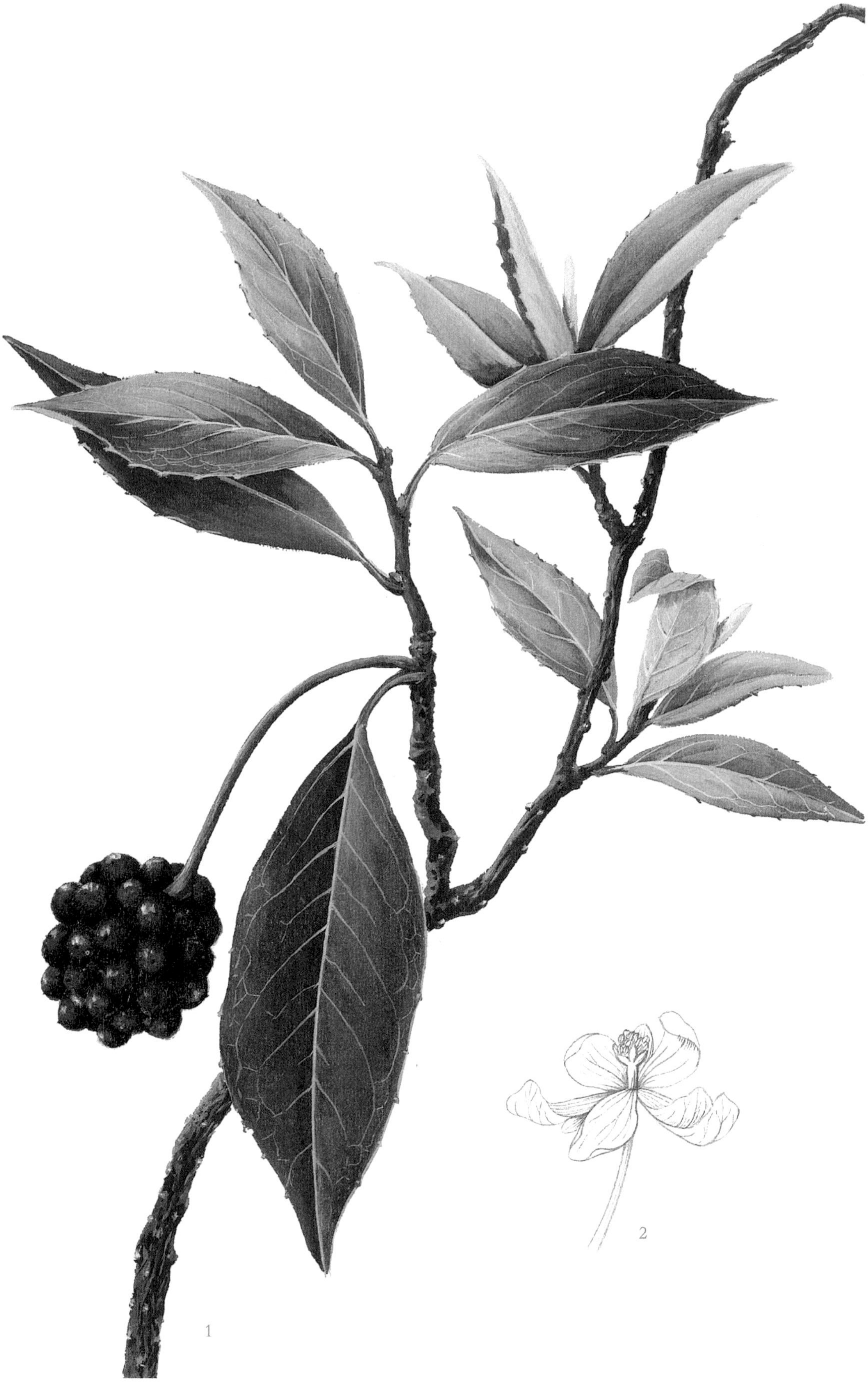

1. 果枝（fruiting stem） 2. 花（flower）

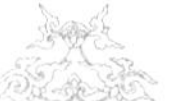

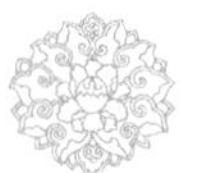

黑老虎

Heilaohu

Kadsura coccinea

基　源　木兰科 Magnoliaceae 南五味子属 *Kadsura* 植物黑老虎 *Kadsura coccinea* (Lem.) A. C. Smith 的干燥根。药材名为“黑老虎”。

形态特征　藤本，全株无毛。叶革质，长圆形至卵状披针形，先端钝或短渐尖，基部宽楔形或近圆形，全缘，侧脉每边 6-7 条，网脉不明显。花单生于叶腋，稀成对，雌雄异株；雄花　花被片红色，10-16 片；雌花　花被片与雄花相似。聚合果近球形，红色或暗紫色，小浆果倒卵形，外果皮革质。种子心形或卵状心形。

生境分布　分布于江西、福建、湖南、广东、广西、四川、贵州、云南等地。生于山地疏林中，常缠绕于大树上。

采收加工　全年均可采，掘起根部及须根，洗净泥沙，切成小段，晒干。

性味功能　温，辛、微苦。行气止痛，散瘀通络。

主治用法　主要用于胃及十二指肠溃疡，慢性胃炎，急性胃肠炎，风湿痹痛，跌打损伤，骨折，痛经，产后瘀血腹痛，疝气痛。

化学成分　根中含有木脂素类成分，如新南五味子木脂宁、乙酰基日本南五味子木脂素 A、丙酰基氧代南五味子烷、乙酰基氧代南五味子烷、苯甲酰氧代南五味子烷、异戊酰氧代南五味子醇、24- 亚甲基环木菠萝烯酮、南五味子酸、黑老虎酸、异南五味子木脂宁、冷饭团素、去氧五味子素、R- 五味子丙素、南五味子木脂宁等成分。

备　注　黑老虎的果实可食，为南方特色水果之一。

Source　It is the dried root of *Kadsura coccinea* (Lem.) A. C. Smith (Magnoliaceae). The medicinal material is called “Heilaohu”.

Distribution　*K. coccinea* is distributed in Jiangxi, Fujian, Hunan, Guangdong, Guangxi, Sichuan, Guizhou, Yunnan and other provinces. It grows in sparse mountain forests, and often twines on big trees.

Indications　It is mainly used to treat gastric and duodenal ulcers, chronic gastritis, acute gastroenteritis, wind–dampness impediment pain, traumatic injury, bone fracture, dysmenorrhea, postpartum abdominal pain due to blood stasis, and pain caused by hernia.

Chemical Constituents　The root contains lignans, such as neokadsuranin, acetylbinankadsurin A, propionyl oxokadsurane, acetoxyl oxokadsurane, benzoyl oxokadsurane, isovaleroyl oxokadsuranol, 24-methylene cycloartenone, kadsuric acid, coccinic acid, isokadsuranin, kadsutherin, deoxyschizandrin, R-schisandrin C, kadsuranin, etc.

Note　The fruit is edible and is a regional specialty in southern China.

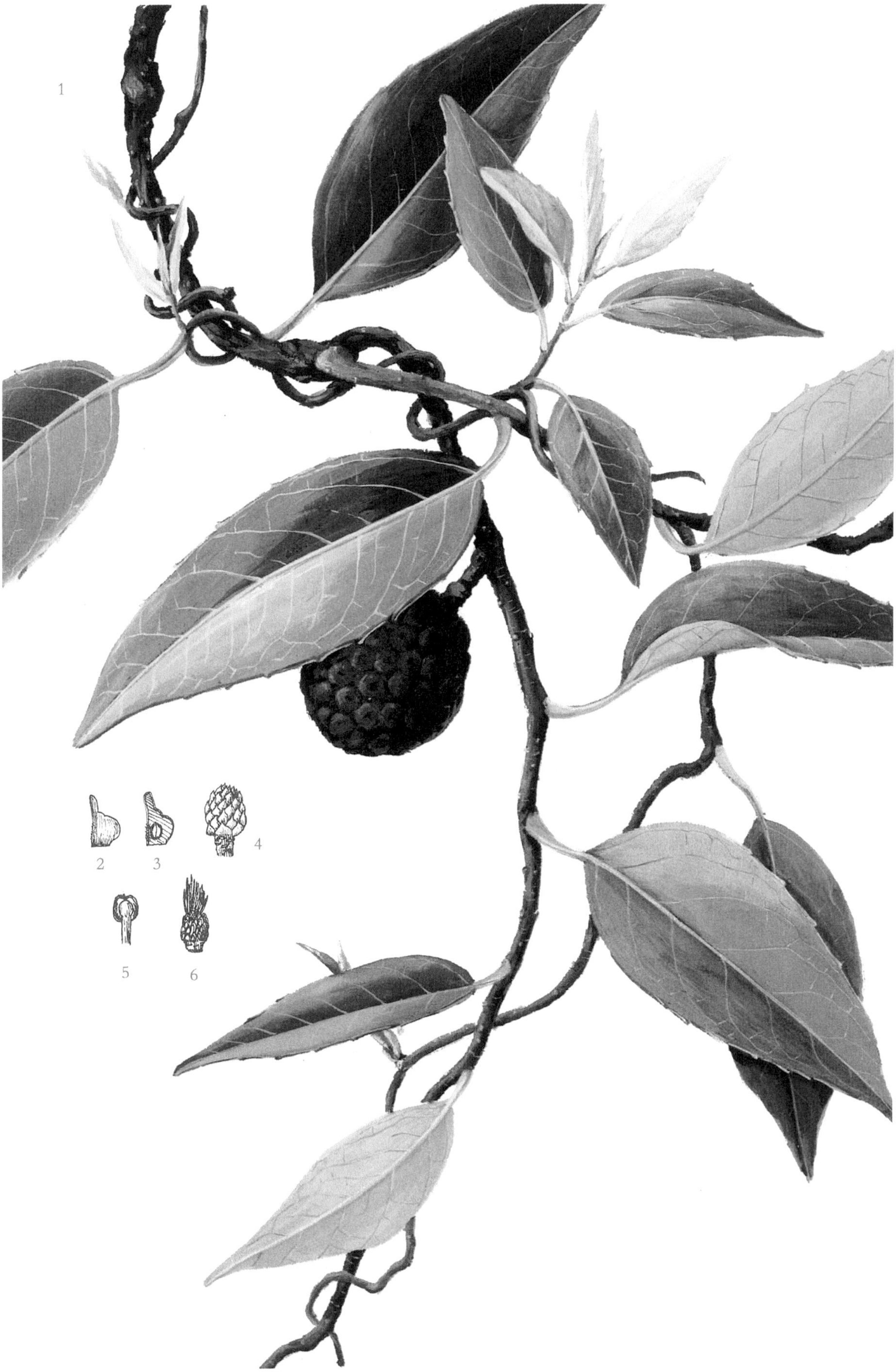

1. 果枝（fruiting stem） 2. 雌蕊（pistil） 3. 雌蕊纵切面（vertical section of pistil） 4. 雌蕊群（gynoecium） 5. 雄蕊（stamen） 6. 雄蕊群（androecium）

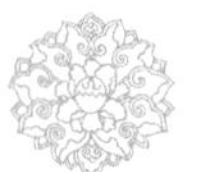

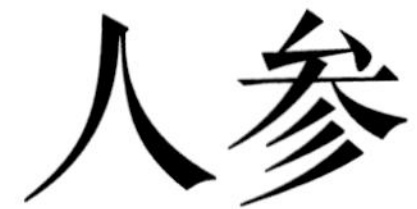

人参

Renshen

Panax ginseng

基　　源　五加科 Araliaceae 人参属 *Panax* 植物人参 *Panax ginseng* C. A. Mey. 的干燥根和根茎。药材名为“人参”，栽培的称“园参”，播种于山林野地状态下自然生长的称“林下山参”，习称“籽海”。

形态特征　多年生草本。主根肥大。茎单生。叶为掌状复叶，3-6 枚轮生茎顶；小叶片 3-5，薄膜质，边缘有锯齿，上面散生少数刚毛，下面无毛。伞形花序单个顶生；总花梗通常较叶长；花淡黄绿色。果实扁球形，鲜红色。种子肾形，乳白色。

生境分布　主要分布于北纬 33° -48° ，即我国东北地区和俄罗斯、日本、韩国、朝鲜等地。生于海拔 300-900 m 的以红松为主的针阔混交林或落叶阔叶林下。如今在我国东北地区栽培面积甚广。

采收加工　园参一般于栽培后的第 6 年于秋季茎叶枯萎时采收。林下山参一般于播种后 15 年以上采收。鲜参除去须根干燥者称“生晒参”，直接干燥者称“全须生晒参”，栽培品经蒸制干燥者称“红参”，商品亦有“糖参”“高丽参”等。

性味功能　温，甘、微苦。大补元气，复脉固脱，补脾益肺，生津养血，安神益智。

主治用法　主要用于体虚欲脱，肢冷脉微，脾虚食少，肺虚喘咳，津伤口渴，内热消渴，气血亏虚，久病虚羸，惊悸失眠，阳痿宫冷。常用量 3-9g，另煎兑服；也可研粉吞服。不宜与藜芦同用。服用期间忌食萝卜与浓茶。

化学成分　人参根中含有人参皂甙和少量挥发油，此外还含有人参多糖、亚油酸、多肽、黄酮、多种维生素等；人参茎叶中主要含有黄酮类、糖类。

备　　注　野山参的经验鉴别为“芦长碗密枣核艼，紧皮细纹珍珠须”。

Source　It is the dried root and rhizome of *Panax ginseng* C. A. Mey. (Araliaceae). The medicinal material is called “Renshen”.

Distribution　*P. ginseng* is mainly distributed between 33°N and 48°N, i.e., in northeastern China, Russian Federation, Japan, Republic of Korea, Democratic People’s Republic of Korea, etc. It grows under the theropencedrymion or deciduous broad–leaf forest dominated by Korean pine at an altitude of 300–900 m. Now, it is widely cultivated in northeastern China.

Indications　It is mainly used to treat weak health with verging on collapse, cold limbs with a faint pulse, spleen deficiency with reduced eating, lung deficiency with cough and panting, body fluid deficiency and thirst, internal heat and wasting thirst, qi–blood deficiency, weak health with enduring illness, palpitation and insomnia, impotence and uterine cold. The usual amount is 3–9 g. It can be taken after separating decoction or as a ground powder. It is not appropriate to use together with Radix et Rhizoma Veratri. Turnip and strong tea should not be taken together with it.

Chemical Constituents　The root contains ginsenoside and a small amount of volatile oil. It also contains ginseng polysaccharide, linoleic acid, polypeptide, flavonoids, and a variety of vitamins. The stem and leaves mainly contain flavonoids and saccharides.

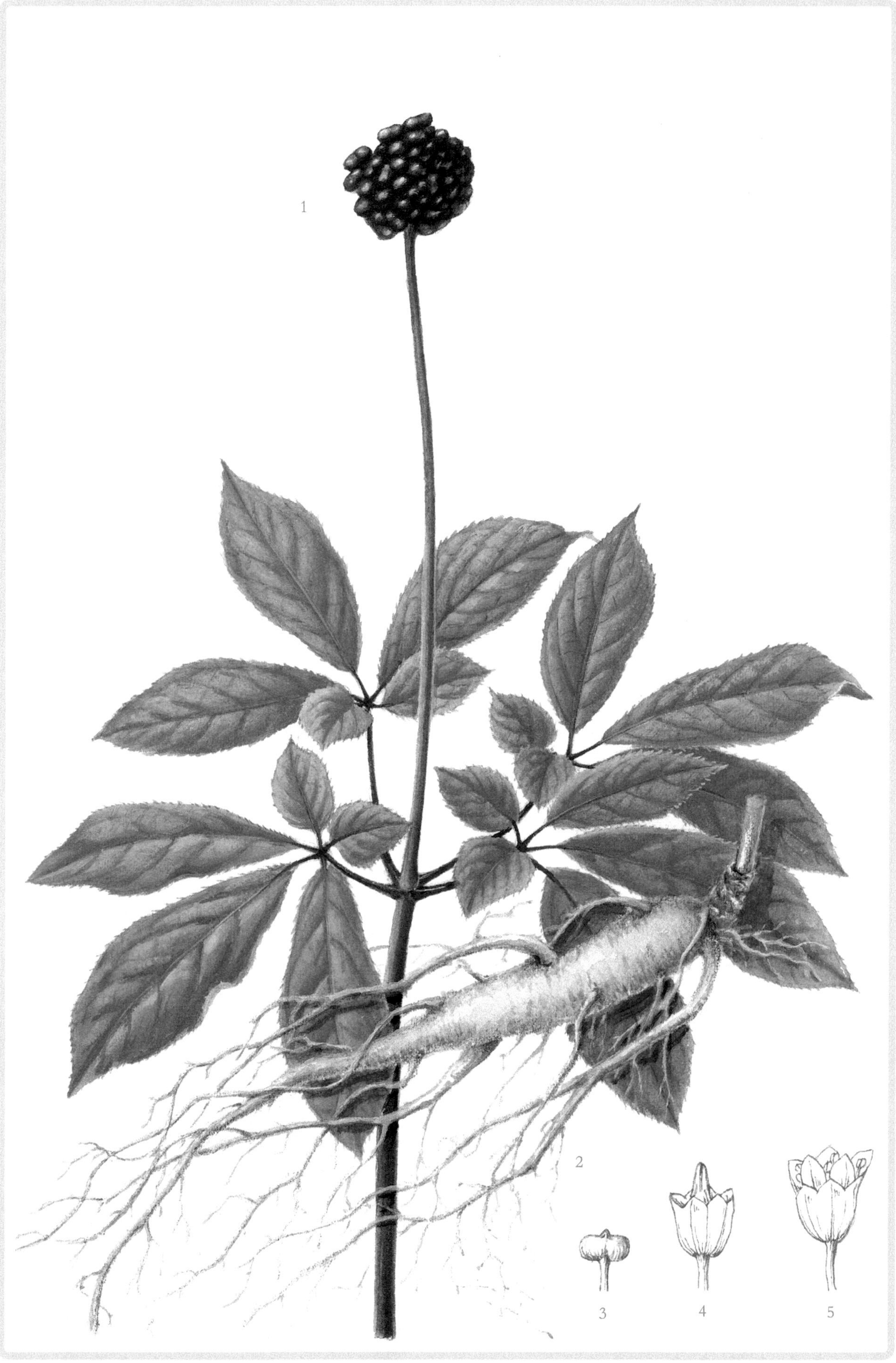

1. 果枝（fruiting stem） 2. 根（root） 3. 果实（fruit） 4. 花萼（calyx） 5. 花（flower）

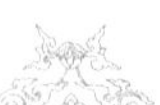

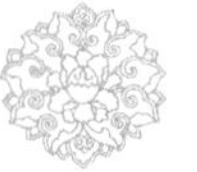

西洋参

Xiyangshen

Panax quinquefolius

基　　源　五加科 Araliaceae 人参属 *Panax* 植物西洋参 *Panax quinquefolius* L. 的干燥根。药材名为“西洋参”。

形态特征　多年生草本。根肉质，纺锤形，时有分枝。茎圆柱形，具纵条纹。掌状复叶，通常 3-4 枚轮生茎顶；小叶通常 5 枚，小叶片倒卵形，先端急尾尖，边缘具粗锯齿，上面叶脉有稀疏细刚毛。伞形花序单一顶生，花萼钟状，绿色；花冠绿白色。核果状浆果，扁球形，成熟时鲜红色。

生境分布　我国东北、山东等地有栽培。原产北美洲。

采收加工　均系栽培品，秋季采挖，洗净，晒干或低温干燥。

性味功能　凉，甘、微苦。补气养阴，清热生津。

主治用法　主要用于气虚阴亏，虚热烦倦，咳喘痰血，内热消渴，口燥咽干。另煎兑服。体质虚寒者慎服；不宜与藜芦同用。服用期间忌食萝卜与浓茶。

化学成分　根茎含有皂苷类，主要是人参皂苷；又含有挥发油、多糖、树脂、有机酸、氨基酸等。

备　　注　国产西洋参因加工方法不同，分为软支与硬支；进口西洋参仅有软支加工方法。

Source　It is the dried root of *Panax quinquefolius* L. (Araliaceae). The medicinal material is called “Xiyangshen”.

Distribution　*P. quinquefolius* is native to North America and cultivated in northeastern China and Shandong Province.

Indications　It is mainly used to treat qi deficiency and yin depletion, deficiency heat with tiredness, cough and panting with phlegm and blood, internal heat and wasting thirst, dry mouth and throat. It should be decocted separately and mixed with the other decoction before taking. People with cold and weak constitution should use this with caution, and it should not be used with Radix et Rhizoma Veratri. Turnip and strong tea should not be taken together with it.

Chemical Constituents　The rhizome contains saponins, mainly ginsenosides. It also contains volatile oils, polysaccharides, resins, organic acids and amino acids.

Note　Radix Panacis Quinquefolii produced in China can be divided into soft branches and hard branches due to different processing methods. Radix Panacis Quinquefolii produced by other countries provides soft branches only.

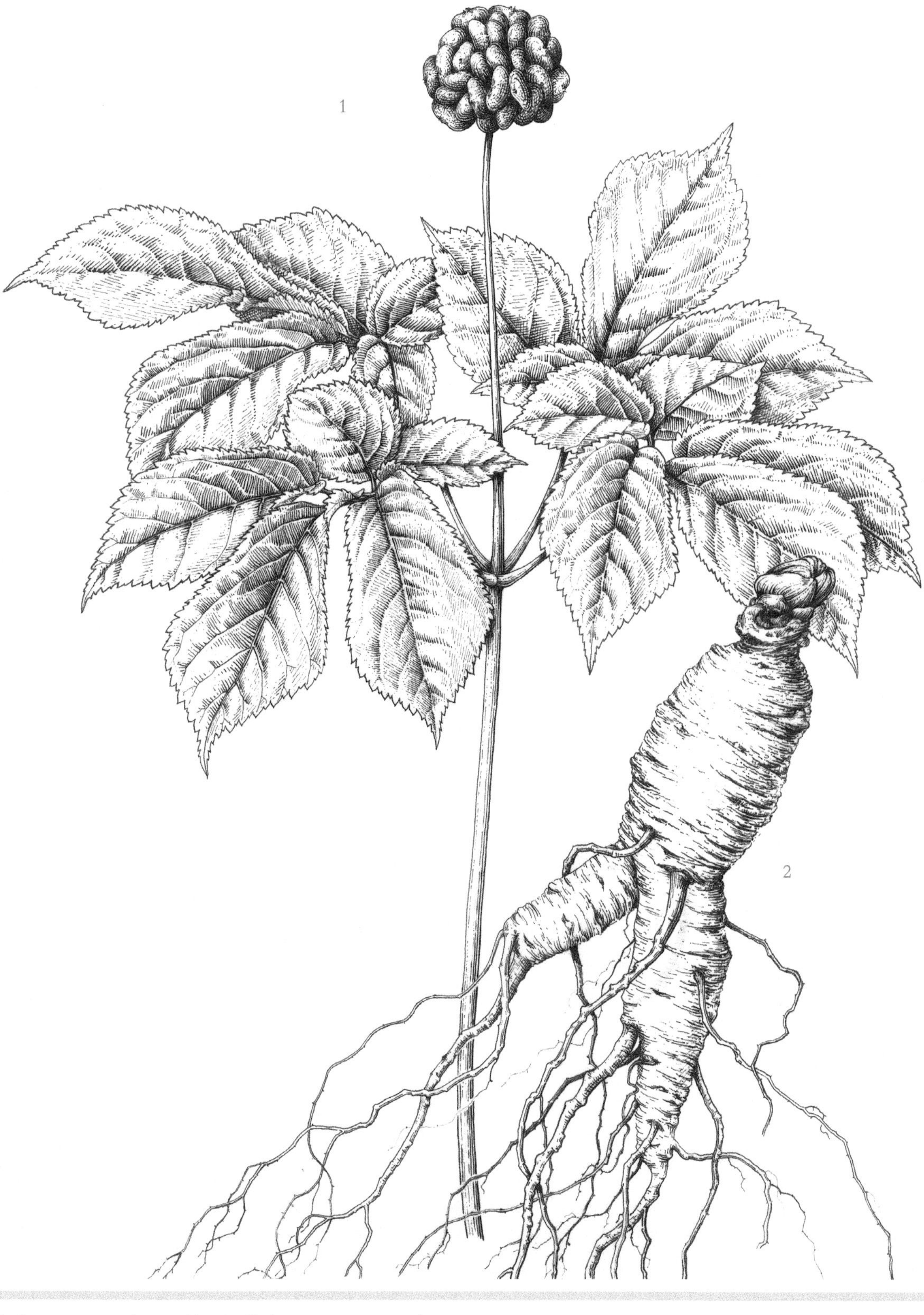

1

2

1. 果枝（fruiting stem）　2. 根及根茎（root and rhizome）

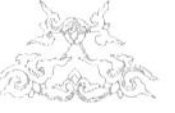

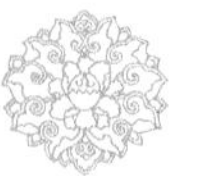

工布乌头

Gongbuwutou

Aconitum kongboense

基　源　毛茛科 Ranunculaceae 乌头属 *Aconitum* 植物工布乌头 *Aconitum kongboense* Lauener 的干燥块根。药材名为“雪上一支蒿”。

形态特征　多年生草本。块根近圆柱形。茎直立，粗壮，高大，上部与花序均密被反曲的短柔毛。叶心状卵形，三全裂，中央全裂片菱形，自中部向上近羽状深裂，侧全裂片斜扇形。总状花序长达 60cm，与分枝的花序形成圆锥花序；萼片白色带紫色或淡紫色，外面被短柔毛，上萼片盔形；花瓣 2，疏被短毛。蓇葖果。种子多数。

生境分布　分布于我国四川西部及西藏。生于海拔 3000-4000 m 的山坡草地或灌丛中。

采收加工　9-10 月采挖根部，除去须根，洗净，晒干。

性味功能　温，苦、辛；有大毒。祛风除湿，止痛。

主治用法　用于风湿关节疼痛，跌打损伤，毒虫咬伤等。未经炮制，严禁内服。

化学成分　块根含有黄草乌碱甲、工布乌头碱、展花乌头碱等。

Source　It is the dried root rhizome of *Aconitum kongboense* Lauener. (Ranunculaceae). The medicinal material is called “Xueshangyizhihao”.

Distribution　*A. kongboense* is distributed in western Sichuan and Tibet and grows on grasslands or shrubs on hillsides at an altitude of 3000–4000 m.

Indications　It is used to treat painful joints caused by wind–dampness, traumatic injury, poisonous insect bite, etc. Oral administration is strictly prohibited before it is processed.

Chemical Constituents　The root rhizome contains vilmorrianine A, kongboenine, chasmaconitine, etc.

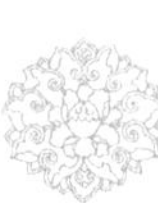

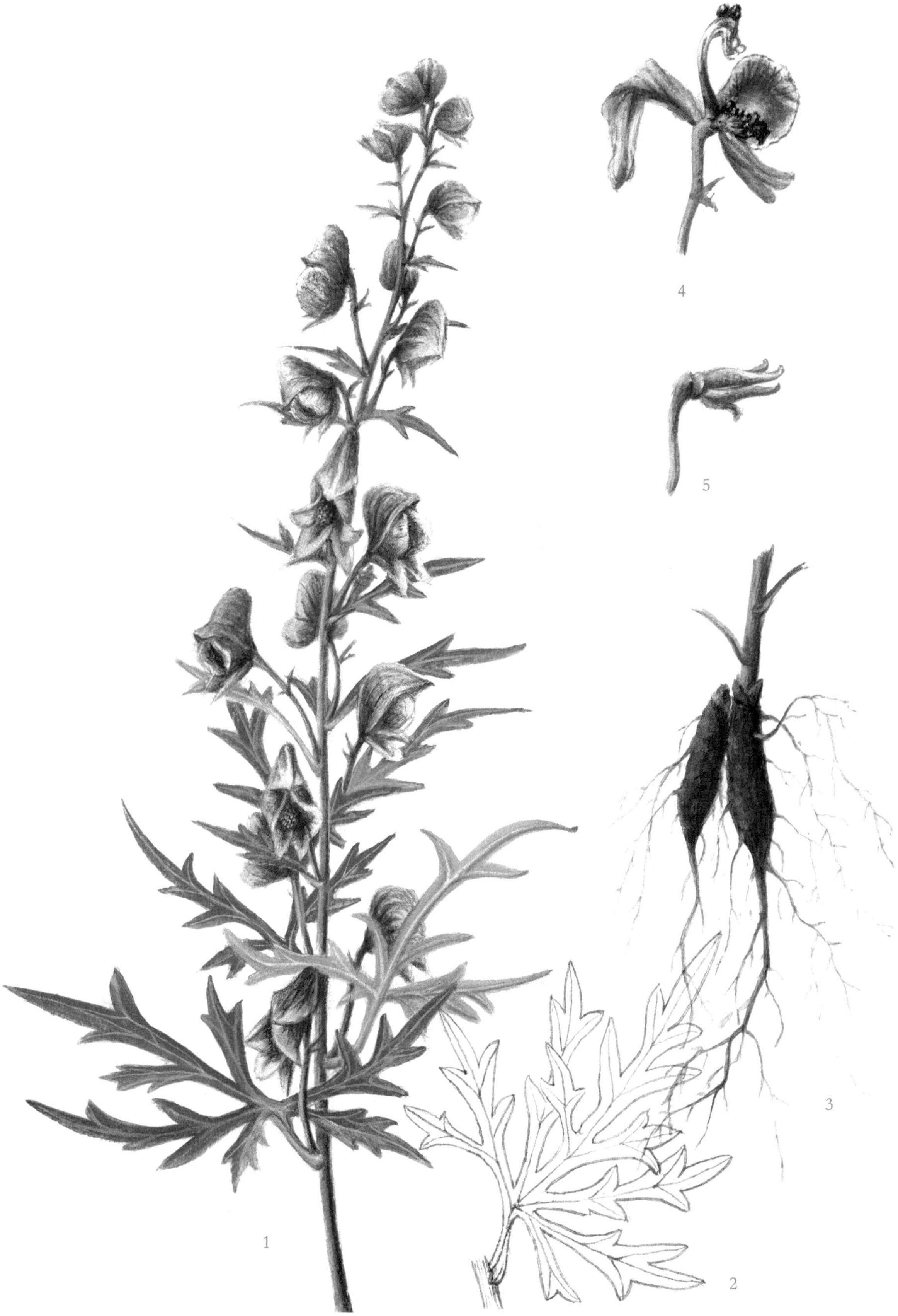

1. 花枝（flowering stem） 2. 叶（leaf） 3. 根（root） 4. 花（flower） 5. 雌蕊（pistil）

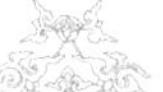

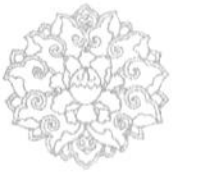

北乌头

Beiwutou

Aconitum kusnezoffii

基　　源　毛茛科 Ranunculaceae 乌头属 *Aconitum* 植物北乌头 *Aconitum kusnezoffii* Reichb. 的干燥块根。药材名为“草乌”。

形态特征　多年生草本。块根圆锥形。茎无毛，茎下部叶在开花时枯萎。叶片纸质，五角形，三全裂。顶生总状花序，通常与其下的腋生花序形成圆锥花序；萼片紫蓝色，上萼片盔形或高盔形。蓇葖果。种子扁椭圆球形，沿棱具狭翅，只在一面生横膜翅。

生境分布　分布于我国东北与华北的山地草坡或疏林中。

采收加工　秋季茎叶枯萎时采挖，除去须根及泥沙，干燥。

性味功能　热，辛、苦；有大毒。祛风除湿，温经止痛。

主治用法　一般经过炮制后用于风寒湿痹，关节疼痛，心腹冷痛，寒疝作痛及麻醉止痛。生品内服宜慎；孕妇禁用；不宜与半夏、瓜蒌、天花粉、贝母、白蔹、白及同用。

化学成分　块根中主要含有生物碱类，如乌头碱、次乌头碱、新乌头碱等；叶中含有生物碱、肌醇、鞣质等。

备　　注　草乌叶为蒙古族习用药材，主要用于清热，解毒，止痛。

Source　It is the dried root rhizome of *Aconitum kusnezoffii* Reichb. (Ranunculaceae). The medicinal material is called “Caowu”.

Distribution　*A. kusnezoffii* is distributed on hillsides covered with grass or in the woodlands in Northern and Northeastern China.

Indications　After processing, it is used to treat wind–cold–dampness arthralgia, joint pain, cold pain in the heart and abdomen, pain caused by cold abdominal colic, as well as narcotherapy to relieve pain. Oral administration of raw medicine should be with caution. Pregnant women are not allowed to use it. It is inappropriate to use with Rhizoma Pinelliae, Fructus Trichosanthis, Radix Trichosanthis, fritillaria, Radix Ampelopsis, Rhizoma Bletillae, etc.

Chemical Constituents　The root rhizome mainly contains alkaloids, such as aconitine, hypaconitine, and mesaconitine. The leaves contain alkaloids, inositol, tannins, etc.

Note　Folium Aconiti Kusnezoffii is a commonly used Mongolian medicine, which is mainly used to clear heat, remove toxins, and relieve pain.

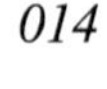

北乌头

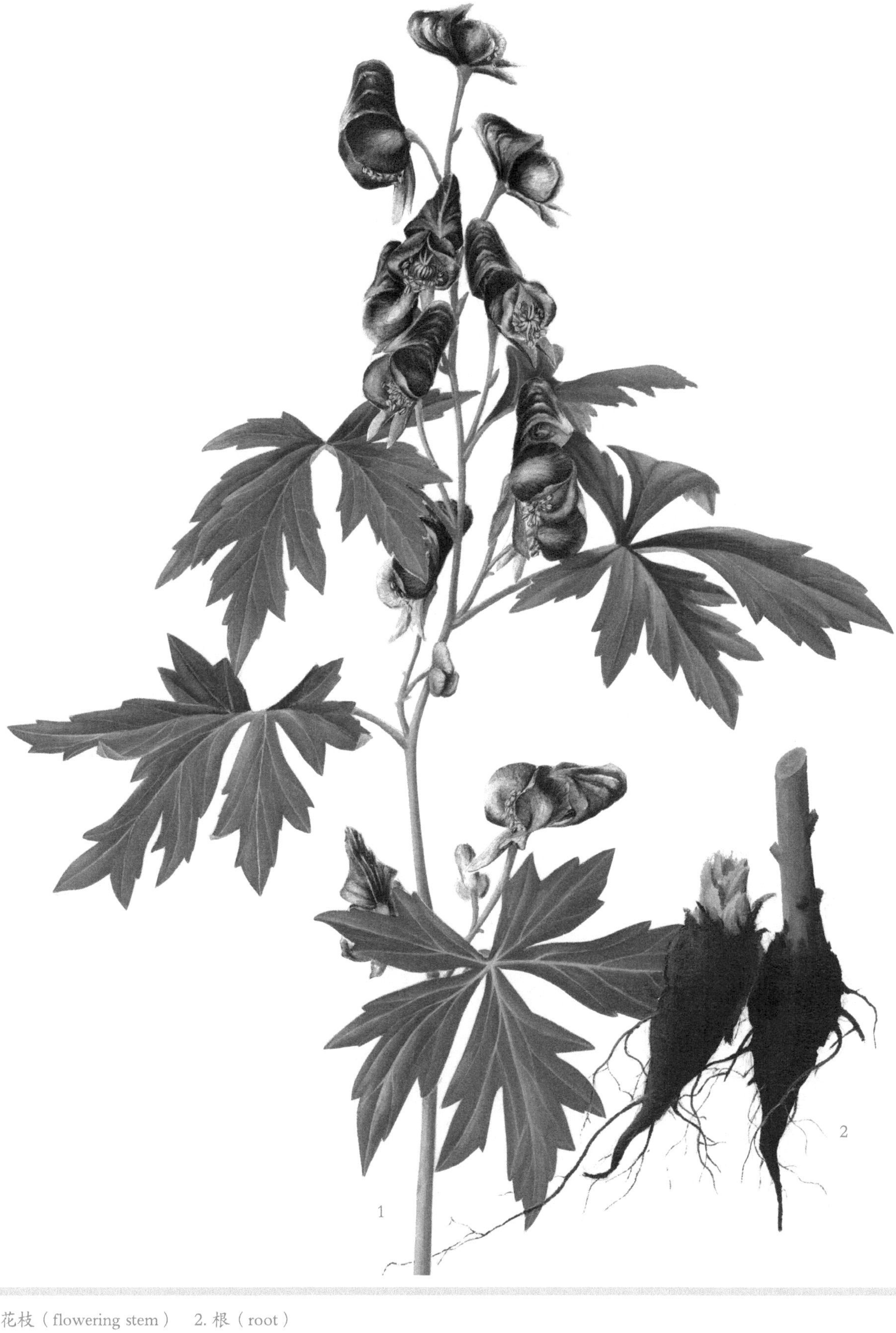

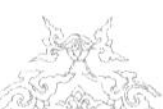

1. 花枝（flowering stem）　2. 根（root）

白头翁

Baitouweng

Pulsatilla chinensis

基　　源　毛茛科 Ranunculaceae 白头翁属 *Pulsatilla* 植物白头翁 *Pulsatilla chinensis* (Bge.) Regel 的干燥根。药材名为“白头翁”。

形态特征　多年生草本。花叶近同期。基生叶 4-6，叶片宽卵形，三全裂，表面疏被毛，背面有长柔毛；叶柄有密长柔毛。花葶 1-2，有柔毛；苞片 3，三深裂，背面密被长柔毛；花直立；萼片蓝紫色，长圆状卵形，背面有密柔毛。瘦果纺锤形，被长柔毛，顶部有羽毛状宿存花柱。

生境分布　分布于我国东北、华北、华中、华东等大多数省区。常生于平原和低山的山坡草丛中、林边或干旱多石的坡地。

采收加工　春、秋二季采挖，除去泥沙，干燥。

性味功能　寒，苦。清热解毒，凉血止痢。

主治用法　用于热毒血痢，阴痒带下。

化学成分　根中主要含有白头翁皂甙、白头翁素、有机酸、葡萄糖、阿拉伯糖等。

备　　注　白头翁为治阿米巴痢疾的要药，其茎叶具有强心作用，有一定毒性。

Source　It is the dried root of *Pulsatilla chinensis* (Bge.) Regel. (Ranunculaceae). The medicinal material is called “Baitouweng”.

Distribution　*P. chinensis* is distributed in most provinces in Northeastern, Northern, Central and Eastern China and commonly grows on grassy hillsides, at the edge of the forests or on dry and rocky slopes of plains and low mountains.

Indications　It is used to treat hemorrhagic dysentery caused by heat toxin, vulval pruritus and leukorrhea.

Chemical Constituents　The root mainly contains anemoside, anemonin, organic acids, glucose, arabinose, etc.

Note　It is an important medicine to treat amoebic dysentery. The stem and leaves have the function of cardiotonic and have moderate toxicity.

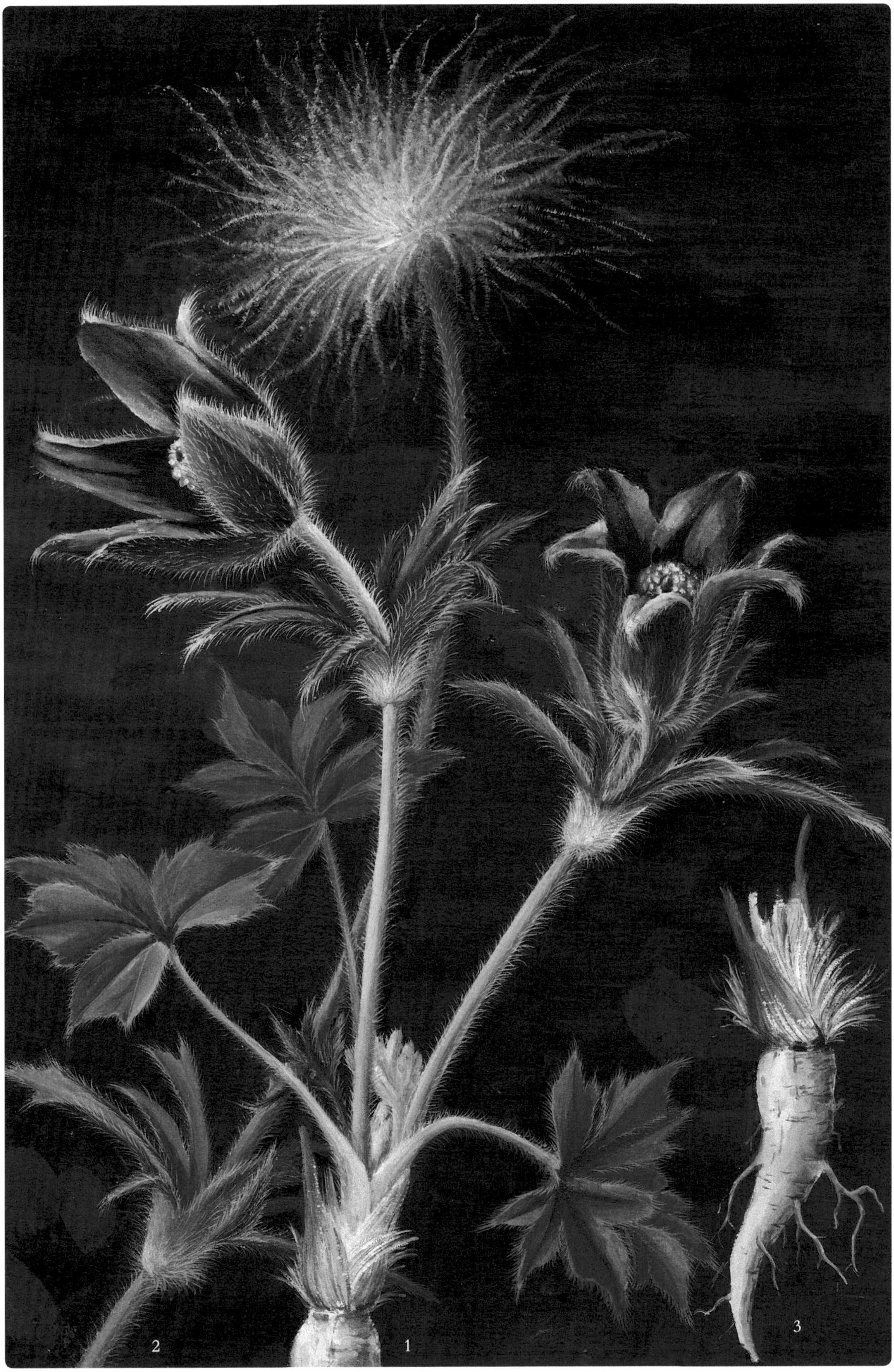

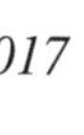

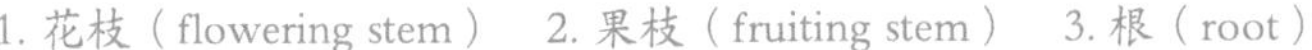

1. 花枝（flowering stem） 2. 果枝（fruiting stem） 3. 根（root）

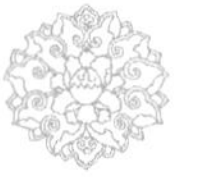

梅叶冬青

Meiyedongqing
Ilex asprella

基　　源　冬青科 Aquifoliaceae 冬青属 *Ilex* 植物梅叶冬青 *Ilex asprella* (Hook. et Arn.) Champ. ex Benth. 的根。药材名为“岗梅根”。

形态特征　落叶灌木。小枝无毛，绿色。叶互生；叶片膜质，卵形或卵状椭圆形，先端渐尖成尾状，基部宽楔形，边缘具钝锯齿。花白色，雌雄异株；雄花 2-3 朵簇生或单生叶腋，花 4-5 数，花萼裂片阔三角形或圆形，基部结合；雌花单生叶腋。果球形，熟时黑紫色，分核 4-6 粒，倒卵状椭圆形，内果皮石质。

生境分布　分布于江西、福建、台湾、湖南、广东、广西等地。常生于海拔 400-1000 m 的山谷路旁灌丛中或阔叶林中。

采收加工　秋、冬采挖，晒干，或切片晒干。

性味功能　寒，苦、甘。清热，生津，散瘀，解毒。

主治用法　可用于感冒头痛，眩晕，热病烦渴，痧气，热泻，肺痈，百日咳，咽喉肿痛，痔血，淋病，疔疮肿毒，跌打损伤等。

化学成分　含有三萜皂苷、香豆素内酯及少量生物碱。

Source　It is the root of *Ilex asprella* (Hook. et Arn.) Champ. ex Benth. (Aquifoliaceae). The medicinal material is called “Gangmeigen”.

Distribution　*I. asprella* is distributed in Jiangxi, Fujian, Chinese Taiwan, Hunan, Guangdong, Guangxi and other places. It commonly grows in the roadside shrubs or broad-leaved forests in valleys at an altitude of 400–1000 m.

Indications　It is commonly used to treat headache caused by cold, dizziness, extreme thirst caused by febrile disease, eruptive disease, diarrhea due to heat, lung abscess, whooping cough, sore swollen throat, hemorrhoidal bleeding, gonorrhea, furuncle, sore, pyogenic infection, traumatic injury, etc.

Chemical Constituents　It contains triterpenoid saponins, coumarin lactone and a small amount of alkaloids.

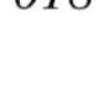

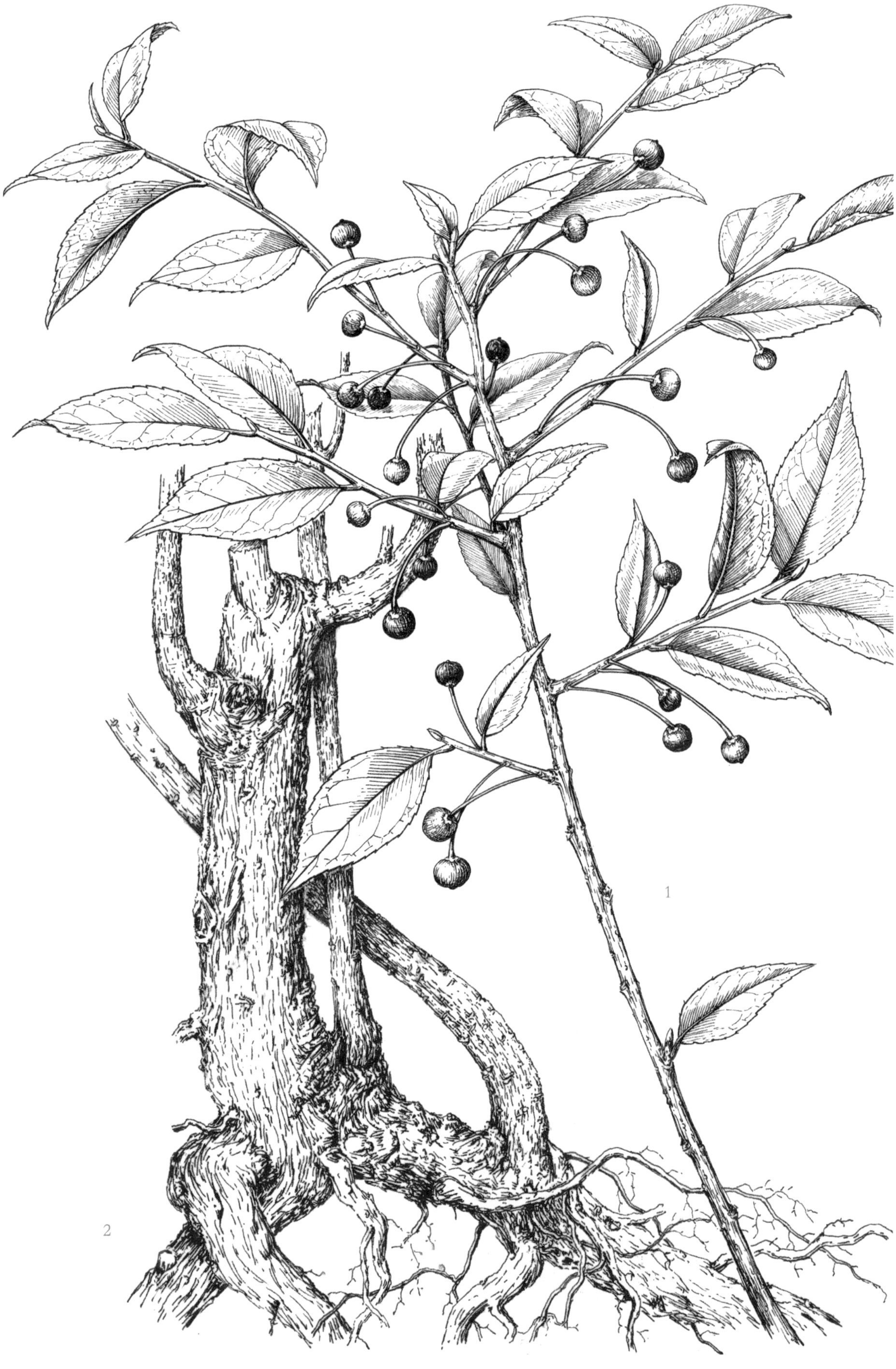

梅叶冬青

1

2

1. 果枝（fruiting stem）　2. 根（root）

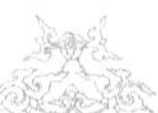

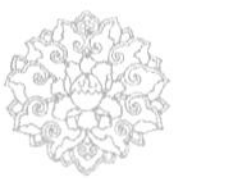

地黄

Dihuang

Rehmannia glutinosa

基　　源　玄参科 Scrophulariaceae 地黄属 *Rehmannia* 植物地黄 *Rehmannia glutinosa* (Gaert.) Libosch. ex Fisch. et Mey. 的干燥块根。药材名为“生地黄”。

形态特征　多年生草本，全株密被灰白色腺毛。根茎肉质，鲜时黄色；茎紫红色。叶在茎基部成莲座状，向上则强烈缩小；基生叶长椭圆形，上面绿色，下面略带紫色，边缘具不规则齿，基部渐狭成柄。花在茎顶部略排列成总状花序；花萼萼齿 5；花冠裂片 5，内面黄紫色，外面紫红色；雄蕊 4 枚。蒴果卵形至长卵形。

生境分布　分布于我国华北、华东、华中各省区，常见生于较低海拔的砂质壤土荒地上。为著名的“四大怀药”之一。

采收加工　秋季采挖，除去芦头、须根及泥沙，将地黄缓缓烘焙至约八成干。

性味功能　寒，甘。清热凉血，养阴生津。

主治用法　用于热入营血，温毒发斑，吐血衄血，热病伤阴，舌绛烦渴，津伤便秘，阴虚发热，骨蒸劳热，内热消渴。地黄亦可鲜用。

化学成分　主要含有萜类及其苷类成分，如梓醇、益母草苷、桃叶珊瑚苷等；另还含有毛蕊花糖苷、棉子糖、葡萄糖、氨基酸、有机酸、甾醇等。

备　　注　鲜地黄与生地黄均可清热凉血，前者偏于生津，后者偏于养阴。生地黄蒸至黑润后为熟地黄，可补血滋阴。

Source　It is the dried root rhizome of *Rehmannia glutinosa* Libosch. (Scrophulariaceae). The medicinal material is called “Shengdihuang”.

Distribution　*R. glutinosa* is distributed in the provinces of North, East and Central China. It commonly grows on the wasteland with sandy loam at low altitudes. It is one of the famous “Four Huai Medicines”.

Indications　It is used to treat an invasion of the nutrient and blood levels by heat, eruption caused by warm toxin, hematemesis and epistaxis, yin damage in febrile diseases, crimson tongue and extreme thirst, constipation caused by depltion of body fluid, yin-deficiency fever, bone-steaming with hectic fever, internal heat and wasting thirst. The fresh herb can also be used.

Chemical Constituents　It mainly contains terpenes and glycosides, such as catalpol, ajugol, and aucubin. It also contains verbascoside, raffinose, glucose, amino acids, organic acids, sterols, etc.

Note　Both fresh and unprocessed Radix Rehmanniae have the function of clearing heat and cooling blood. Fresh Radix Rehmanniae has more effect in generating body fluids, while raw rehmannia is more potent in nourishing yin. Unprocessed Radix Rehmanniae can be steamed to black color, which is called Radix Rhemanniae Praeparata. Radix Rhemanniae Praeparata can nourish blood and nourish yin.

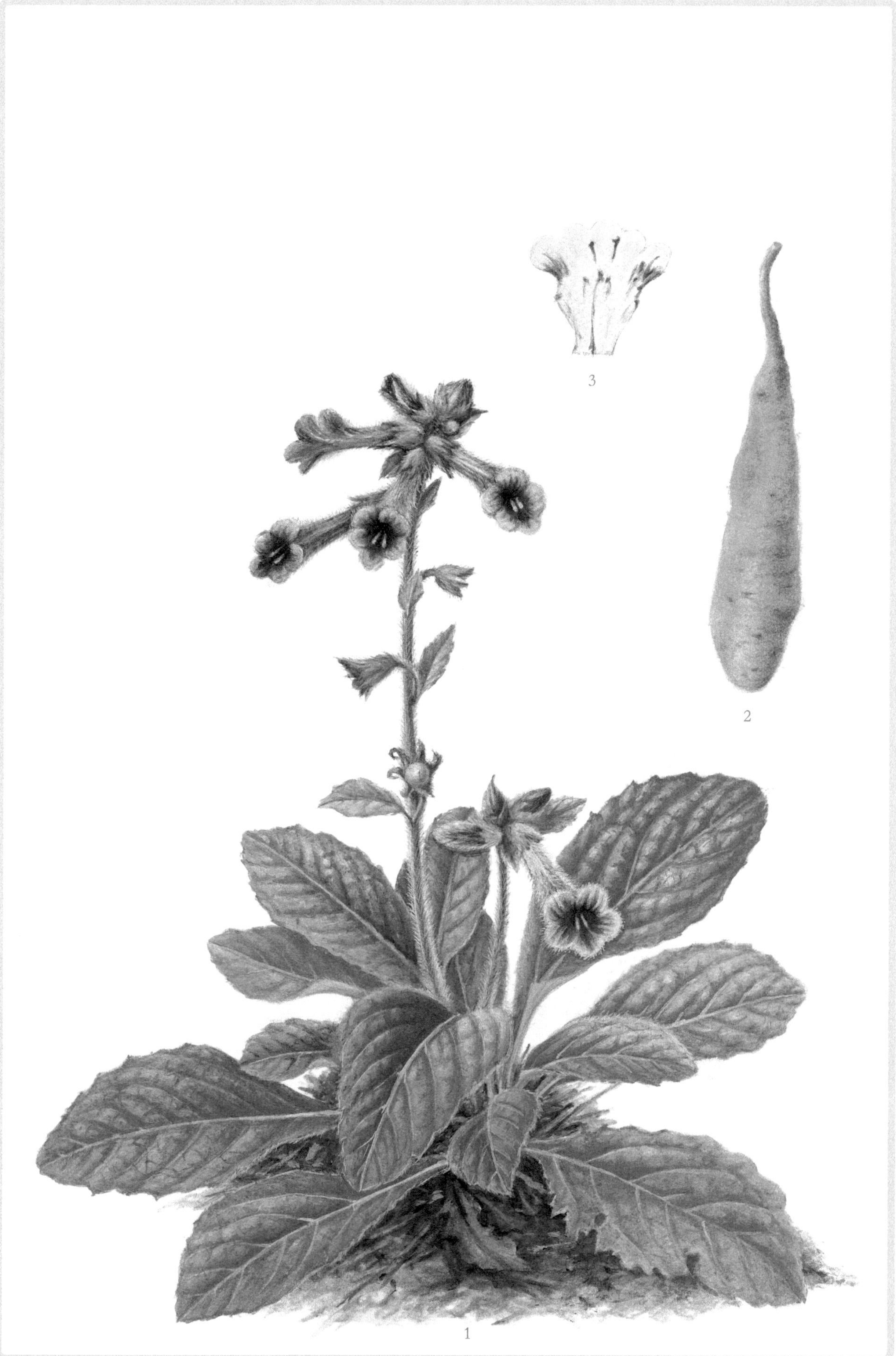

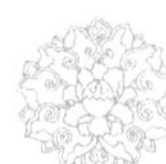

1. 植株（plant） 2. 根（root） 3. 花内面及雄蕊（flower open showing stamens）

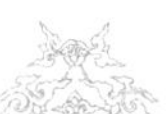

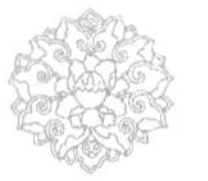

天麻

Tianma

Gastrodia elata

基　源　兰科 Orchidaceae 天麻属 *Gastrodia* 植物天麻 *Gastrodia elata* Bl. 的干燥块茎。药材名为“天麻”。

形态特征　腐生草本。植株高大。块茎椭圆形至近哑铃形，肉质，具较密的节，节上被许多三角状宽卵形的鞘；茎直立，橙黄色多见，无叶，下部被数枚膜质鞘。总状花序；花扭转，橙黄色，近直立；唇瓣基部贴生于蕊柱足末端与花被筒内壁上并有一对肉质胼胝体。蒴果倒卵状椭圆形。

生境分布　主要分布于我国东北、华东、西南部分省区。常生于海拔 400-3200 m 的疏林下、林中空地、林缘、灌丛边缘。

采收加工　春季 4-5 月间采挖为“春麻”；立冬前 9-10 月间采挖的为“冬麻”，质量较好。挖起后趁鲜洗去泥土，刮去外皮，水煮或蒸透心，切片，摊开晾干。

性味功能　平，甘。息风止痉，平抑肝阳，祛风通络。

主治用法　主要用于小儿惊风，癫痫抽搐，破伤风，头痛眩晕，手足不遂，肢体麻木，风湿痹痛。

化学成分　天麻中含量较高的主要成分是天麻苷，也称天麻素，另含有天麻多糖、β-谷甾醇、胡萝卜苷、柠檬酸、维生素 A、腺嘌呤等。

备　注　天麻又名赤箭，不能进行光合作用，须与蜜环菌和紫萁小菇共生，紫萁小菇为种子萌发提供营养，蜜环菌为天麻块茎生长提供营养。

Source　It is the dried rhizome of *Gastrodia elata* Bl. (Orchidaceae). The medicinal material is called “Tianma”.

Distribution　*G. elata* is distributed in northeastern, eastern, and southwestern China. It commonly grows in the woodland, in open spaces in forests, at the edge of forests on shrubs at an altitude of 400–3200 m.

Indications　It is used to treat infantile convulsions, epilepsy and convulsion, tetanus, headache and dizziness, paralysis and nunbness of limbs wind–dampness impediment pain.

Chemical Constituents　The main constituent with a high level is gastrodin. It also contains polysaccharide, β-gusterol, daucosterol, citric acid, vitamin A, adenine, etc.

Note　Photosynthesis cannot be performed in *G. elata*. It must co-exist with the *Armillaria mellea* and the *Mycena osmundicola*. *M. osmundicola* and *A. mellea* provide nutrients for seed germination and growth of *G. elata* tuber respectively.

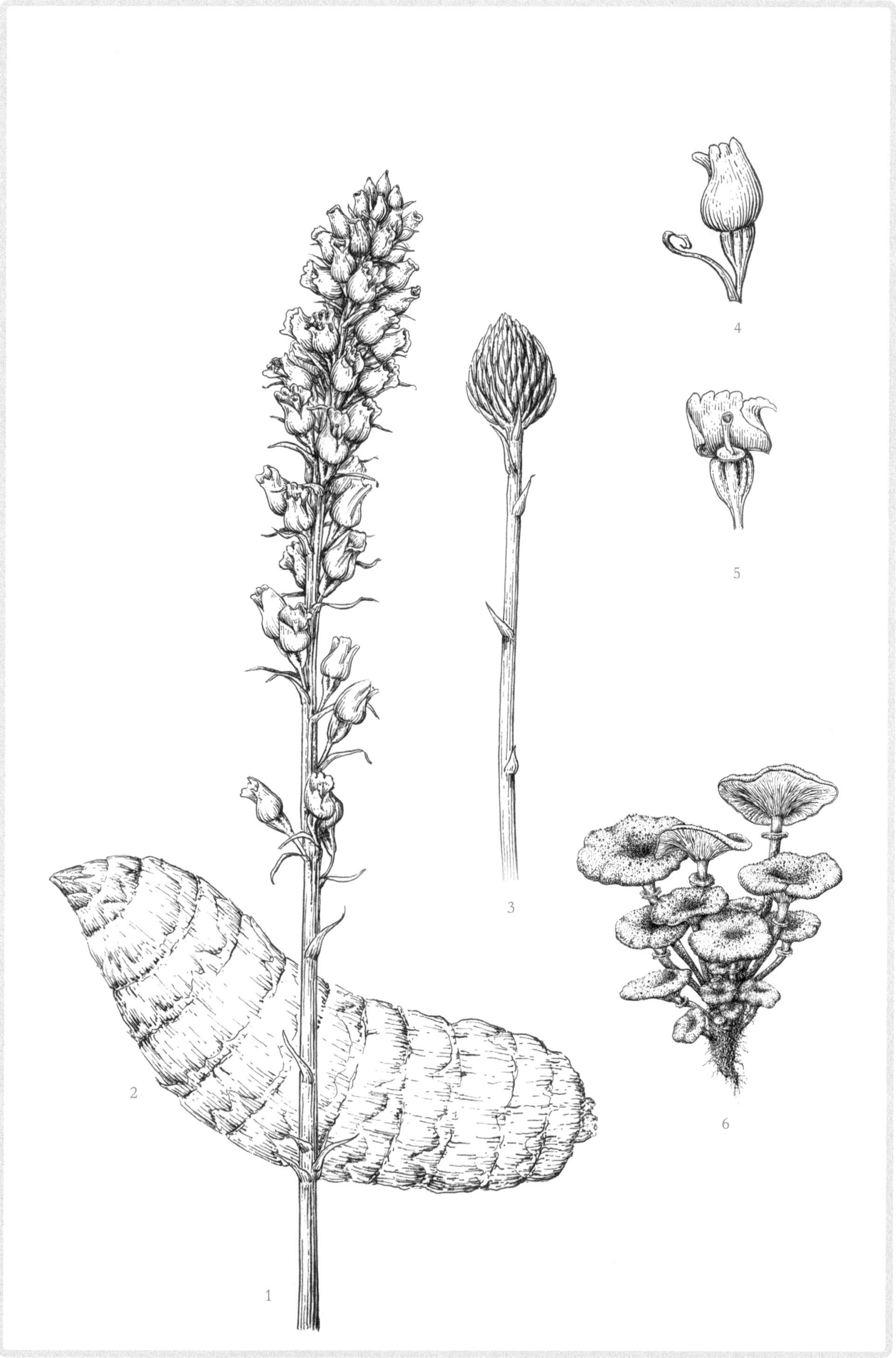

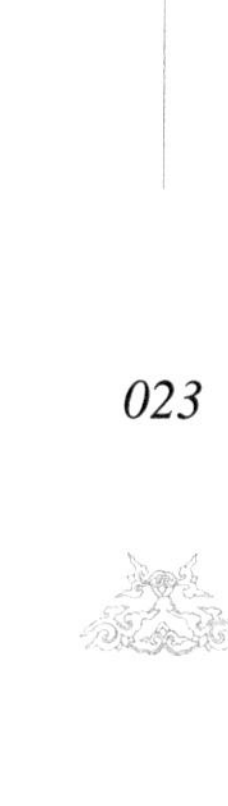

1. 花枝（flowering stem）　2. 块茎（tuber）　3. 幼花序（inflorescence）　4. 花（flower）　5. 雌蕊（pistil）
6. 蜜环菌（*Armillaria mellea*）

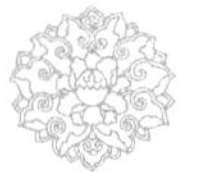

大百合

Dabaihe

Cardiocrinum giganteum

基　源　百合科 Liliaceae 大百合属 *Cardiocrinum* 植物大百合 *Cardiocrinum giganteum* (Wall.) Makino 的干燥鳞茎。药材名为“水百合”。

形态特征　小鳞茎卵形。茎直立，中空，高大。叶纸质，网状脉；基生叶卵状心形或近宽矩圆状心形，茎生叶卵状心形，向上渐小。总状花序有花 10-16 朵；花狭喇叭形，白色，里面具淡紫红色条纹。蒴果近球形，顶端有 1 小尖突，基部有粗短果柄，具 6 钝棱和多数细横纹，3 瓣裂。种子呈扁钝三角形，红棕色，周围具淡红棕色半透明的膜质翅。

生境分布　主要分布于我国西南各省。生海拔 1450-2300 m 的林下草丛中。国外分布于印度、尼泊尔、不丹等地。

采收加工　春、夏采挖，洗净，鲜用或晒干。

性味功能　凉，苦、微甘。清肺止咳，解毒消肿。

主治用法　主要用于治疗感冒，肺热咳嗽，咯血，鼻渊，聤耳，乳痈，无名肿毒。外用适量，捣烂绞汁，滴鼻、耳；或捣敷。

化学成分　主要含有甾体生物碱类、黄酮类等成分。

Source　It is the dried bulbs of *Cardiocrinum giganteum* (Wall.) Makino (Liliaceae). The medicinal material is called “Shuibaihe”.

Distribution　*C. giganteum* is mainly distributed in southwest China and grows in the underbrush of the forest at an altitude of 1450–2300 m. It is also distributed in the Republic of India, Kingdom of Nepal, Kingdom of Bhutan, etc.

Indications　It is mainly used to treat colds, cough with lung heat, hemoptysis, sinusitis, cerumen, acute mastitis, and innominate pyogenic infection. The crushed liquid formula can be applied externally with appropriate amounts in the nose and ear.

Chemical Constituents　It mainly contains steroid alkaloids, flavonoids, etc.

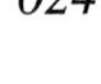

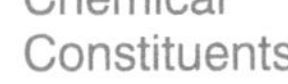

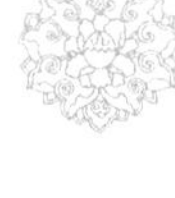

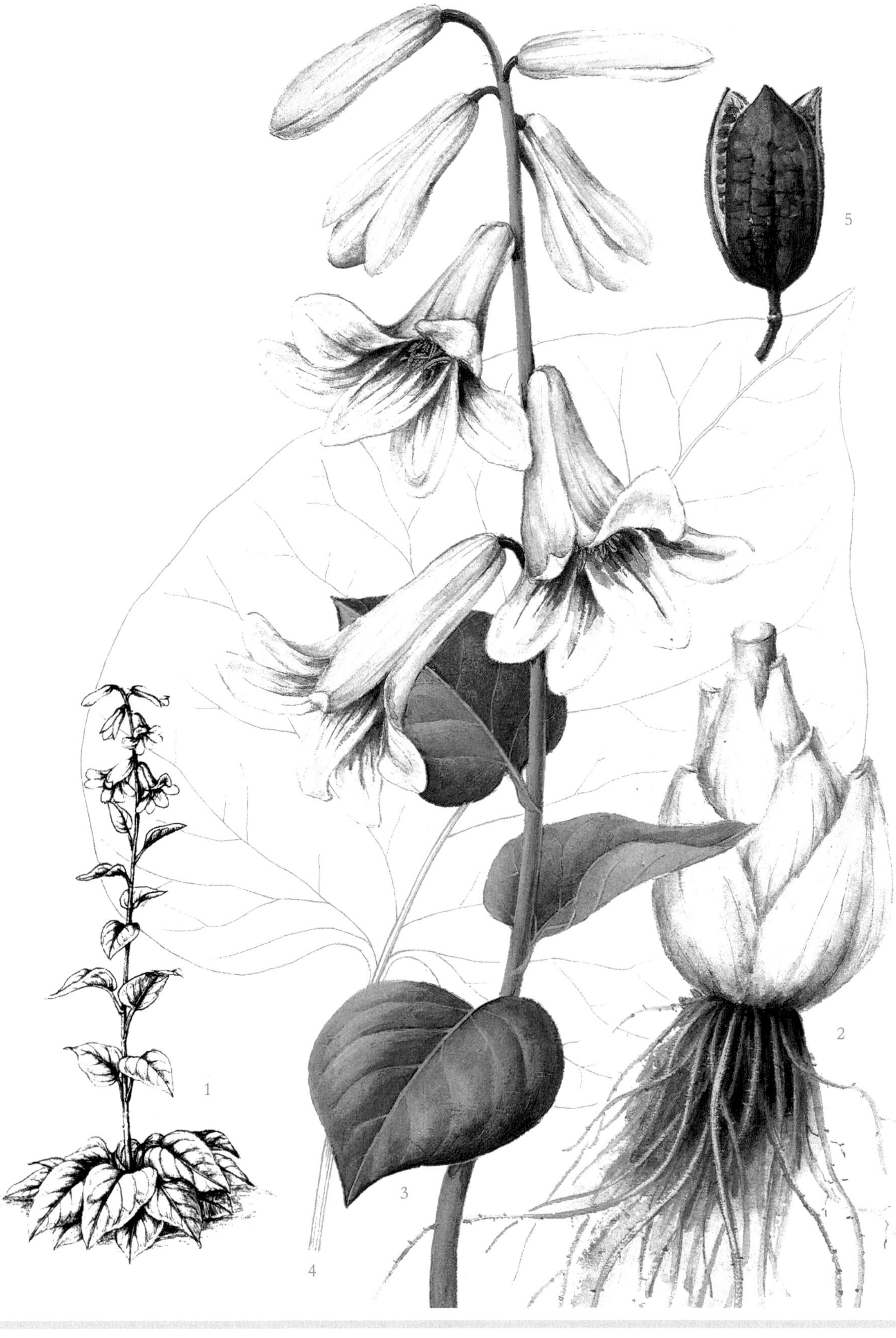

大百合

1. 植株（plant） 2. 鳞茎（bulb） 3. 花枝（flowering stem） 4. 叶（leaf） 5. 果实（fruit）

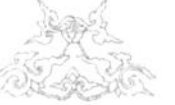

浙贝母

Zhebeimu

Fritillaria thunbergii

基　源　百合科 Liliaceae 贝母属 *Fritillaria* 植物浙贝母 *Fritillaria thunbergii* Miq. 的干燥鳞茎。药材名为“浙贝母”。

形态特征　多年生草本。鳞茎由 2(-3) 枚鳞片组成。最下面的叶对生或散生，向上常兼有散生、对生和轮生的，近条形至披针形。花 1-6 朵，淡黄色，顶端的花具 3-4 枚叶状苞片，其余的具 2 枚苞片；苞片先端卷曲。蒴果，有棱，棱上有宽约 6-8 mm 的翅。

生境分布　主要分布于江苏、安徽、浙江等省；日本也有分布。生于海拔较低的山丘荫蔽处或竹林下。为著名的道地药材“浙八味”之一。

采收加工　初夏植株枯萎时采挖，洗净。大小分开，大者除去芯芽，习称“大贝”；小者不去芯芽，习称“珠贝”。分别撞擦，除去外皮，拌以煅过的贝壳粉，吸去擦出的浆汁，干燥；或取鳞茎，大小分开，洗净，除去芯芽，趁鲜切成厚片，洗净，干燥，习称“浙贝片”。

性味功能　寒，苦。清热化痰止咳，解毒散结消痈。

主治用法　主要用于风热咳嗽，痰火咳嗽，肺痈，乳痈，瘰疬，疮毒。不宜与乌头类中药同用。

化学成分　鳞茎含有浙贝母碱（浙贝甲素）和去氢浙贝母碱（浙贝乙素）等多种生物碱。其它还含有脂肪酸和贝母醇等。

Source　It is the dried bulb of *Fritillaria thunbergii* Miq. (Liliaceae). The medicinal material is called “Zhebeimu”.

Distribution　*F. thunbergii* is distributed in Jiangsu, Anhui, Zhejiang and other provinces, and can be found in Japan as well. It grows in the shade of hills or under bamboo groves at a low altitudes. It is one of the famous authentic medicinal materials—“Eight Tastes of Zhejiang”.

Indications　It is used to treat cough due to wind–heat, phlegm–fire–induced cough, lung abscess, acute mastitis, scrofula, and sore toxin. It should not be used with medicinal materials of *Aconitum* spp.

Chemical Constituents　The bulb contains many alkaloids, e.g., peimine and verticinone. It also contains fatty acids and propeimine.

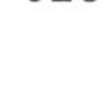

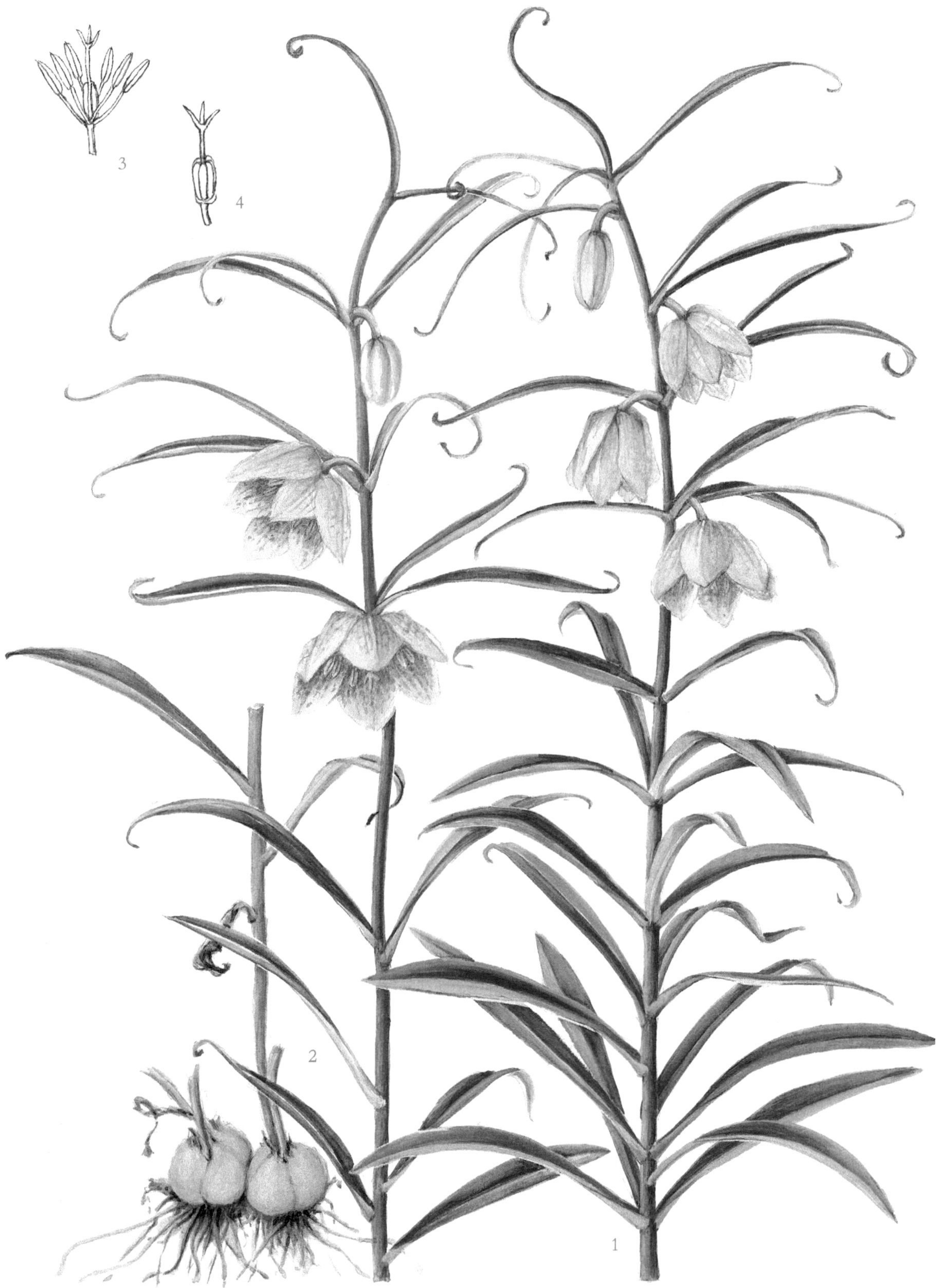

浙贝母

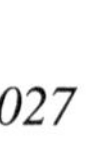

1. 花枝（flowering stem） 2. 鳞茎（bulb） 3. 雄蕊及雌蕊（stamen and pistil） 4. 雌蕊（pistil）

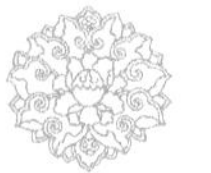

梭砂贝母

Suoshabeimu

Fritillaria delavayi

基　　源　百合科 Liliaceae 贝母属 *Fritillaria* 植物梭砂贝母 *Fritillaria delavayi* Franch. 的干燥鳞茎。药材名为“川贝母”，习称“炉贝”。

形态特征　多年生草本。鳞茎由 2-3 枚鳞片组成。叶 3-5 枚（包括叶状苞片），较紧密地生于植株中部或上部，全部散生或最上面 2 枚对生，卵状椭圆形，先端不卷曲。花 1-2 朵，钟形，浅黄色至黄褐色，具红褐色斑点或小方格。蒴果有棱，棱上具狭翅，宿存花被常多少包住蒴果。

生境分布　主要分布于我国西藏、云南、四川等省区。生于海拔 4000 m 以上的流石滩缝隙中。

采收加工　夏、秋二季或积雪融化时采挖，除去须根、粗皮及泥沙，晒干或低温干燥。

性味功能　微寒，苦、甘。清热润肺，化痰止咳，散结消痈。

主治用法　主要用于肺热燥咳，干咳少痰，阴虚劳嗽，痰中带血。瘰疬，乳痈，肺痈。研粉冲服。不宜与乌头类中药同用。

化学成分　鳞茎含有生物碱，如梭砂贝母碱、梭砂贝母酮碱等。

备　　注　梭砂贝母的鳞茎习称“炉贝”。

Source　It is the dried bulb of *F. delavayi* Franch. (Liliaceae). The medicinal material is called “Chuanbeimu”.

Distribution　It is mainly distributed in Tibet, Yunnan, Sichuan and other rigions. It grows in stone crevices on rocky beaches at altitudes above 4000 m.

Indications　It is used to treat irritating dry cough due to lung heat, dry cough with less sputum, consumptive cough due to yin deficiency, phlegm containing blood, scrofula, acute mastitis, and lung abscess. It should be ground into powder and taken after mixed with water. It should not be used with medicinal materials of *Aconitum* spp.

Chemical Constituents　The bulb contains alkaloids, e.g., delavine and delavinone.

Note　The bulb is commonly called Bulbus Fritillariae Delavayi.

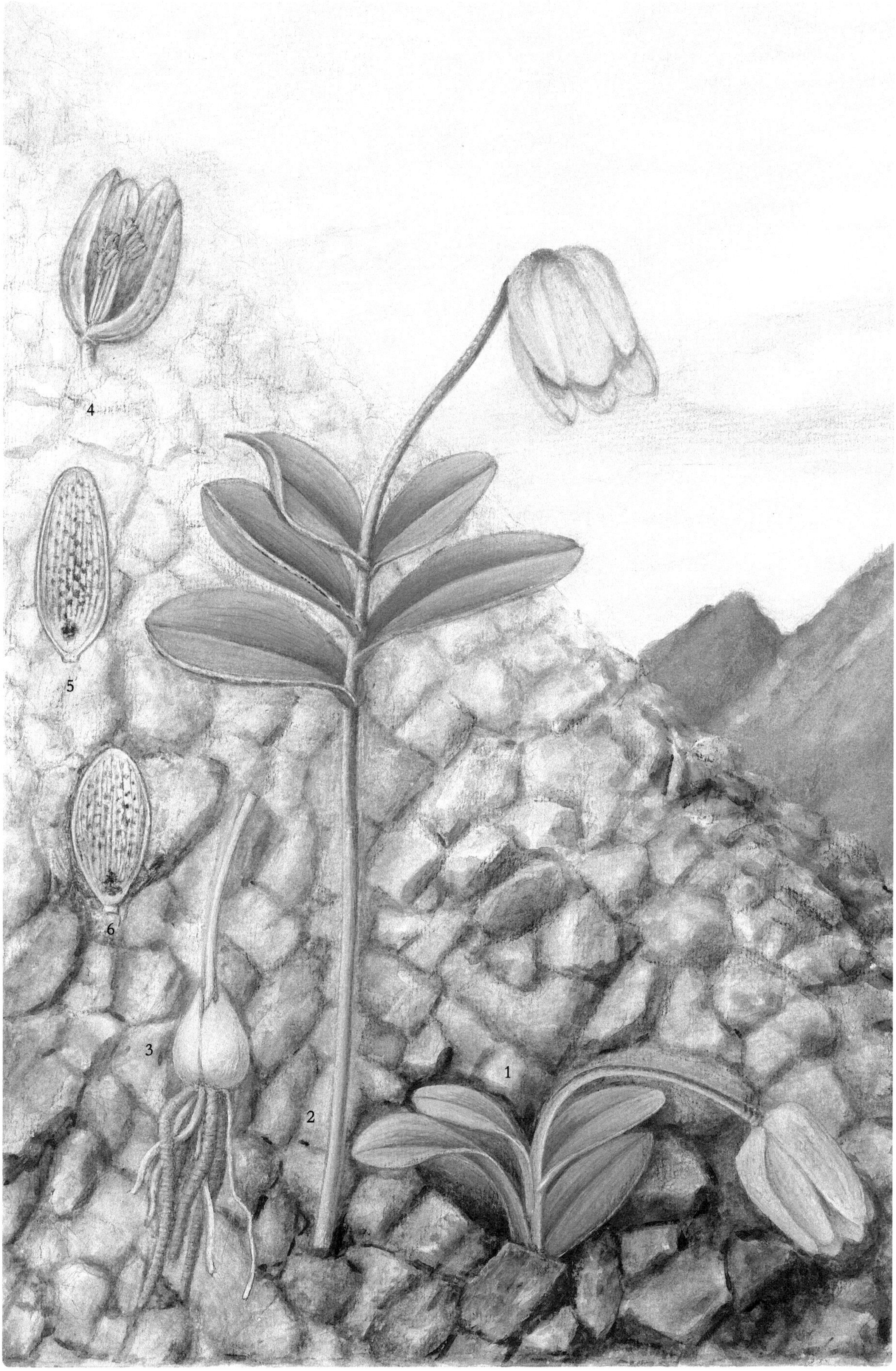

梭砂贝母

1. 植株及生境（plant and habitat） 2. 花枝（flowering stem） 3. 鳞茎（bulb） 4. 花（flower） 5. 外轮花被片（outer tepal） 6. 内轮花被片（inner tepal）

暗紫贝母

Anzibeimu

Fritillaria unibracteata

基　　源　百合科 Liliaceae 贝母属 *Fritillaria* 植物暗紫贝母 *Fritillaria unibracteata* Hsiao et K.C.Hsia 的干燥鳞茎。药材名为“川贝母”。

形态特征　多年生草本。鳞茎由 2 枚鳞片组成。最下面的 1-2 对叶为对生，上面的叶散生或对生，条形或条状披针形。花单朵，钟形；外面深紫色，内有黄褐色小方格。叶状苞片 1 枚，先端不卷曲。蒴果有棱，棱上翅狭。

生境分布　主要分布于我国四川西北部、青海东南部。生于海拔 2800-4200 m 的草地灌丛中。

采收加工　夏、秋二季或积雪融化时采挖，除去须根、粗皮及泥沙，晒干或低温干燥。

性味功能　微寒，苦、甘。清热润肺，化痰止咳，散结消痈。

主治用法　主要用于肺热燥咳，干咳少痰，阴虚劳嗽，痰中带血，瘰疬，乳痈，肺痈。研粉冲服。不宜与乌头类中药同用。

化学成分　鳞茎含有生物碱类，如松贝辛、松贝甲素等；还含有蔗糖、硬脂酸、棕榈酸、β - 谷甾醇等。

备　　注　暗紫贝母按性状不同分别习称“松贝”和“青贝”。松贝性状鉴别习称“怀中抱月”。

Source　It is the dried bulb of *Fritillaria unibracteata* Hsiao et K.C.Hsia (Liliaceae). The medicinal material is called “Chuanbeimu”.

Distribution　*F. unibracteata* is mainly distributed in northwestern Sichuan and southeastern Qinghai. It grows in the grassland thickets at an altitude of 2800–4200 m.

Indications　It is used to treat irritating dry cough due to lung heat, dry cough with less sputum, consumptive cough due to yin deficiency, sputum containing blood, scrofula, acute mastitis, and lung abscess. It should be ground into powder and taken after mixed with water. It should not be used with medicinal materials of *Aconitum* spp.

Chemical Constituents　The bulb contains alkaloids, e.g., songbeisine and songbeinine. It also contains sucrose, stearic acid, palmitic acid, β-sitosterol, etc.

Note　*F. unibracteata* can be differentiated according to their different traits with the names “Songbei” and “Qingbei”. The characteristic of the former is known as “embracing the moon”.

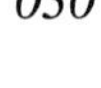

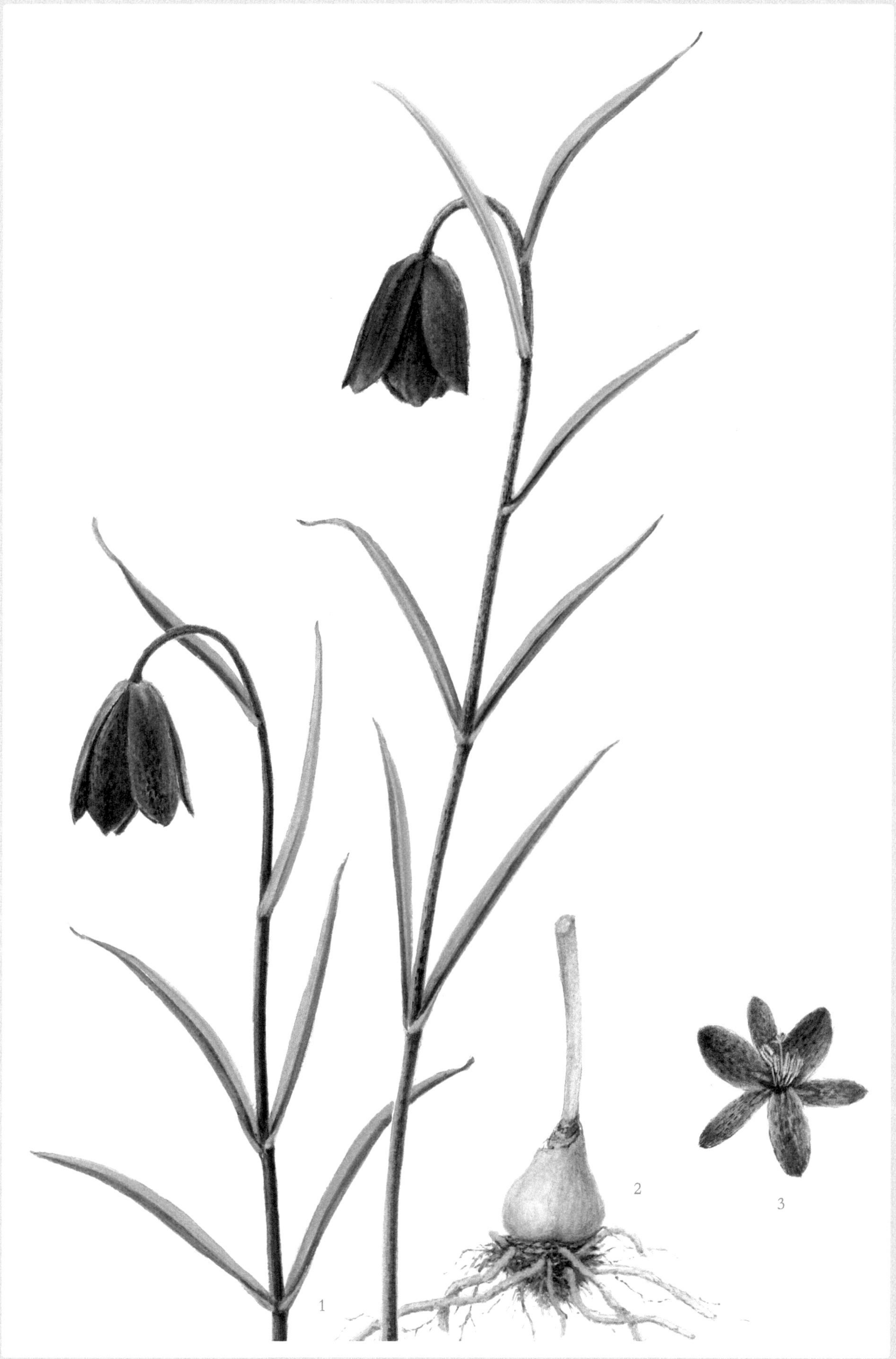

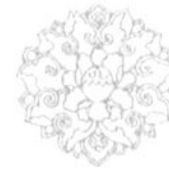

1. 花枝（flowering stem） 2. 鳞茎（bulb） 3. 花内面（inner flower）

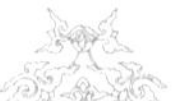

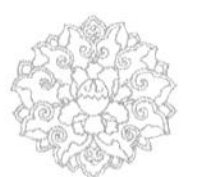

山丹

Shandan

Lilium pumilum

基　　源　百合科 Liliaceae 百合属 *Lilium* 植物山丹（细叶百合）*Lilium pumilum* DC. 的干燥肉质鳞叶。药材名为“百合”。

形态特征　多年生草本。鳞茎卵形；鳞片矩圆形，白色；茎有小乳头状突起。叶散生于茎中部，条形。花单生或数朵排成总状花序，鲜红色，通常无斑点，下垂；花被片反卷。蒴果矩圆形。

生境分布　主要分布于我国华北与西北的部分省区。生于山坡、草地或林缘。

采收加工　秋季采挖，洗净，剥取鳞叶，置沸水中略烫，干燥。

性味功能　寒，甘。养阴润肺，清心安神。

主治用法　主要用于阴虚燥咳，劳嗽咳血，虚烦惊悸，失眠多梦，精神恍惚。

化学成分　鳞叶主要含有多糖、皂苷、生物碱、酚类和甾类糖苷等成分。

备　　注　药食两用。花美丽，可栽培供观赏，也含挥发油，可提取做香料用。

Source　It is the dried succulent scale leaf of *L. pumilum* DC. (Liliaceae). The medicinal material is called “Baihe”.

Distribution　*L. pumilum* is mostly distributed in several provinces of North’and Northeastern China. It grows on the hillsides, grassland, or at forest edges.

Indications　It is used to treat irritating dry cough due to yin deficiency, consumptive cough and hemoptysis, deficient dysphoria and palpitation due to fright, insomnia and dreaminess sleep, and absentmindedness.

Chemical Constituents　The succulent scale leaf contains polysaccharides, saponins, alkaloids, phenols and steroid glycosides.

Note　Bulbus Lilii (*L. pumilum* DC.) can be used as both medicinal material and food. The flower is beautiful and can be cultivated for viewing. The flower also contains volatile oils, which can be extracted and used in spices.

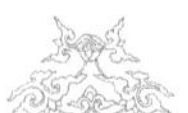

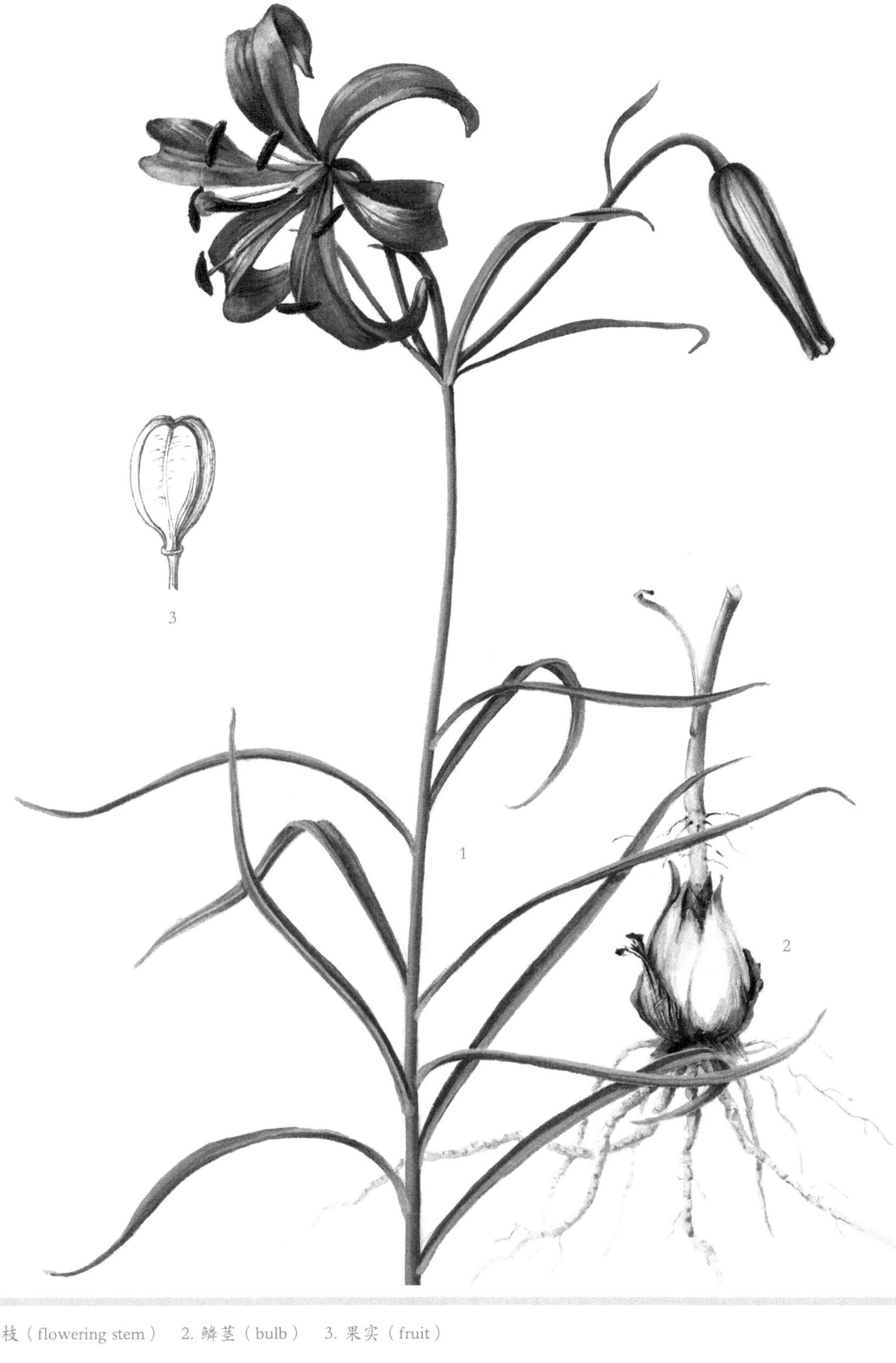

3

1

2

1. 花枝（flowering stem）　2. 鳞茎（bulb）　3. 果实（fruit）

百合

Baihe

Lilium brownii var. *viridulum*

基　　源　百合科 Liliaceae 百合属 *Lilium* 植物百合 *Lilium brownii* F. E. Brown var. *viridulum* Baker 的干燥肉质鳞叶。药材名为“百合”。

形态特征　多年生草本。鳞茎球形，鳞片披针形，白色。茎直立。叶散生，倒披针形至倒卵形，全缘，两面无毛。花单生或几朵排成近伞形；花喇叭形，有香气，乳白色，外面稍带紫色，无斑点，向外张开；雄蕊向上弯，花柱柱头三裂。蒴果矩圆形，有棱。种子多数。

生境分布　主要分布于我国华中及华南的部分省区。生于山坡草丛中、疏林下、山沟旁、地边或村旁。也有栽培。

采收加工　秋季采挖，洗净，剥取鳞叶，置沸水中略烫，干燥。

性味功能　寒，甘。养阴润肺，清心安神。

主治用法　主要用于阴虚燥咳，劳嗽咳血，虚烦惊悸，失眠多梦，精神恍惚。

化学成分　主要含有酚酸甘油酯、丙酸酯衍生物、酚酸的糖苷、甾体糖苷、甾体生物碱、微量元素、淀粉、蛋白质、脂肪等成分。

备　　注　药食两用。湖南省隆回县的特产“龙牙百合”即为此种。

Source　It is the dried succulent scale leaf of *Lilium brownii* F. E. Brown var. *viridulum* Baker (Liliaceae). The medicinal material is called “Baihe”.

Distribution　*L. brownii* is mainly distributed in provinces in Central and South China. It grows on underbrush on hillsides, under sparse forests, and beside ravines, farmlands or villages. It also can be cultivated.

Indications　It is used to treat irritating dry cough due to yin deficiency, consumptive cough and hemoptysis, deficient dysphoria and palpitation due to fright, insomnia and dreaminess, and absentmindedness.

Chemical Constituents　It contains phenolic acid glyceride, propionate derivative, glycoside of phenolic acid, steroid glycoside, steroid alkaloids, trace elements, starch, protein, fat and other components.

Note　It can be used as both medicine and food. “Longyabaihe”, a speciality product of Longhui County, Hunan Province belongs to this category.

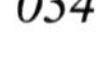

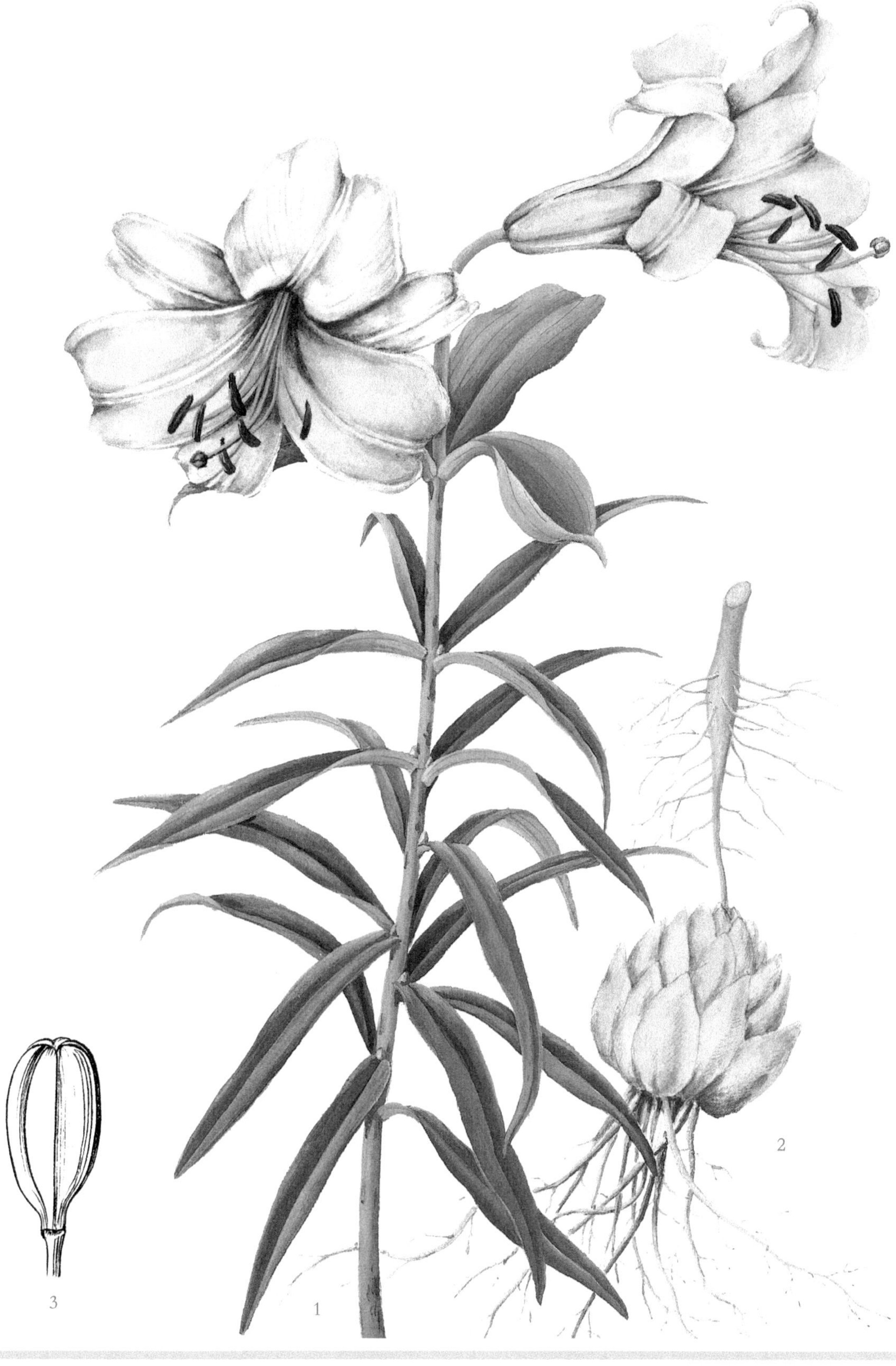

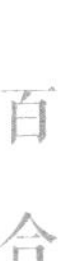

百合

1. 花枝（flowering stem） 2. 鳞茎（bulb） 3. 果实（fruit）

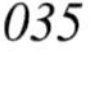

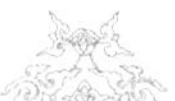

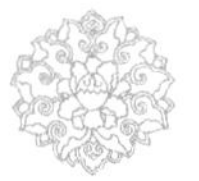

麦冬

Maidong

Ophiopogon japonicus

基　　源　百合科 Liliaceae 沿阶草属 *Ophiopogon* 植物麦冬 *Ophiopogon japonicus* (L. f.) Ker-Gawl. 的干燥块根。药材名为“麦冬”。

形态特征　多年生草本。根近末端常膨大成纺锤形的小块根；地下走茎细长，节上具膜质的鞘。茎短，叶基生成丛，禾叶状，边缘具细锯齿。花葶通常比叶短；总状花序；花单生或成对着生于苞片腋内；花被片常稍下垂而不展开，披针形，白色或淡紫色。种子球形。

生境分布　主要分布于我国中部和南部大部分省区。生于海拔 2000 m 以下的山坡阴湿处、林下或溪旁。现广为栽培。为著名道地药材“浙八味”之一。

采收加工　夏季采挖，洗净，反复暴晒、堆置，至七八成干，除去须根，干燥。

性味功能　微寒，甘、微苦。养阴生津，润肺清心。

主治用法　主要用于肺燥干咳，阴虚痨嗽，喉痹咽痛，津伤口渴，内热消渴，心烦失眠，肠燥便秘。

化学成分　块根中主要含有皂苷类、黄酮类、挥发油类；另还含有龙脑葡萄糖苷、维生素、β-谷甾醇等。

Source　It is the dried root rhizome of *Ophiopogon japonicus* (L. f.) Ker-Gawl. (Liliaceae). The medicinal material is called “Maidong”.

Distribution　*O. japonicus* is mainly distributed in most provinces of the middle and southern part of China. It grows on shady hillsides, on the forests or beside streams below 2000 m above sea level and is widely cultivated at present. Radix Ophiopogonis is one of the famous authentic medicinal materials—“Eight Tastes of Zhejiang”.

Indications　It is used to treat dry cough due to dryness in the lung, consumptive cough due to yin deficiency, pharyngitis and sore throat, fluid damaging and thirst, internal heat and wasting thirst, vexation and insomnia, intestinal dryness with constipation.

Chemical Constituents　The root rhizome mainly contains saponins, flavonoids, volatile oils, borneol-2-*O*-glucopyranoside, vitamins, β-sitosterol, etc.

麦冬

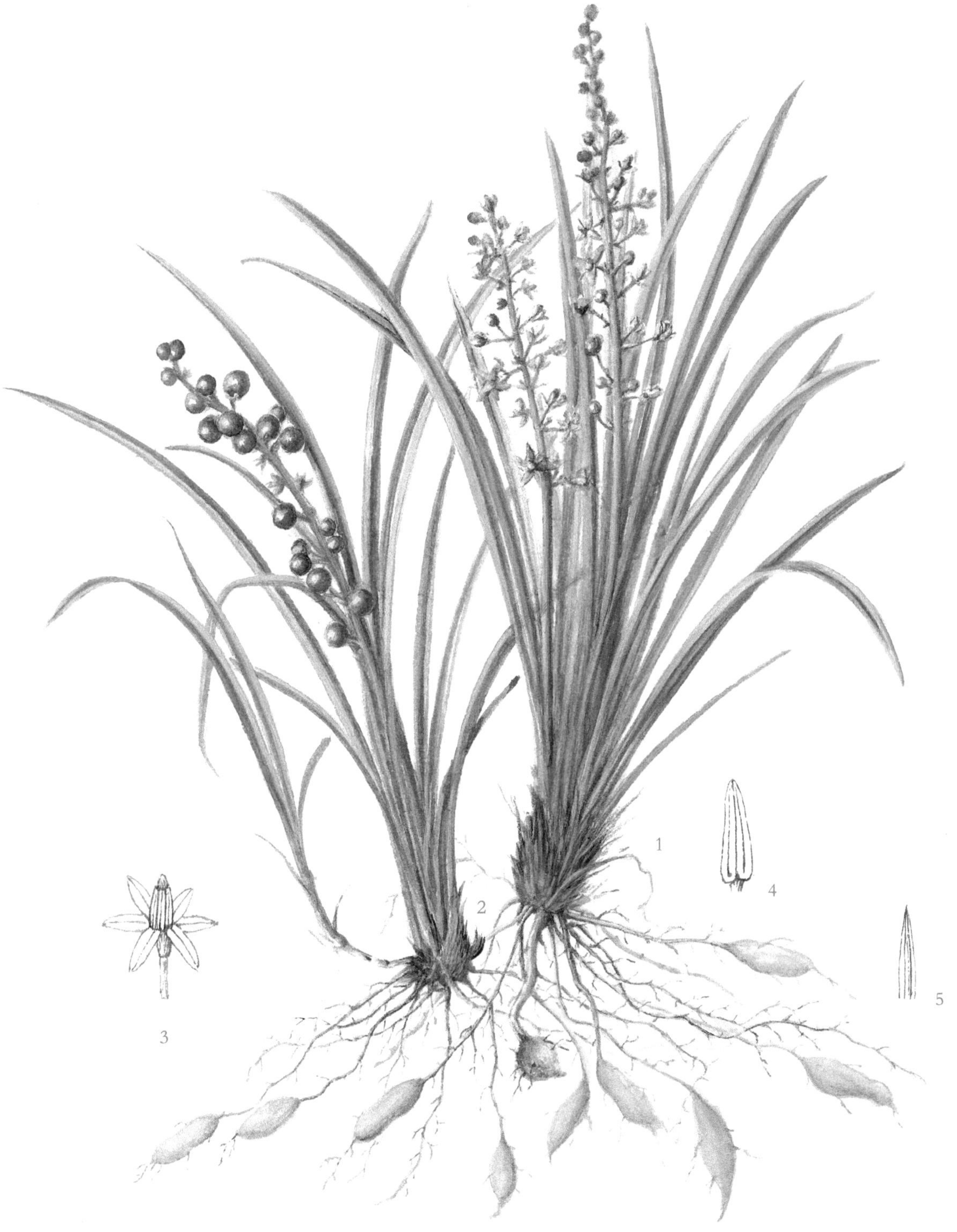

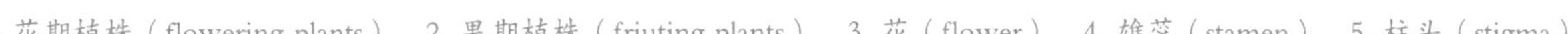

1. 花期植株（flowering plants） 2. 果期植株（friuting plants） 3. 花（flower） 4. 雄蕊（stamen） 5. 柱头（stigma）

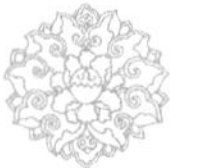

七叶一枝花

Qiyeyizhihua

Paris polyphylla var. *chinensis*

基　　源　百合科 Liliaceae 重楼属 *Paris* 植物七叶一枝花 *Paris polyphylla* Smith var. *chinensis* (Franch.) Hara 的干燥根茎。药材名为“重楼”。

形态特征　多年生草本。根状茎粗厚，密生多数环节和须根；茎常带紫红色，基部有干膜质的鞘。叶通常 7 枚，倒卵状披针形，基部通常楔形。花被片两轮，近披针形；雄蕊 8-10 枚，花药长为花丝的 3-4 倍，药隔略突出；子房近球形，具棱，顶端具一盘状花柱基。蒴果紫色。种子乳白色，具红色多浆汁的外种皮。

生境分布　分布于我国南方大部分省区。常生于海拔 600 m 以上的林下阴湿处或竹林中。

采收加工　秋季采挖，除去须根，洗净，晒干。

性味功能　微寒，苦；有小毒。清热解毒，消肿止痛，凉肝定惊。

主治用法　主要用于疔疮痈肿，咽喉肿痛，蛇虫咬伤，跌扑伤痛，惊风抽搐。

化学成分　主要含有重楼皂苷；另还含有甾酮、蜕皮激素，以及黄酮类成分。

备　　注　重楼属多种植物均在民间作为清热解毒的良药使用，其中北重楼 *Paris verticillata* M. Bieb. 入药称“王孙”。近年来，由于无节制的采挖，野生资源破坏极其严重。

Source　It is the dried rhizome of *Paris polyphylla* Smith var. *chinensis* (Franch.) Hara (Liliaceae). The medicinal material is called “Chonglou”.

Distribution　*P. polyphylla* var. *chinensis* is distributed in most provinces of southern China. It generally grows in the understory or bamboo groves at an altitude of over 600 m.

Indications　It is mainly used to treat boil, sore, swollen welling-abscess, swollen sore throat, snake and insect bites, traumatic injury, infantile convulsion and convulsion.

Chemical Constituents　It mainly contains polyphyllins, as well as sterone, ecdyone and flavonoids.

Note　Many species of the *Paris* genus are used as an effective medicine for clearing heat and removing toxin. Among them, *P. verticillata* M. Bieb. used as medicine is called “Wangsun”. In recent years, due to uncontrolled harvesting, the destruction of wild resources is severe.

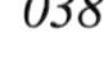

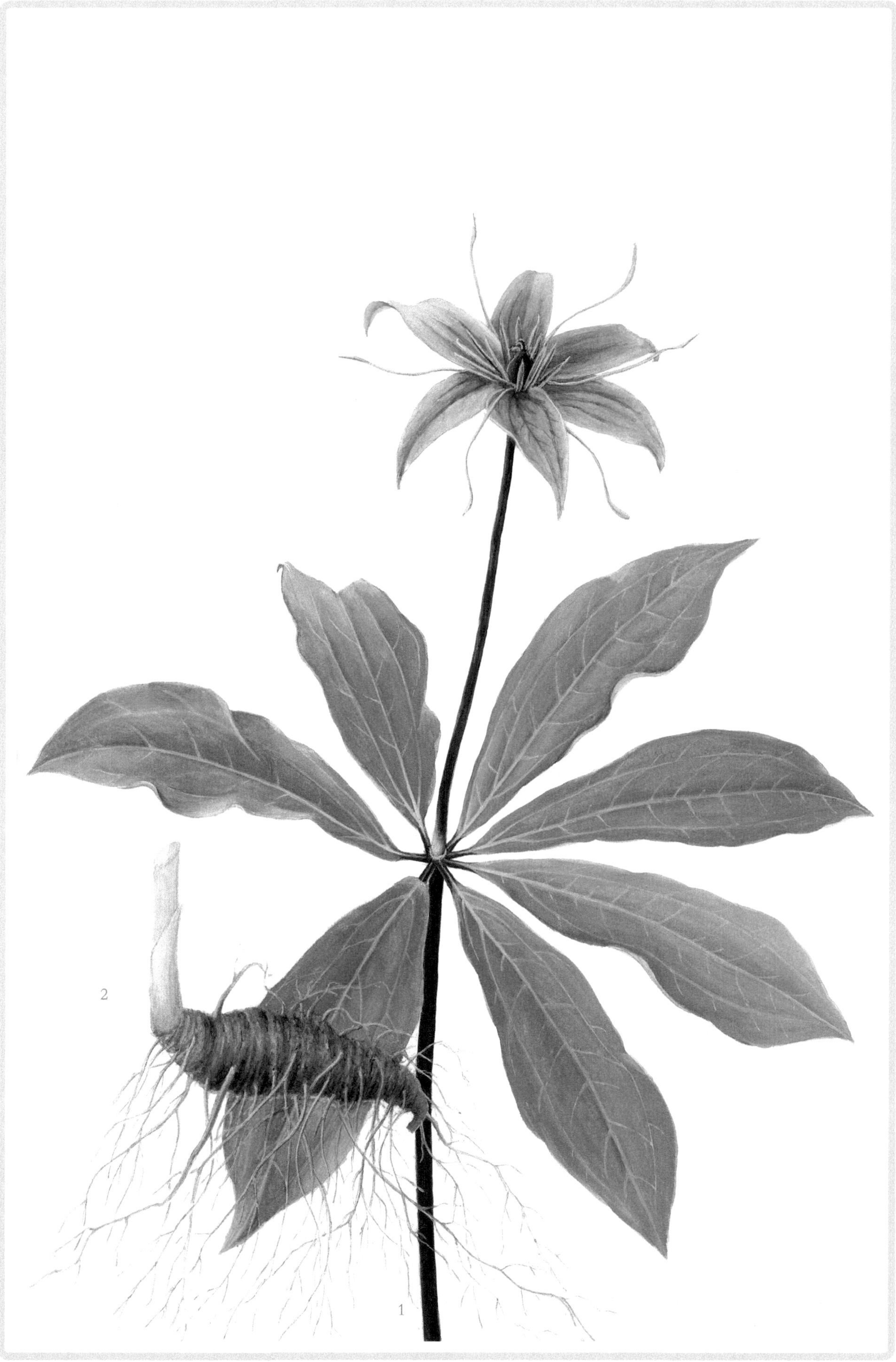

2

1

1. 花枝（flowering stem） 2. 根状茎（rhizome）

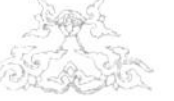

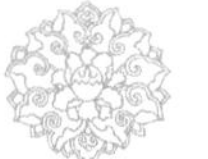

当归

Danggui

Angelica sinensis

基　　源　伞形科 Apiaceae 当归属 *Angelica* 植物当归 *Angelica sinensis* (Oliv.) Diels 的干燥根。药材名为“当归”。

形态特征　多年生草本。根圆柱状，有浓郁香气。茎直立，具纵深沟纹。叶三出式二至三回羽状分裂，基部膨大成薄膜质鞘，常为紫色；基生叶及茎下部叶卵形，边缘有缺刻状锯齿；茎上部叶简化成囊状的鞘和羽状分裂的叶片。复伞形花序；花白色。果实椭圆形，背棱线形，隆起，侧棱成宽而薄的翅。

生境分布　栽培于陕西、甘肃、湖北、四川、云南、贵州等地。甘肃岷县当归量大质优，久负盛名，为道地药材。

采收加工　秋末采挖，除去须根和泥沙，待水分稍蒸发后，捆成小把，上棚，用烟火慢慢熏干。

性味功能　温，甘、辛。补血活血，调经止痛，润肠通便。

主治用法　用于血虚萎黄，眩晕心悸，月经不调，经闭痛经，虚寒腹痛，风湿痹痛，跌扑损伤，痈疽疮疡，肠燥便秘。酒当归活血通经。用于经闭痛经，风湿痹痛，跌扑损伤。

化学成分　主要含有糖类，如当归多糖、蔗糖、果糖等；另还含有阿魏酸、苯酞、苯酚、腺嘌呤、尿嘧啶等。

备　　注　传统中医认为当归的根头部称“归头”，主根称“归身”，支根及支根梢部称“归尾”，功效略有不同。

Source　It is the dried root of *Angelica sinensis* (Oliv.) Diels. (Apiaceae). The medicinal material is called “Danggui”.

Distribution　*A. sinensis* is cultivated in Shaanxi, Gansu, Hubei, Sichuan, Yunnan, Guizhou provinces, etc. Radix Angelicae Sinensis produced in Mianxian County, Gansu has large production and good quality, which is the authentic medicinal material.

Indications　It is used to treat shallow yellow due to blood deficiency, dizziness and palpitation, menstrual irregularities, amenorrhea and dysmenorrhea, abdominal pain due to cold deficiency, wind–dampness impediment pain, traumatic injury, carbuncle, cellulitis, sore, and ulcer, intestinal dryness and constipation. Radix Angelicae Sinensis processed with rice wine can be used for promoting blood circulation to regulate menstruation, which can be used to treat amenorrhea and dysmenorrhea, wind–dampness impediment pain, as well as traumatic injury.

Chemical Constituents　It mainly contains saccharides, e.g., angelica polysaccharide, sucrose, and fructose. It also contains ferulic acid, phthalide, phenol, adenine, uracil, etc.

Note　In traditional Chinese medicine (TCM), the head part of Radix Angelicae Sinensis is called “Guitou”; the main root “Guishen”, and the rootlet part “Guiwei”. Each part has slightly different effects.

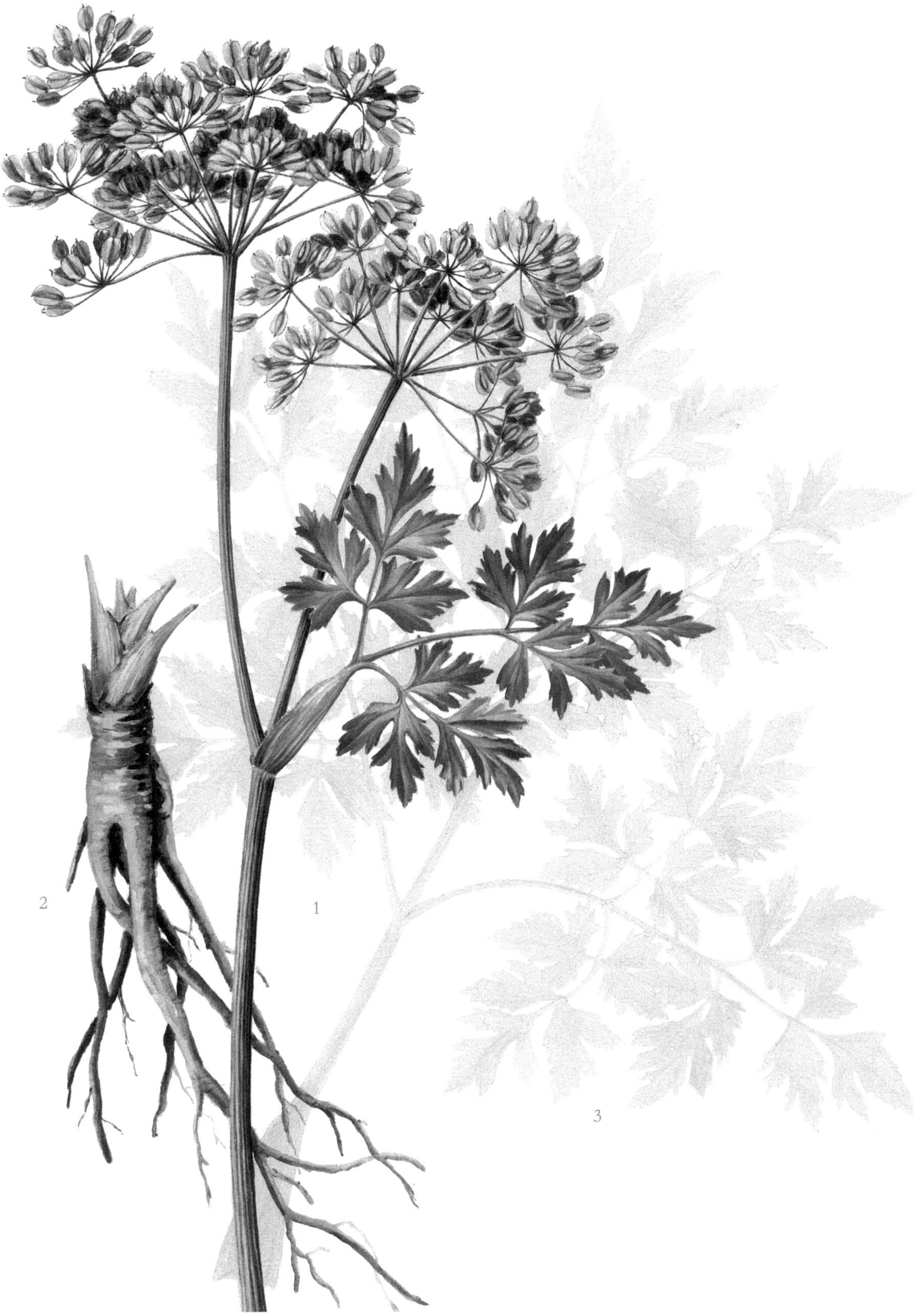

1. 果枝（fruiting stem） 2. 根（root） 3. 茎生叶（stem leaf）

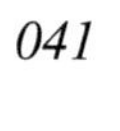

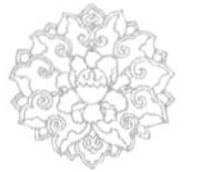

狭叶柴胡

Xiayechaihu

Bupleurum scorzonerifolium

基　　源　伞形科 Apiaceae 柴胡属 *Bupleurum* 植物狭叶柴胡 *Bupleurum scorzonerifolium* Willd. 的干燥根。药材名为“柴胡”，习称“南柴胡”。

形态特征　多年生草本。主根发达，上端有横环纹。茎基部密覆叶柄残余纤维，茎呈之字形弯曲。叶细线形，顶端长渐尖，基部抱茎，质厚，稍硬挺，常内卷。伞形花序自叶腋间抽出，花序多，形成较疏松的圆锥花序；小伞形花序有花 9-11；花瓣黄色。果实椭圆形，深褐色，每棱槽中油管 5-6，合生面 4-6。

生境分布　分布于我国东北、华北、华东、华中各省区。生于干燥的草地及向阳的山坡灌丛边缘。

采收加工　春、秋二季采挖，除去茎叶和泥沙，干燥。

性味功能　微寒，辛、苦。疏散退热，疏肝解郁，升举阳气。

主治用法　用于感冒发热，寒热往来，胸胁胀痛，月经不调，子宫脱垂，脱肛。

化学成分　主要含有柴胡皂苷类成分。还含有挥发油类，如柠檬烯、月桂烯、葎草烯等；黄酮类，如槲皮素、山奈苷等；以及有机酸和 β-谷甾醇等。

Source　It is the dried root of *Bupleurum scorzonerifolium* Willd. (Apiaceae). The medicinal material is called “Chaihu”.

Distribution　*B. scorzonerifolium* is distributed in the provinces of Northeast, North, East and Central China. It grows on dry grasslands and the edge of the shrubs on hillsides with sun exposure.

Indications　It is used to treat cold and fever, alternating chills and fever, distending pain in the chest and hypochondrium, menstrual irregularities, and prolapse of the uterus and rectum.

Chemical Constituents　It mainly contains saikosaponins. It also contains volatile oils (e.g., limonene, myrcene, humulene), flavonoids (e.g., quercetin, kaempferitrin), organic acids, and β-sitosterol.

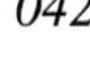

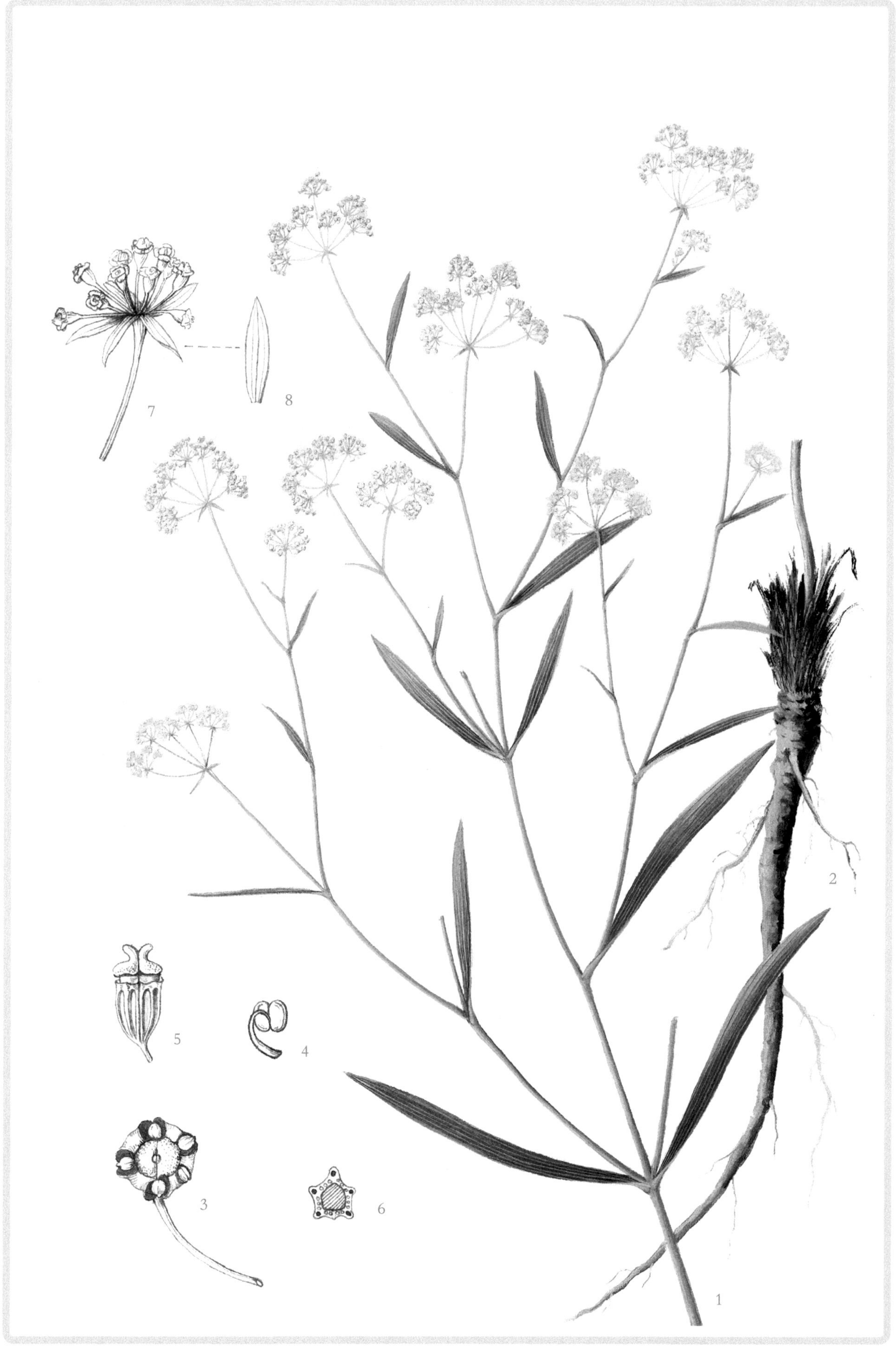

1. 花枝（flowering stem） 2. 根（root） 3. 花（flower） 4. 雄蕊（stamen） 5. 果实（fruit） 6. 果实横切（cross section of fruit） 7. 花序（inflorescence） 8. 苞片（bract）

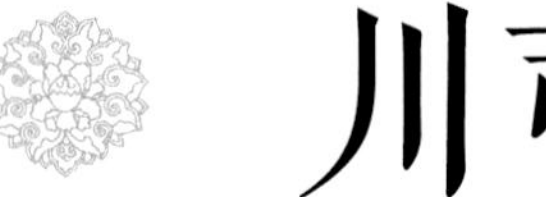

川芎

Chuanxiong

Ligusticum sinense 'Chuanxiong'

基　　源　伞形科 Apiaceae 藁本属 *Ligusticum* 植物川芎 *Ligusticum sinense* 'Chuanxiong' 的干燥根茎。药材名为“川芎”。

形态特征　多年生草本。根状茎为结节状拳形团块，具浓烈香气；茎直立，圆柱形，具纵条纹，上部多分枝，下部茎节膨大呈盘状；茎下部叶具柄，基部扩大成鞘。叶片轮廓卵状三角形，二至三回羽状复叶，羽片卵状披针形；茎上部叶渐简化。复伞形花序顶生或侧生；花瓣白色。双悬果卵圆形，五棱，有窄翅。

生境分布　主产四川都江堰、彭州。栽培植物。

采收加工　夏季当茎上的节盘显著突出，并略带紫色时采挖，除去泥沙，晒后烘干，再去须根。

性味功能　温，辛。活血行气，祛风止痛。

主治用法　主要用于胸痹心痛，胸胁刺痛，跌扑肿痛，月经不调，经闭痛经，癥瘕腹痛，头痛，风湿痹痛。

化学成分　主要含有挥发油类成分，如藁本内酯、3- 丁叉苯酞、香桧烯等；此外还含有苯酞衍生物，如川芎内酯、川芎酚等；生物碱类，如川芎嗪、盐酸胆碱等；有机酸类及酯类，如阿魏酸、叶酸、苯乙酸甲酯等；另还含有香草醛、维生素 A 等。

备　　注　川芎为血中之气药。

Source　It is the dried rhizome of *Ligusticum sinense* 'Chuanxiong' (Apiaceae). The medicinal material is called “Chuanxiong”.

Distribution　*L. sinense* is a cultivated plant and is mainly produced in Dujiangyan and Pengzhou, Sichuan.

Indications　It is used to treat heart pain due to chest impediment, stabbing pain and distending pain in the chest and hypochondrium, painful swelling with traumatic injury, menstrual irregularities, amenorrhea and dysmenorrhea, abdominal mass and pain, headache, wind–dampness impediment pain.

Chemical Constituents　It mainly contains volatile oils, e.g., ligustilide, 3-butylidenephthalide and sabinene. Besides, it contains phthalide derivatives (e.g., cnidilide, chuanxingol), alkaloids (e.g., ligustrazine, choline hydrochloride), organic acids and esters (e.g., ferulic acid, folate, methyl phenylacetate). It also contains vanillin, vitamin A, etc.

Note　It is a medicine used to facilitate the movement of blood by moving qi.

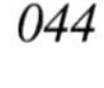

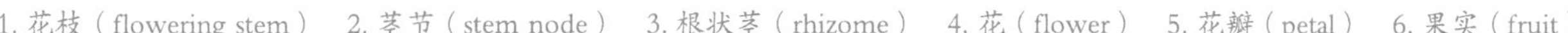
1. 花枝（flowering stem） 2. 茎节（stem node） 3. 根状茎（rhizome） 4. 花（flower） 5. 花瓣（petal） 6. 果实（fruit）

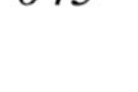

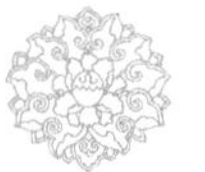

粉防己

Fenfangji

Stephania tetrandra

基　源　防己科 Menispermaceae 千金藤属 *Stephania* 植物粉防己 *Stephania tetrandra* S.Moore 的干燥根。药材名为“防己”。

形态特征　草质藤本。主根肉质。叶柄盾状着生，长与叶片相等；叶互生，纸质，阔三角形，顶端有凸尖，两面或仅下面被贴伏短柔毛；掌状脉 9-10 条，较纤细，网脉甚密，明显。花序头状，于腋生、长而下垂的枝条上作总状式排列；花小，雌雄异株。核果成熟时近球形，红色。

生境分布　分布于我国华东及华南部分省区。常见于路边灌丛中。

采收加工　秋季采挖，洗净，除去粗皮，晒至半干，切段，个大者再纵切，干燥。

性味功能　寒，苦。祛风止痛，利水消肿。

主治用法　用于风湿痹痛，水肿脚气，小便不利，湿疹疮毒。

化学成分　主要含有生物碱类成分，如粉防己碱、防己诺林碱、门尼新碱、氧化防己碱、防己菲碱等；另还含有黄酮苷类、有机酸类、酚类、挥发油类等。

备　注　广防己曾作为防己入药，因含有马兜铃酸，现已取消入药标准。

Source　It is the dried root of *Stephania tetrandra* S.Moore (Menispermaceae). The medicinal material is called as “Fangji”.

Distribution　*S. tetrandra* is distributed in East China and parts of South China. It is commonly found in road-side thickets.

Indications　It is used to treat wind–dampness impediment pain, edema and beriberi, dysuria, eczema and sore toxin.

Chemical Constituents　It mainly contains alkaloids, e.g., tetrandrine, fangchinoline, menisine, oxofangchirine and stephanthrine. It also contains flavonoid glycosides, organic acids, phenols and volatile oils.

Note　*Isotrema fangchi* was previously used as medicine. However, since it contains aristolochic acid, it has been eliminated from medicinal standards at present.

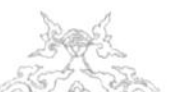

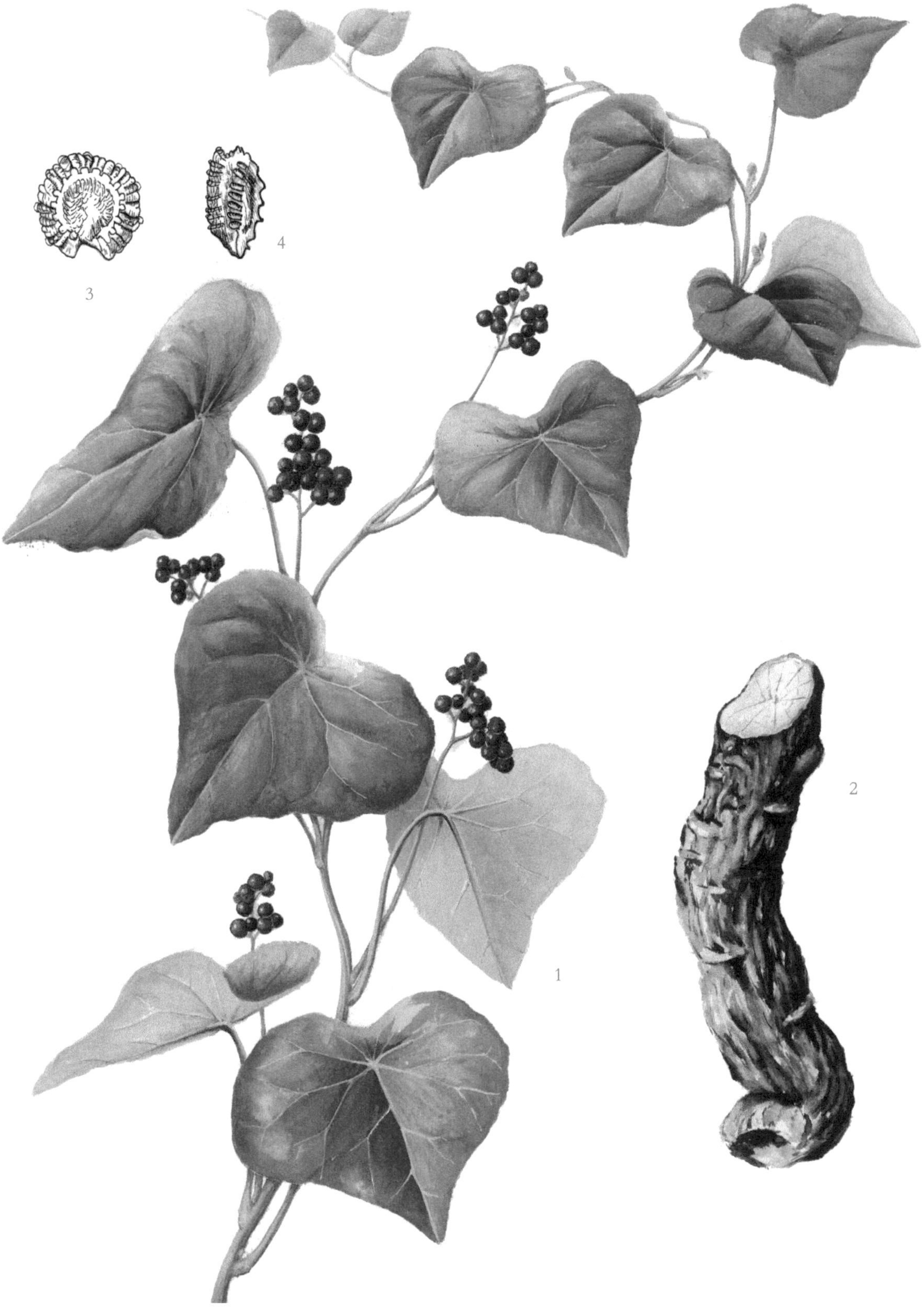

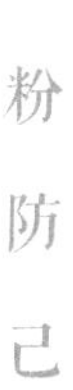

粉防己

1. 果枝（fruiting stem） 2. 根（root） 3. 种子（seed） 4. 种子侧面观（lateral view of the seed）

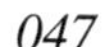

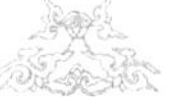

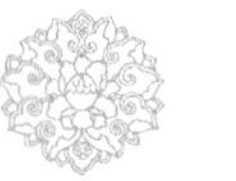

青牛胆

Qingniudan

Tinospora sagittata

基　　源　防己科 Menispermaceae 青牛胆属 *Tinospora* 植物青牛胆 *Tinospora sagittata* (Oliv.) Gagnep. 的干燥块根。药材名为“金果榄”。

形态特征　多年生草质藤本，具连珠状块根，黄色。枝纤细，常被柔毛。叶纸质，披针状箭形，先端渐尖，基部弯缺，上面或两面近无毛；掌状脉 5 条，连同网脉均在下面凸起。单性异株；花序腋生，成总状或圆锥花序；雄花序常簇生，雌花序常单生。核果红色，近球形；果核近半球形。

生境分布　沿四川东部、湖北西部分布至我国中南大部分地区。常散生于林下、林缘、竹林下等。

采收加工　秋、冬二季采挖，除去须根，洗净，晒干。

性味功能　寒，苦。清热解毒，利咽，止痛。

主治用法　主要用于咽喉肿痛，痈疽疔毒，泄泻，痢疾，脘腹疼痛。

化学成分　主要含有生物碱类成分，如防己碱、药根碱；还含有古伦宾等萜类和甾醇类等成分。

Source　It is the dried root rhizome of *Tinospora sagittata* (Oliv.) Gagnep. (Menispermaceae). The medicinal material is called as “Jinguolan”.

Distribution　*T. sagittata* is distributed in the regions within eastern Sichuan, western Hubei to south–central China. It commonly grows dispersively in forest, forest margins, bamboo groves, etc.

Indications　It is used to treat sore swollen throat, abscess, carbuncle, boil and toxin, diarrhea, dysentery, epigastric pain.

Chemical Constituents　It mainly contains alkaloids, e.g., tetrandrine and jatrorrhizine. It also contains terpenoids (e.g., furanodiene) and sterols.

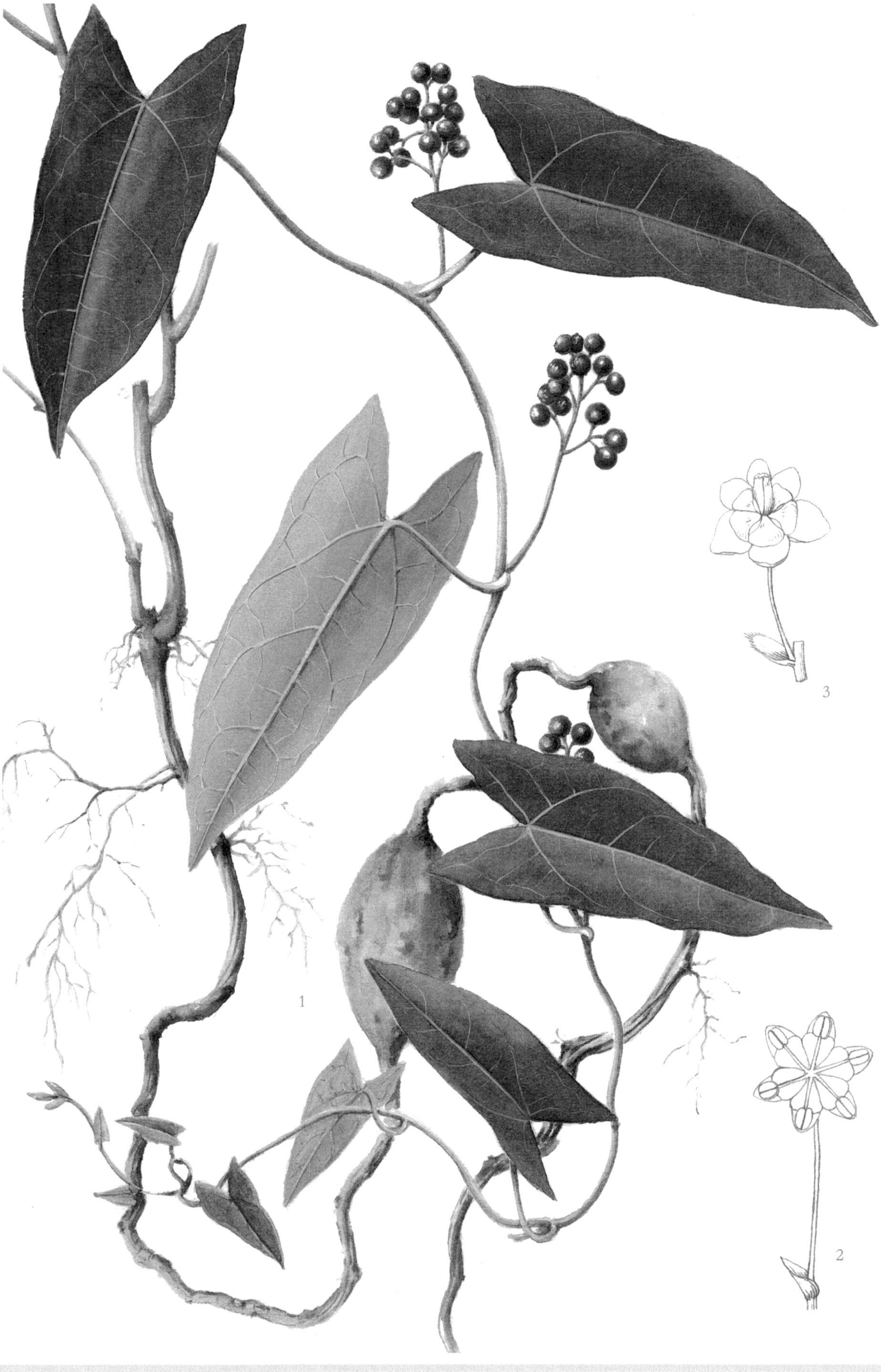

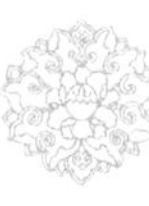

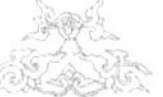

1. 植株（plant） 2. 雄花（male flower） 3. 雌花（female flower）

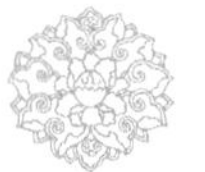

远志

Yuanzhi

Polygala tenuifolia

基　源　远志科 Polygalaceae 远志属 *Polygala* 植物远志 *Polygala tenuifolia* Willd. 的干燥根。药材名为“远志”。

形态特征　多年生草本。主根粗壮，韧皮部肉质。茎多数丛生，被短柔毛。单叶互生，叶片纸质，线形，先端渐尖，全缘。总状花序；萼片 5，宿存，里面 2 枚花瓣状；花瓣 3，紫色，侧瓣斜长圆形，基部与龙骨瓣合生，龙骨瓣具流苏状附属物。蒴果圆形，顶端微凹，具狭翅。种子卵形，黑色，密被白色柔毛。

生境分布　分布于我国东北、华北、西北和华中以及四川。常生于海拔 200-2000 m 的草地、山坡草地、灌丛中、杂木林下。

采收加工　春、秋二季采挖，除去须根和泥沙，晒干。

性味功能　温，苦、辛。安神益智，交通心肾，祛痰，消肿。

主治用法　用于心肾不交引起的失眠多梦、健忘惊悸、神志恍惚，咳痰不爽，疮疡肿毒，乳房肿痛。

化学成分　主要含有皂苷（远志皂苷）、呫酮、寡糖酯和生物碱等。

Source　It is the dried root of *Polygala tenuifolia* Willd. (Polygalaceae). The medicinal material is called as “Yuanzhi”.

Distribution　*P. tenuifolia* is distributed in Northeast China, North China, Northwest China, Central China and Sichuan Province. It commonly grows in grassland, grassy hillside, shrub and mixed wood forests at an altitude of 200–2000 m.

Indications　It is used to treat insomnia and dreaminess due to no interaction between heart and kidney, amnesia and palpitation due to fright, absent–minded, expectoration, sore, ulcer, pyogenic infection, mammary distending pain.

Chemical Constituents　It mainly contains saponins (onjisaponin), xanthones, oligosaccharides and alkaloids.

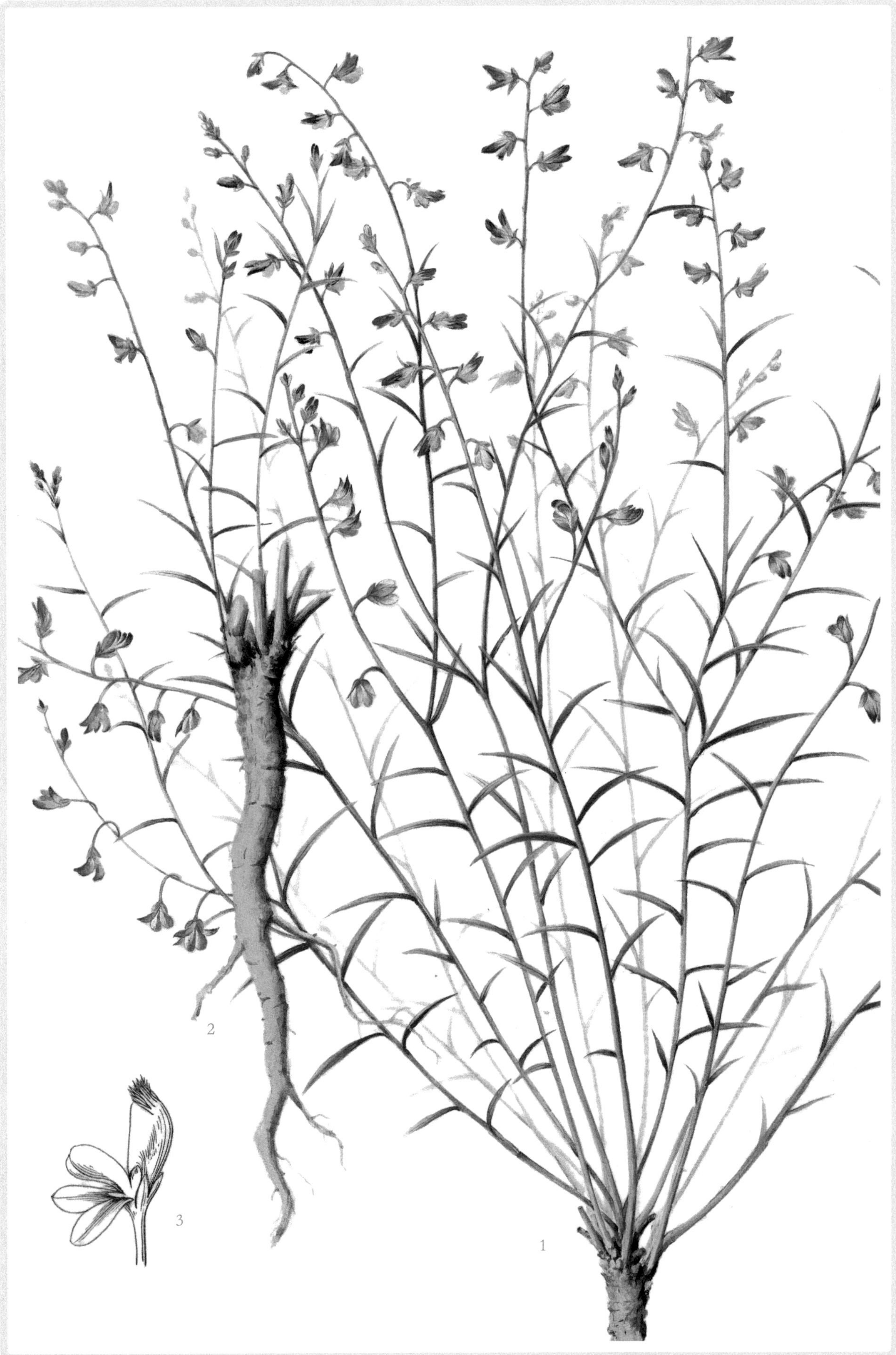

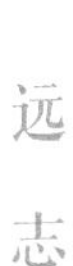

1. 花枝（flowering stem）　2. 根（root）　3. 花（flower）

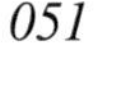

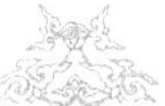

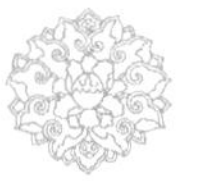

甘草

Gancao

Glycyrrhiza uralensis

基 原 豆科 Fabaceae 甘草属 *Glycyrrhiza* 植物甘草 *Glycyrrhiza uralensis* Fisch. 的干燥根和根茎。药材名为“甘草”。

形态特征 多年生草本。根与根状茎粗壮，具甜味。茎直立，多分枝，密被鳞片状腺点和绒毛。复叶，小叶 5-17 枚，常为卵形，两面均密被腺点及短柔毛，边缘多少反卷。总状花序腋生，花多数；苞片褐色，膜质；花萼基部偏斜并膨大呈囊状；花冠常为淡紫色。荚果弯曲，密集成球，密生瘤状突起和刺毛状腺体。

生境分布 分布于我国东北、华北、西北各省区。常生于干旱沙地、河岸砂质地、山坡草地及盐渍化土壤中。

采收加工 春、秋二季采挖，除去须根，晒干。

性味功能 平，甘。补脾益气，清热解毒，祛痰止咳，缓急止痛，调和诸药。

主治用法 主要用于脾胃虚弱，倦怠乏力，心悸气短，咳嗽痰多，脘腹、四肢挛急疼痛，痈肿疮毒，缓解药物毒性、烈性。

化学成分 主要含有皂苷类成分，如甘草酸、甘草皂苷 A3、甘草皂苷 B2、甘草皂苷 C2 等；黄酮类成分，如甘草素、异甘草素、甘草醇；另还含有生物碱和多糖等。

备 注 甘草为国家二级重点保护野生药材。

Source It is the dried root and rhizome of *Glycyrrhiza uralensis* Fisch. (Fabaceae). The medicinal material is called as “Gancao”.

Distribution *G. uralensis* is distributed in provinces of Northeast, North and Northwest China. It commonly grows on dry sand, sandy land on river banks, grasslands on the hillside and salinized land.

Indications It is used to treat spleen–stomach weakness, fatigue and lack of strength, palpitations and shortness of breath, cough with copious sputum, hypertonicity and pain of the limbs and abdomen, swollen abscess, sore and toxin. It can also counteract drug toxicity and potentency.

Chemical Constituents It mainly contains saponins (e.g., glycyrrhizic acid, glycyrrhizin A3, glycyrrhizin B2, glycyrrhizin C2), flavonoids (e.g., liquiritigenin, isoliquiritigenin, glycyrol), alkaloids and polysaccharides.

Note It is considered a level II national key protected wild medicinal species.

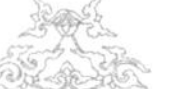

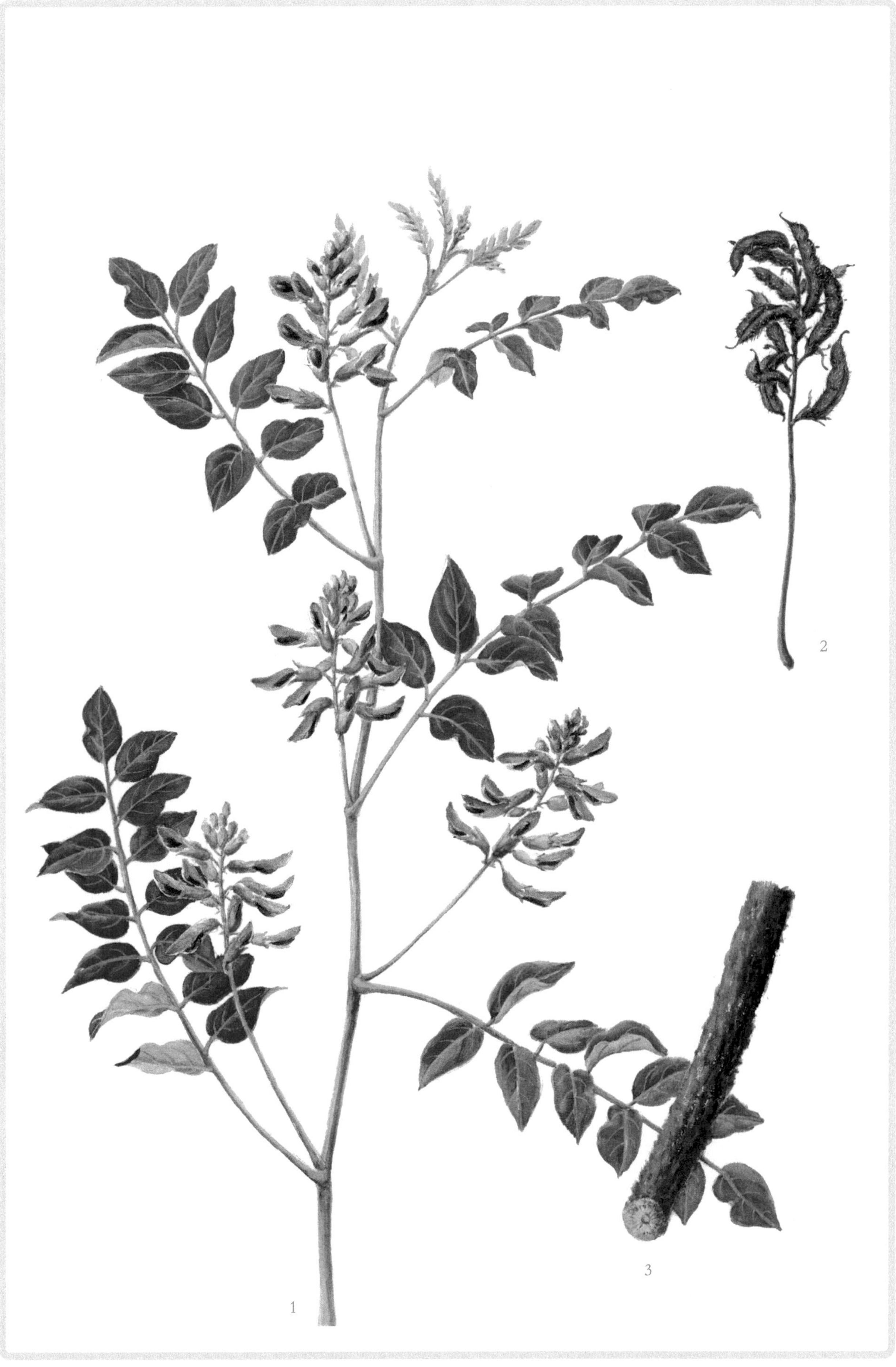

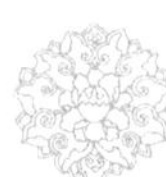

1. 花枝（flowering stem） 2. 果序（infructescence） 3. 根（root）

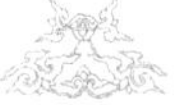

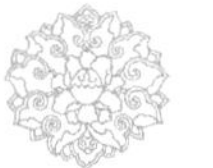

蒙古黄芪

Mengguhuangqi

Astragalus membranaceus var. *mongholicus*

基　　源　豆科 Fabaceae 黄芪属 *Astragalus* 植物蒙古黄芪 *Astragalus membranaceu*s (Fisch.) Bge. var. *mongholicus* (Bge.) Hsiao. 的干燥根。药材名为“黄芪”。

形态特征　多年生草本。根直而长，圆柱形。茎直立，上部有分支，被长柔毛。奇数羽状复叶，互生；托叶披针形；小叶 25-37 片，宽椭圆形，全缘，两面被白色长柔毛。总状花序腋生，排列疏松；花冠黄色，蝶形，翼瓣和龙骨瓣均具长爪。荚果膜质，膨胀，卵状长圆形，表面有显著网状纹理。种子 5-6 粒，肾形，黑色。

生境分布　分布于我国东北及华北等部分省区。生于山坡、疏林或沟边。

采收加工　春、秋二季采挖，除去须根和根头，晒干。

性味功能　微温，甘。补气升阳，固表止汗，利水消肿，生津养血，行滞通痹，托毒排脓，敛疮生肌。

主治用法　用于气虚乏力，食少便溏，中气下陷，久泻脱肛，便血崩漏，表虚自汗，气虚水肿，内热消渴，血虚萎黄，半身不遂，痹痛麻木，痈疽难溃，久溃不敛。

化学成分　主要含有皂苷类成分，如黄芪皂苷甲、黄芪皂苷乙、黄芪皂苷丙、大豆皂苷Ⅰ、异黄芪皂苷Ⅱ等；黄酮类成分，如芒柄花素、毛蕊异黄酮等；另还含有氨基酸类和多糖类成分等。

Source　It is the dried root of *Astragalus membranaceu*s (Fisch.) Bge. var. *mongholicus* (Bge.) Hsiao. (Fabaceae). The medicinal material is called as “Huangqi”.

Distribution　*A. membranaceu*s is distributed in some provinces of Northeast and North China. It grows on hillsides, sparse forests or ditch edges.

Indications　It is used to treat qi deficiency and lack of strength, poor appetite and loose stools, sunken middle qi syndrone, chronic diarrhea and prolapse of rectum, bloody stool, metrorrhagia and metrostaxis, spontaneous perspiration in an exterior deficiency syndrome, edema due to qi deficiency, internal heat and wasting thirst, shallow yellow due to blood deficiency, hemiplegia, impediment and numbness, carbuncle-abscess with difficulty to collapse, enduring collapse without healing.

Chemical Constituents　It mainly contains saponins (e.g., astragaloside A, B, C, soyasaponin I, isoastragaloside II), flavonoids (e.g., formononetin, calycosin), amino acids and polysaccharides.

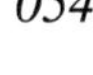

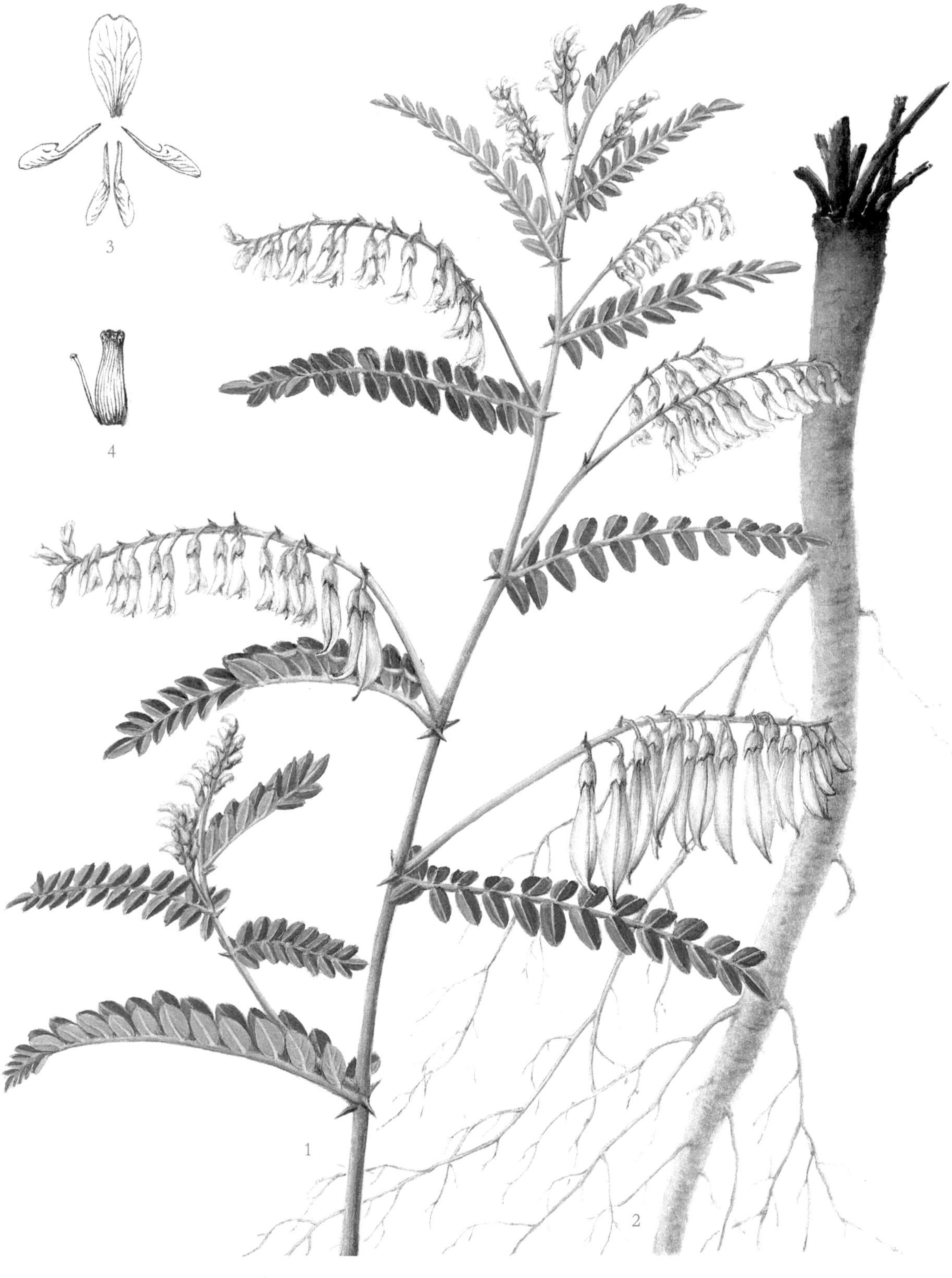

3

4

1

2

1. 花果枝（flowering and fruiting stem） 2. 根（root） 3. 花冠解剖（separate corolla） 4. 雄蕊（stamen）

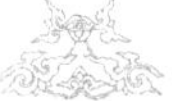

越南槐

Yuenanhuai

Sophora tonkinensis

基　源　豆科 Fabaceae 槐属 *Sophora* 植物越南槐 *Sophora tonkinensis* Gagnep. 的干燥根和根茎。药材名为“山豆根”。

形态特征　灌木。根粗壮。茎枝圆柱形，分枝多。羽状复叶；小叶 5-9 对，革质，对生，椭圆形，叶轴下部的叶渐小，顶生小叶先端钝，骤尖，基部圆形。总状花序顶生，被短而紧贴的柔毛；花萼杯状；花冠黄色，旗瓣近圆形，翼瓣比旗瓣稍长，龙骨瓣背部明显龙骨状，基部具 1 个三角形耳。荚果串珠状。种子卵形，黑色。

生境分布　分布于广西、贵州、云南。生于海拔 1000-2000 m 的亚热带或温带的石灰岩山地的灌木林中。

采收加工　秋季采挖，除去杂质，洗净，干燥。

性味功能　寒，苦；有毒。清热解毒，消肿利咽。

主治用法　主要用于火毒蕴结，乳蛾喉痹，咽喉肿痛，齿龈肿痛，口舌生疮。

化学成分　主要含有生物碱类，如苦参碱、氧化苦参碱、槐果碱、山豆根碱等；黄酮类，如柔枝槐酮、柔枝槐素、柔枝槐酮色烯等；苯丙素类，如紫檀素、红车轴草根苷等；另还含有蛇麻脂醇、甾醇、咖啡酸等。

Source　It is the dried root and rhizome of *Sophora tonkinensis* Gagnep. (Fabaceae). The medicinal material is called as “Shandougen”.

Distribution　*S. tonkinensis* is distributed in Guangxi, Guizhou and Yunnan province. It grows in the shrub of limestone mountains in the subtropical or temperate zone at an altitude of 1000–2000 m.

Indications　It is used to treat fire toxin accumulation and binding, tonsillitis and pharyngitis, sore swollen throat, gingivitis, and mouth and tongue sores.

Chemical Constituents　It mainly contains alkaloids (e.g., matrine, oxymatrine, sophocarpine, dauricine), flavonoids (e.g., sophoranone, sophoradin, sophoranochromene), phenylpropanoids (e.g., pterocarpin, trifolirhizin), lupeol, sterols, caffeic acid, etc.

越南槐

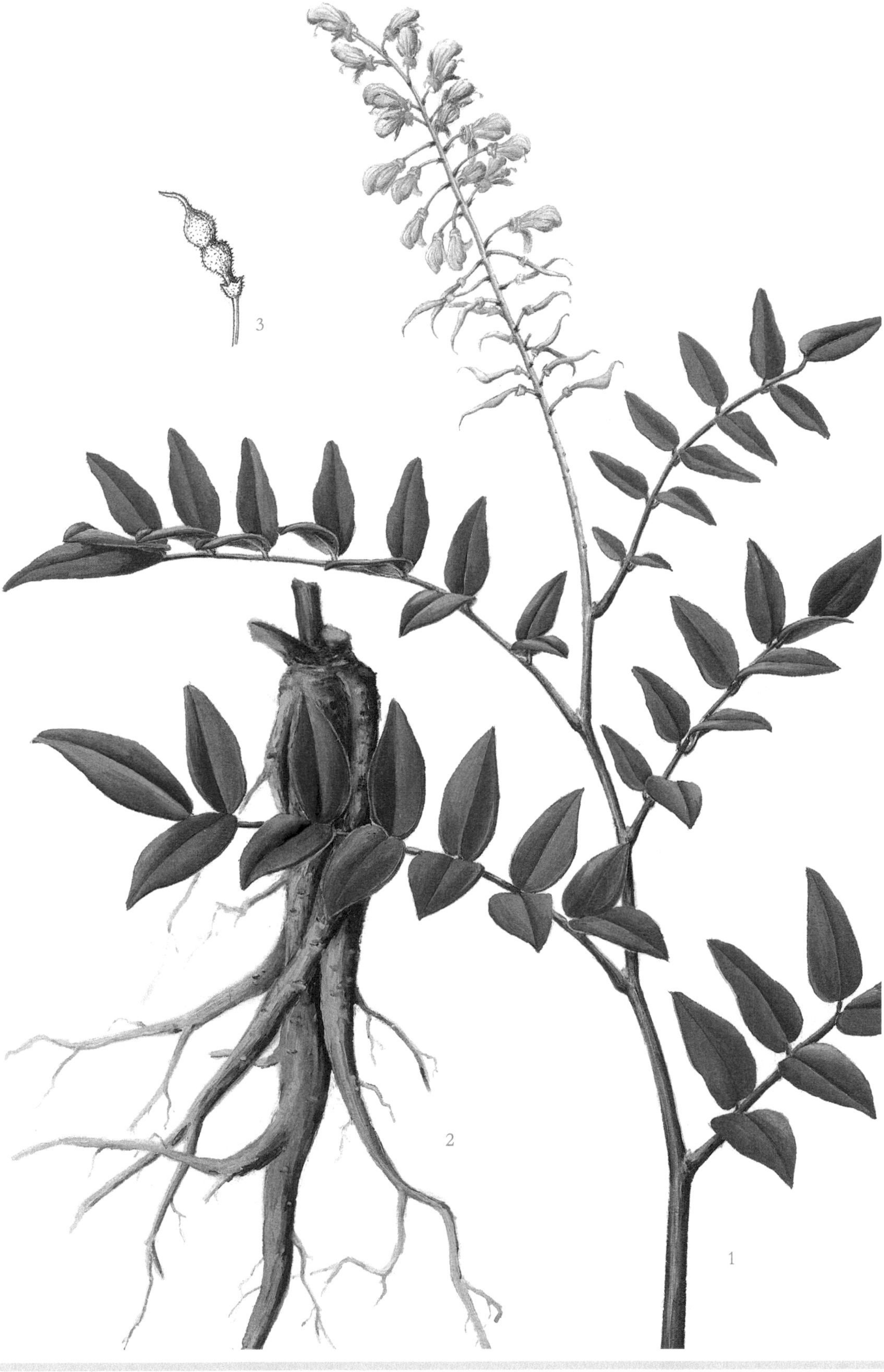

1. 花果枝（flowering and fruiting stem） 2. 根（root） 3. 果实（fruit）

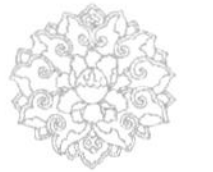

鬼箭锦鸡儿

Guijianjinjier

Caragana jubata

基　　源　豆科 Fabaceae 锦鸡儿属 *Caragana* 植物鬼箭锦鸡儿 *Caragana jubata* (Pall.) Poir. 的根。药材名为“鬼箭锦鸡儿”。

形态特征　灌木，基部多分枝。偶数羽状复叶，小叶 4-6 对；叶轴宿存并硬化成刺，长 5-7cm；叶密生于枝上部，小叶长椭圆形至线状长椭圆形，两面疏生柔毛；托叶与叶柄基部贴生，不硬化成刺。花单生，花梗极短，基部有关节；花萼筒状，密生长柔毛；花冠蝶形，淡红色或近白色。荚果长椭圆形，密生丝状长柔毛。

生境分布　主要分布于我国华北、西北地区。生于较高海拔的干旱山地。

采收加工　秋季采挖根部，洗净，切片，晒干。

性味功能　微寒，辛、苦、涩。清热解毒，降压。

主治用法　主要用于乳痈，疮疖肿痛，高血压病。

化学成分　根中主要含有生物碱、鞣质、皂苷、黄酮、挥发油和糖类成分；嫩枝中含有杨梅树皮素、槲皮素、异鼠李素等化合物。

备　　注　枝叶亦可入药，可接筋续断，祛风除湿，活血通络，消肿止痛。

Source　It is the root of *Caragana jubata* (Pall.) Poir. (Fabaceae). The medicinal material is called as “Guijianjinjier”.

Distribution　*C. jubata* is distributed in the arid mountains with a high altitude in North and Northwest China.

Indications　It is used to treat acute mastitis, swelling and pain of sore and boil, and hypertension.

Chemical Constituents　The root mainly contains alkaloids, tannins, saponins, flavonoids, volatile oils, and saccharides. The twig contains myricetin, quercetin, isorhamnetin, etc.

Note　Both the twig and leaves can be used as medicine to reinforce fractures, expel wind–dampness, promote blood circulation to remove the obstruction from meridians, as well as disperse swelling and relieve pain.

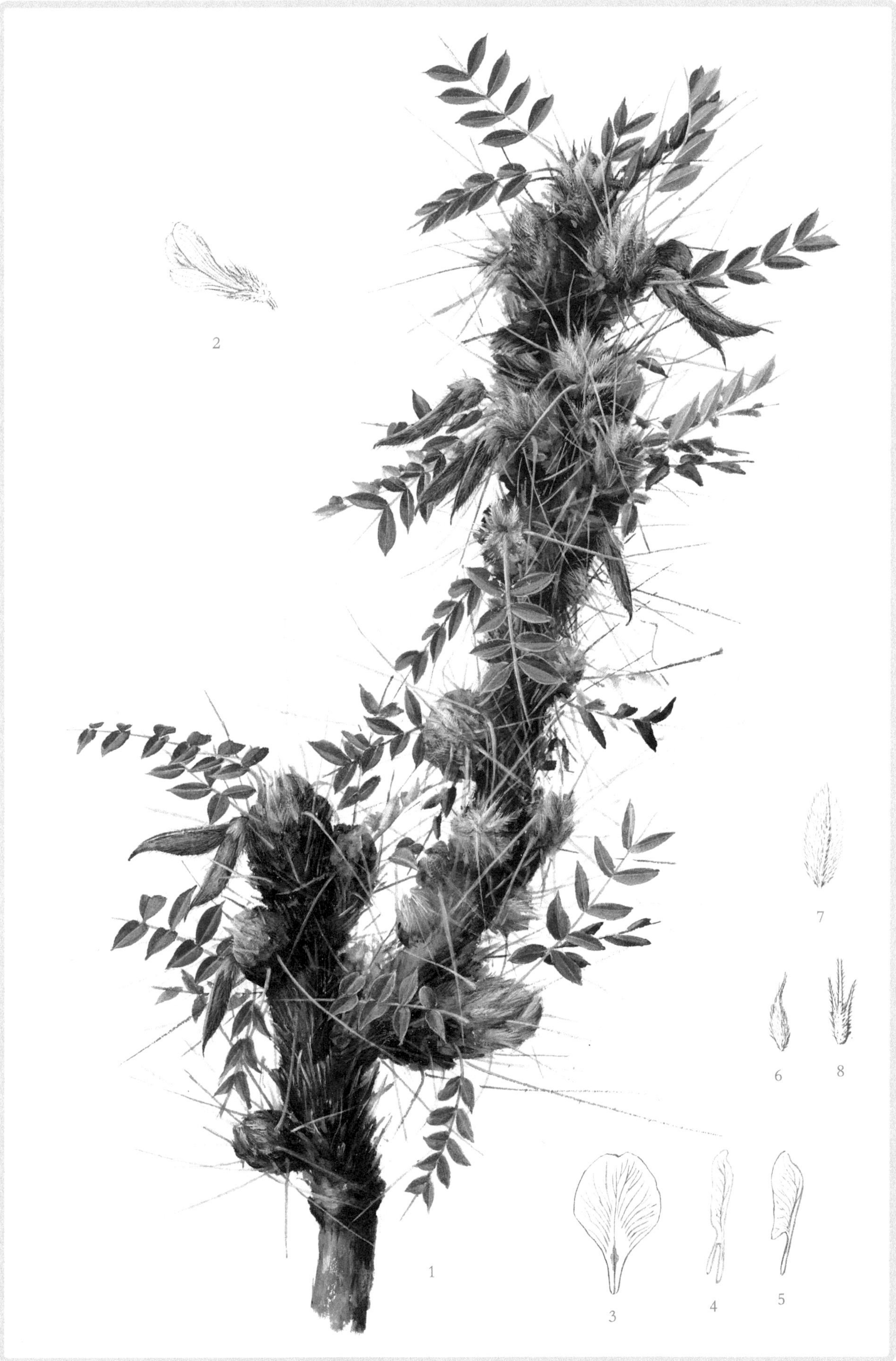

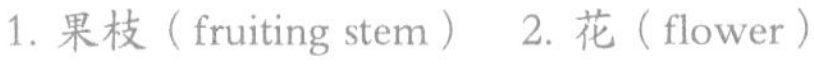

1. 果枝（fruiting stem） 2. 花（flower） 3. 旗瓣（banner） 4. 翼瓣（wing） 5. 龙骨瓣（keel structures of corolla）
6. 苞片（bract） 7. 小叶（small lamina） 8. 托叶（stipule）

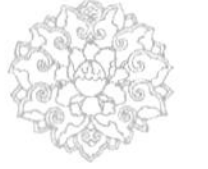

漏斗泡囊草

Loudoupaonangcao

Physochlaina infundibularis

基　源　茄科 Solanaceae 泡囊草属 *Physochlaina* 植物漏斗泡囊草 *Physochlaina infundibularis* Kuang 的干燥根。药材名为“华山参”。

形态特征　多年生草本。植株除叶片外全体被腺质短柔毛。根状茎短而粗壮；茎分枝，细瘦。叶互生，叶片草质，三角形，顶端常急尖，基部骤然狭缩较长的叶柄，边缘有少数大牙齿。花生茎顶或着生于腋生伞形式聚伞花序上；花萼和花冠漏斗状钟形，花冠绿黄色，筒部略带淡紫色，五浅裂；雄蕊伸至花冠喉部。蒴果。种子肾形。

生境分布　主要分布于秦岭中部到东部、河南西南部的山谷或林下。

采收加工　春季采挖，除去须根，洗净，晒干。

性味功能　温，甘、微苦；有毒。温肺祛痰，平喘止咳，安神镇惊。

主治用法　用于寒痰喘咳，惊悸失眠。不宜多服，以免中毒；青光眼患者禁服；孕妇及前列腺重度肥大者慎用。

化学成分　主要含有生物碱类成分，如东莨菪碱、莨菪碱等；还含有香豆素类成分，如东莨菪内酯；另含有黄酮类、氨基酸类、多糖类、甾醇类等。

备　注　为提取莨菪烷类生物碱的重要资源植物。

Source　It is the dried root of *Physochlaina infundibularis* Kuang (Solanaceae). The medicinal material is called as “Huashanshen”.

Distribution　*P. infundibularis* is mainly distributed in the valley or under the forest from central to eastern Qinling Mountains and the southwest of Henan Province.

Indications　It is used to treat panting with coughing due to cold phlegm, palpitation due to fright and insomnia. It should not be an overdose to avoid poisoning. It is prohibited for glaucoma patients. Pregnant women and people with severe prostatic hypertrophy should use it with caution.

Chemical Constituents　It mainly contains alkaloids (e.g., scopolamine, hyoscyamine), and coumarins (e.g., scopoletin). It also contains flavonoids, amino acids, polysaccharides, sterols, etc.

Note　It is an important botanical source for extracting tropane alkaloids.

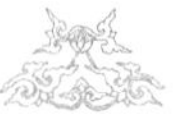

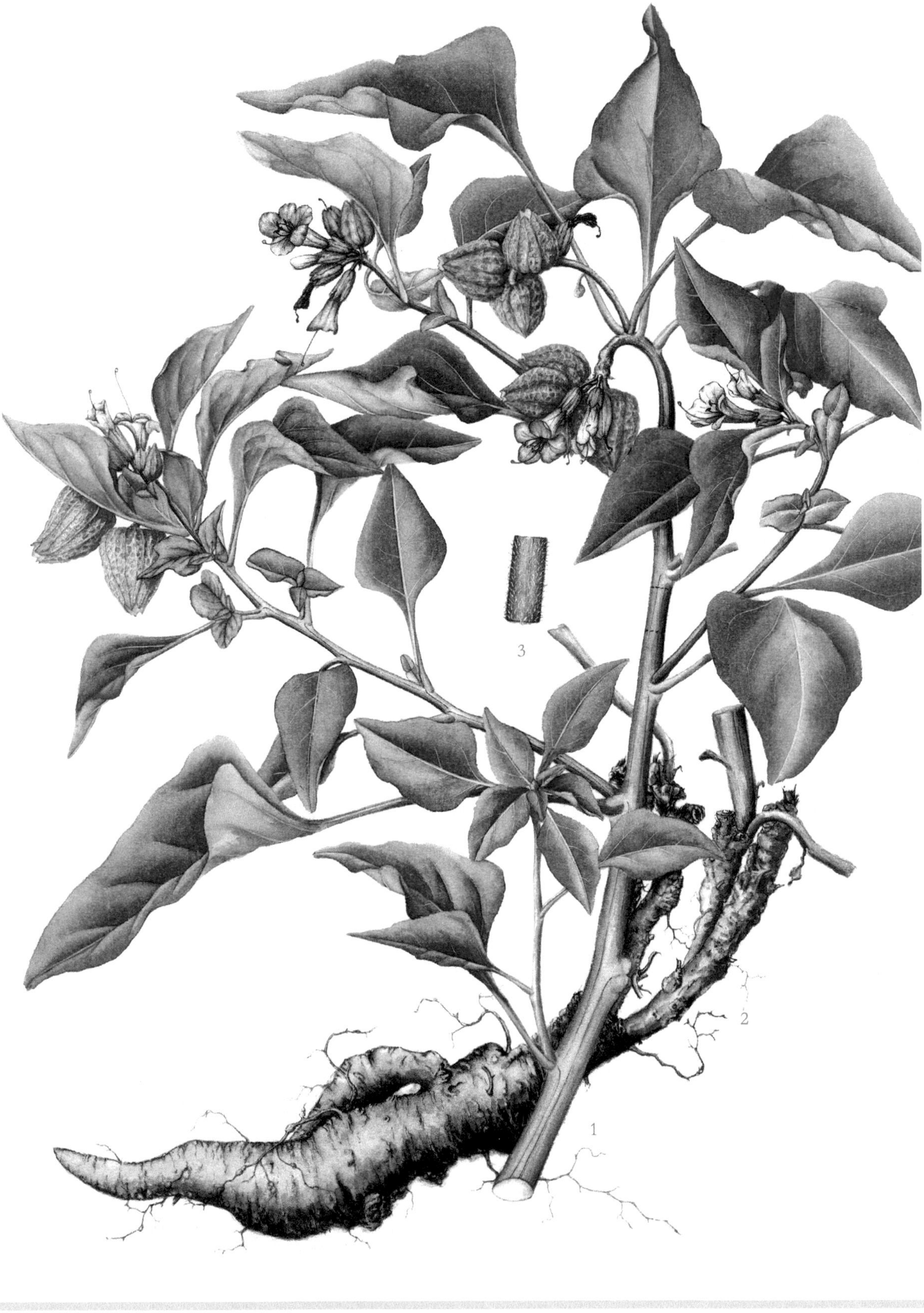

漏斗泡囊草

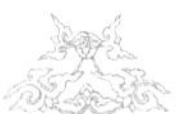

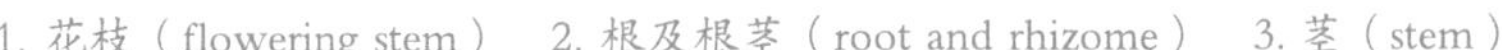

1. 花枝（flowering stem） 2. 根及根茎（root and rhizome） 3. 茎（stem）

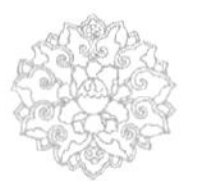

鸢尾

Yuanwei

Iris tectorum

基　　源　鸢尾科 Iridaceae 鸢尾属 *Iris* 植物鸢尾 *Iris tectorum* Maxim. 的干燥根茎。药材名为“川射干”。

形态特征　多年生草本。基部有膜质叶鞘及纤维；根状茎粗壮。叶基生，黄绿色，稍弯曲，中部略宽，宽剑形，基部鞘状。花茎光滑，中下部有叶 1-2 枚；花蓝紫色；花被管上端膨大，外花被裂片宽卵形，中脉上有鸡冠状附属物，内花被花盛开时向外平展。蒴果长椭圆形，成熟时三瓣裂。种子黑褐色，梨形。

生境分布　分布于我国中东部、西南部各省。常生于向阳坡地、林缘及水边湿地。

采收加工　全年均可采挖，除去须根及泥沙，干燥。

性味功能　寒，苦。清热解毒，祛痰，利咽。

主治用法　主要用于热毒痰火郁结，咽喉肿痛，痰涎壅盛，咳嗽气喘。

化学成分　根茎中主要含有黄酮类、三萜类、醌类、酮类、酚类。

备　　注　鸢尾可作为园林绿化植物使用。对氟化物敏感。

Source　It is the dried rhizome of *Iris tectorum* Maxim. (Iridaceae). The medicinal material is called as “Chuanshegan”.

Distribution　*I. tectorum* is distributed in the central–eastern and southwestern provinces of China. It commonly grows on slopes with sun exposure, forest edges and waterfront wetlands.

Indications　It is used to treat stagnation of heat, toxin, phlegm and fire, sore swollen throat, excessive phlegm, coughing and panting.

Chemical Constituents　The rhizome mainly contains flavonoids, triterpenoids, quinones, ketones and phenols.

Note　Rhizoma Iridis Tectori can be used as a landscaping plant. It is sensitive to fluoride.

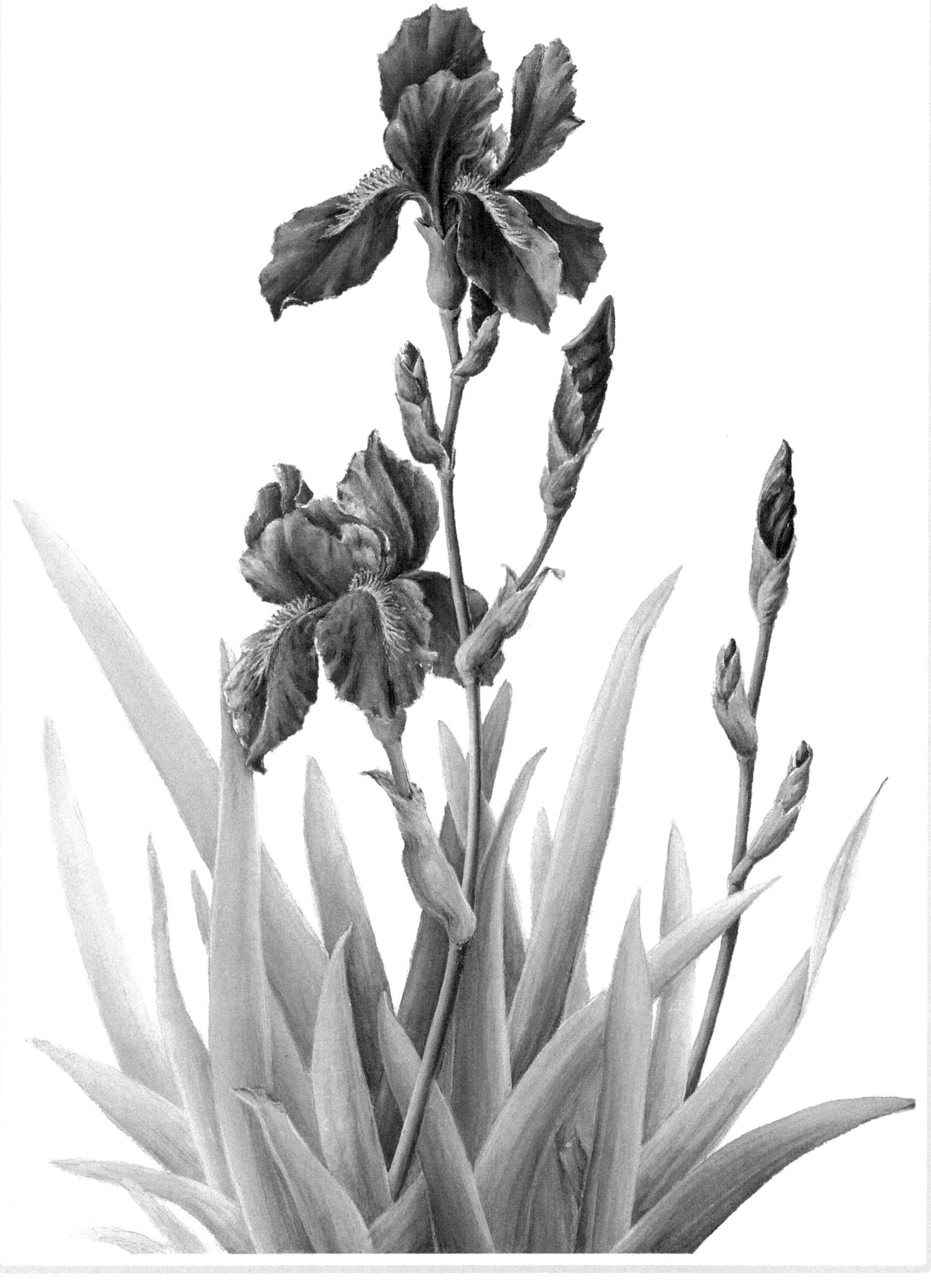

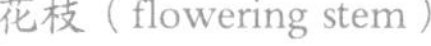

花枝（flowering stem）

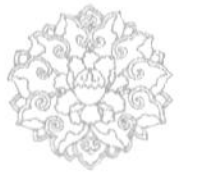

射干

Shegan

Belamcanda chinensis

基　　源　鸢尾科 Iridaceae 射干属 *Belamcanda* 植物射干 *Belamcanda chinensis* (L.) DC. 的干燥根茎。药材名为“射干”。

形态特征　多年生草本。根状茎团块状；须根多数；茎高约 1m，实心。叶互生，嵌迭状排列，剑形，基部鞘状抱茎。花序顶生，叉状分枝，分枝的顶端生数朵花；分枝处均包有膜质的苞片；花橙红色，散生紫褐色的斑点；花被片 6，2 轮排列。蒴果倒卵形，常有花被残存，室背开裂。种子圆球形，黑紫色，有光泽。

生境分布　分布于我国大部分省区。除西南分布海拔较高外，多生于海拔较低的林缘和山坡草地。

采收加工　春初刚发芽或秋末茎叶枯萎时采挖，除去须根和泥沙，干燥。

性味功能　寒，苦。清热解毒，消痰，利咽。

主治用法　用于热毒痰火郁结，咽喉肿痛，痰涎壅盛，咳嗽气喘。

化学成分　主要含有黄酮类，如次野鸢尾黄素、鸢尾苷、野鸢尾苷等；萜类，如射干醛、异德国鸢尾醛等；还含有罗布麻宁、射干酮等。

备　　注　射干可作为园林绿化植物使用。

Source　It is the dried rhizome of *Belamcanda chinensis* (L.) DC. (Iridaceae). The medicinal material is called as “Shegan”.

Distribution　*B. chinensis* is distributed in most provinces in China. It commonly grows on the edge of forests and grassy hillsides at low altitudes and in several areas of high altitudes in the southwest.

Indications　It is used to treat stagnation of heat, toxin, phlegm and fire, sore swollen throat, excessive phlegm, and coughing and panting.

Chemical Constituents　It mainly contains flavonoids (e.g., irisflorentin, tecoridin, iridin), terpenes (e.g., belamcandal, isoiridogermanal), acetovanillone, sheganone, etc.

Note　*B. chinensis* can also be used for landscaping.

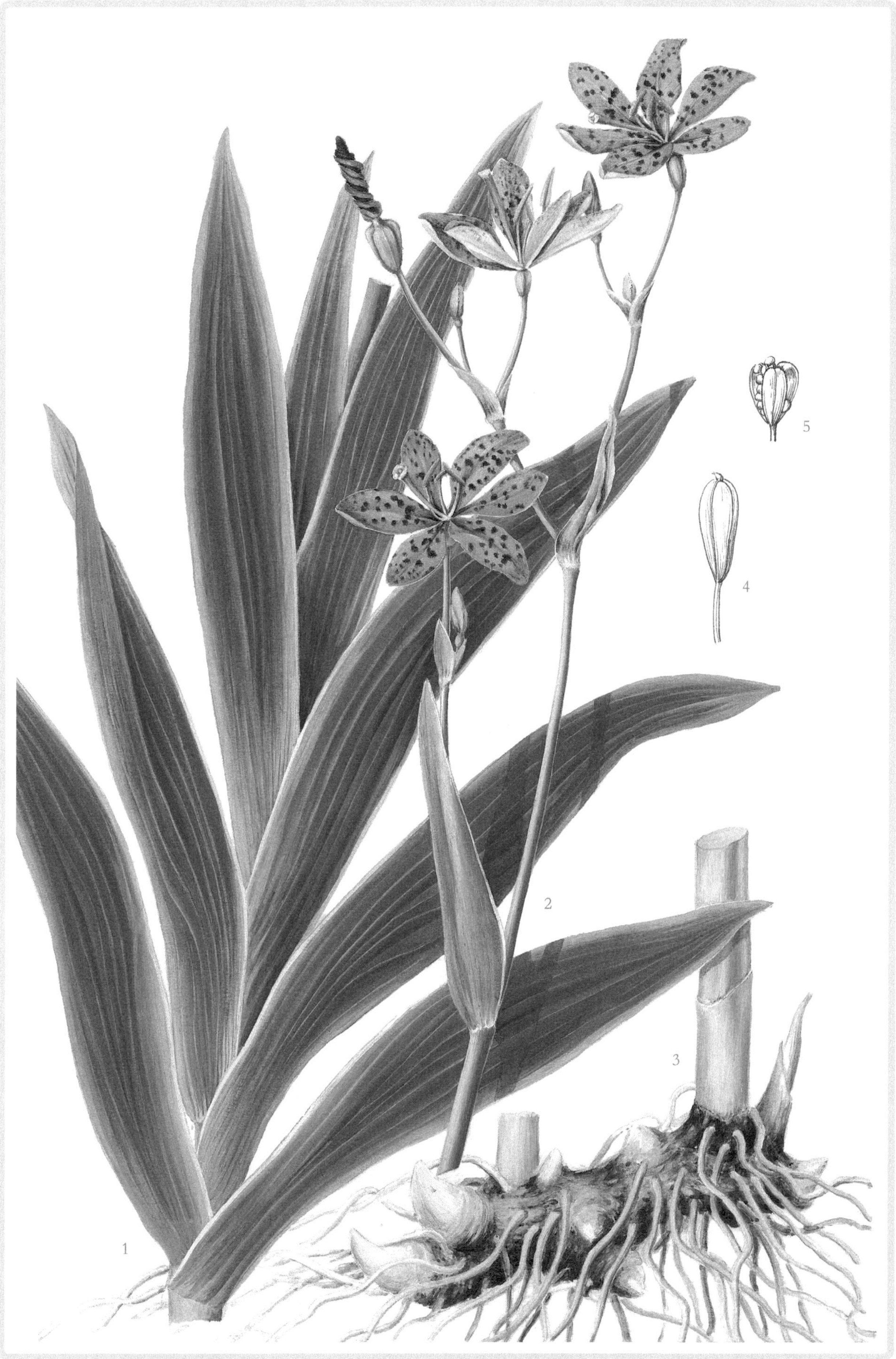

射干

1. 叶（leaf）　2. 花枝（flowering stem）　3. 根状茎（rhizome）　4、5. 果实（fruit）

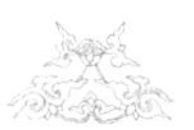

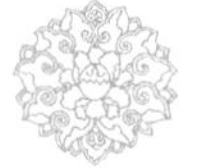

东方泽泻

Dongfangzexie

Alisma orientale

基　　源　泽泻科 Alismataceae 泽泻属 *Alisma* 植物东方泽泻 *Alisma orientale* (Samuel.) Juz. 的干燥块茎。药材名为“泽泻”。

形态特征　多年生沼生草本。叶多数；挺水叶宽披针形、椭圆形。花葶高大。花序具 3-9 轮分枝；花两性；花梗不等长；外轮花被片卵形，边缘窄膜质；内轮花被片近圆形，比外轮大，白色或淡红色，边缘波状。瘦果椭圆形，背部具 1-2 条浅沟，腹部自果喙处凸起，呈膜质翅，两侧果皮纸质。种子紫红色。

生境分布　分布于我国华北、华东、华中各地。生于湖泊、水塘、沟渠、沼泽中。

采收加工　冬季茎叶开始枯萎时采挖，洗净，干燥，除去须根和粗皮。

性味功能　寒，甘、淡。利水渗湿，泄热，化浊降脂。

主治用法　用于小便不利，水肿胀满，泄泻尿少，痰饮眩晕，热淋涩痛，高脂血症。

化学成分　主要含有萜类，如泽泻醇、泽泻醇 A 单乙酸酯。另外还含有氨基酸、有机酸、胆碱、糖类、糠醛等。

Source　It is the dried rhizome of *Alisma orientale* (Samuel.) Juz. (Alismataceae). The medicinal material is called as “Zexie”.

Distribution　*A. orientale* is distributed in North China, East China and Central China. It grows in lakes, ponds, ditches and marshes.

Indications　It is used to treat dysuria, edema with distention and fullness, diarrhea with oliguria, dizziness due to retention of phlegm and fluid, unsmooth and painful urination seen in stranguria due to heat, and hyperlipidaemia.

Chemical Constituents　It mainly contains terpenes (e.g., alisol, alisol A monoacetate). It also contains amino acids, organic acids, choline, saccharides, furfural, etc.

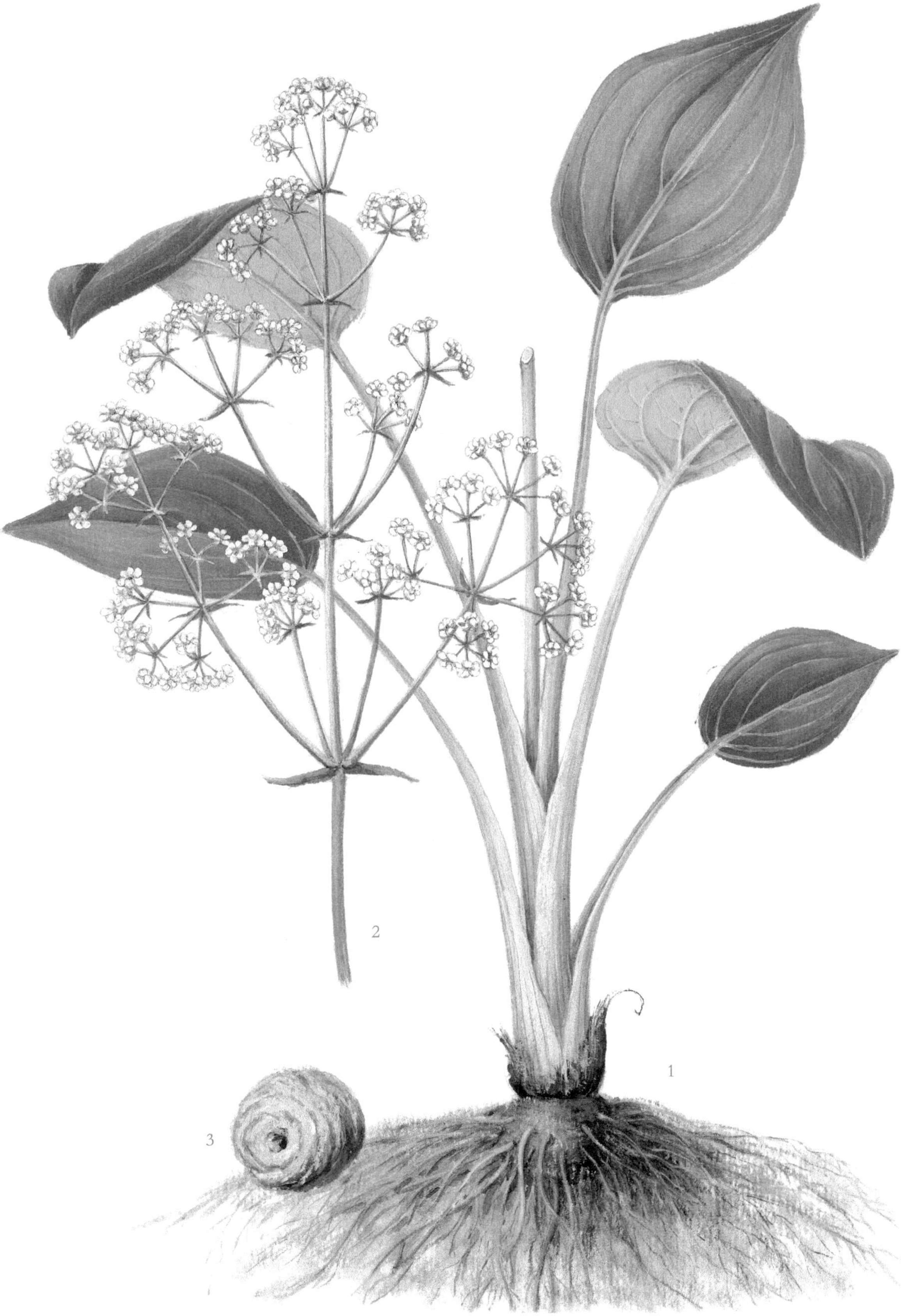

东方泽泻

1. 植株（plant） 2. 花枝（flowering stem） 3. 块茎（rhizome）

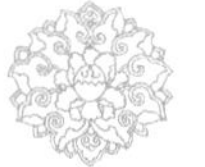

海巴戟

Haibaji
Morinda citrifolia

基　源　茜草科 Rubiaceae 巴戟天属 *Morinda* 植物海巴戟 *Morinda citrifolia* L. 的根。药材名为“橘叶巴戟”。

形态特征　灌木至小乔木。茎枝近四棱柱形。叶交互对生，长圆形、椭圆形或卵圆形，具光泽，全缘。头状花序每隔一节一个，与叶对生；花多数；萼管彼此间多少粘合；花冠白色，漏斗形，喉部密被长柔毛，顶部五裂，裂片卵状披针形。聚花核果浆果状，卵形，幼时绿色，熟时白色。种子长圆形，扁，下部有翅。

生境分布　分布于北自印度和斯里兰卡，南至澳大利亚北部等广大地区及其海岛；我国分布于台湾、海南，以及西沙群岛。生于海滨疏林下。

采收加工　秋季挖根，洗净，晒干。

性味功能　凉，苦。清热解毒。

主治用法　主要用于治疗痢疾，肺结核。

化学成分　根中主要含有蒽醌类成分。

备　注　海巴戟又名诺丽果，果实可供食用。

Source　It is the root of *Morinda citrifolia* L. (Rubiaceae). The medicinal material is called as “Juyebaji”.

Distribution　*M. citrifolia* is distributed widely on island areas from Republic of India and the Democratic Socialist Republic of Sri Lanka to northern Australia. It is also found in Chinese Taiwan, Hainan and the Xisha Islands of China. It grows in coastal forests.

Indications　It is used to treat dysentery and tuberculosis.

Chemical Constituents　The root contains anthraquinones.

Note　The fruit is edible, which is also known as “Noni”.

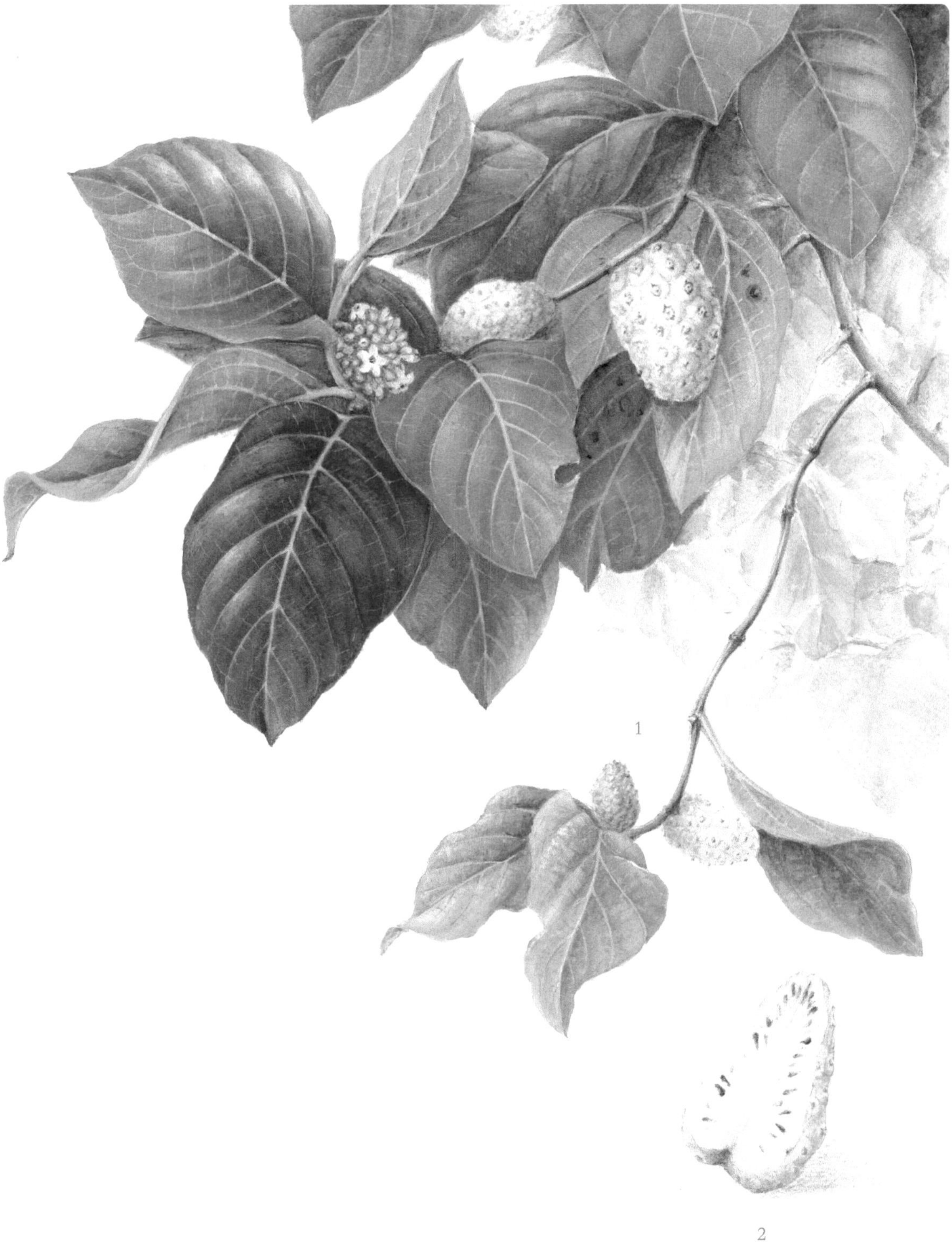

1

2

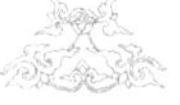

1. 果枝（fruiting stem） 2. 果实及种子（fruit and seed）

广西莪术

Guangxiezhu

Curcuma kwangsiensis

基　　源　姜科 Zingiberaceae 姜黄属 *Curcuma* 植物广西莪术 *Curcuma kwangsiensis* S. G. Lee et C. F. Liang 的干燥根茎。药材名为“莪术”。

形态特征　多年生草本。根状茎卵圆形，节上有残存叶鞘；须根末端常成近纺锤形块根。春季抽叶；叶基生，直立，椭圆状披针形；叶舌边缘有长柔毛；叶鞘被柔毛。穗状花序从根部抽出；花生于下部和中部的苞片腋内。花萼白色，先端呈兜状；唇瓣近圆形，淡黄色，先端三浅圆裂。

生境分布　分布于我国广西。生于阴处的山坡草地及灌木丛中，现多栽培。

采收加工　冬季茎叶枯萎后采挖，洗净，蒸或煮至透心，晒干或低温干燥后除去须根和杂质。

性味功能　温，辛、苦。行气破血，消积止痛。

主治用法　用于癥瘕痞块，瘀血经闭，胸痹心痛，食积胀痛。

化学成分　主要含有挥发油类成分，如姜黄烯、莪术酮、姜黄酮等；另含有姜黄素类成分。

Source　It is the dried root rhizome of *C. kwangsiensis* S. G. Lee et C. F. Liang. (Zingiberaceae). The medicinal material is called as “Ezhu”.

Distribution　*C. kwangsiensis* is distributed in Guangxi, China. It grows on grasslands on shady hillsides and bushes. It is commonly cultivated at present.

Indications　It is used to treat abdominal mass, static blood and amenorrhea, heart pain due to chest impediment, food accumulation and distending pain.

Chemical Constituents　It mainly contains volatile oils, e.g., curcumene, curzerenone, turmerone. It also contains curcumins.

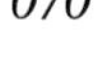

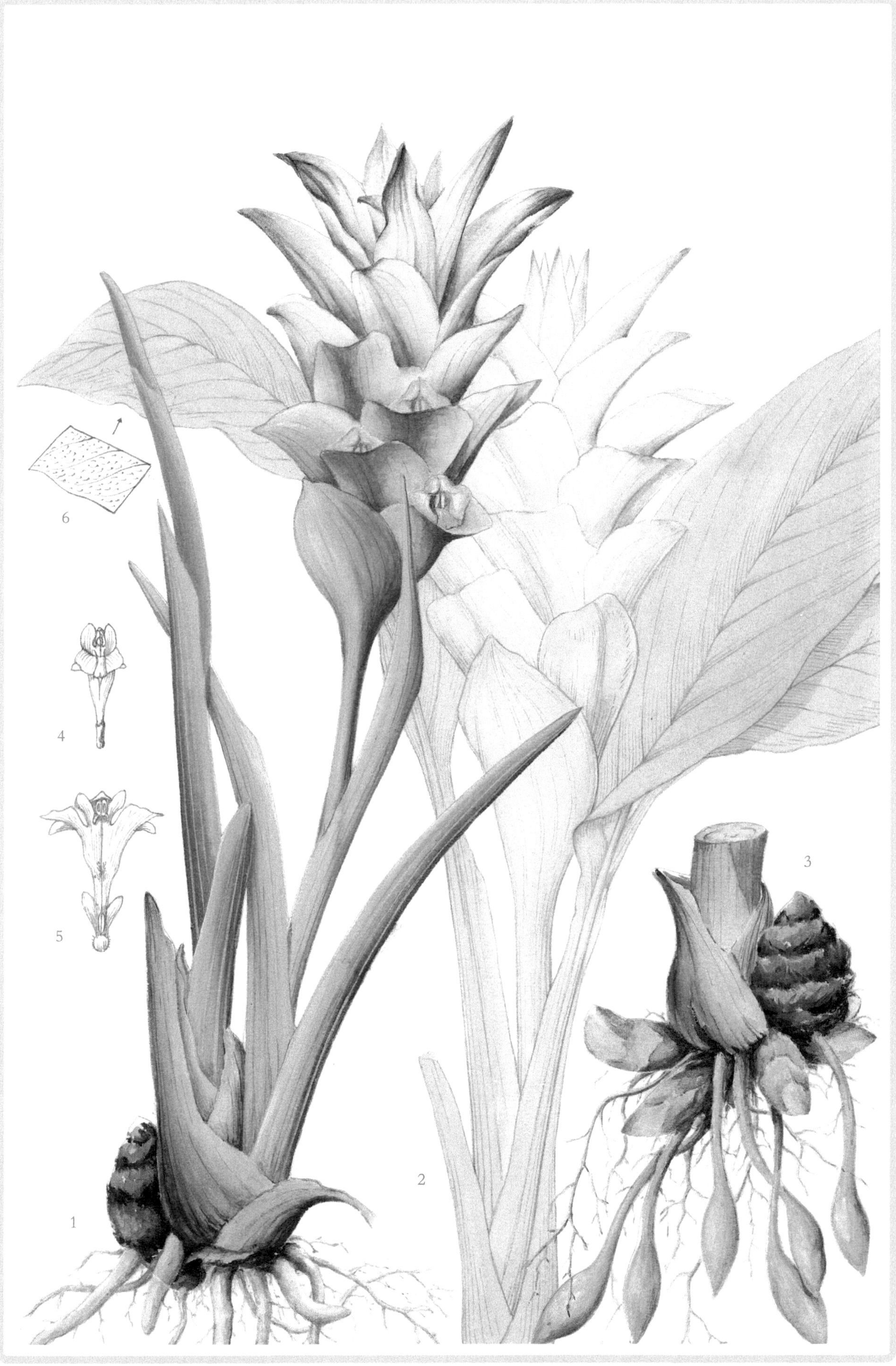

1. 植株（plant） 2. 花枝（flowering stem） 3. 根状茎及块根（rhizome and root tuber） 4、5. 花（flower）
6. 叶表面（leaf surface）

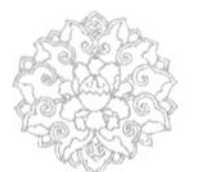

姜黄

Jianghuang

Curcuma longa

基　源　姜科Zingiberaceae姜黄属*Curcuma*植物姜黄*Curcuma longa* L.的干燥根茎。药材名为“姜黄”。

形态特征　多年生草本。根茎发达，橙黄色；根末端膨大成块根。叶基生，二列；叶片长圆形，先端渐尖，基部楔形，下延至叶柄，上面黄绿色，下面浅绿色，无毛。花葶由叶鞘中抽出，穗状花序圆柱状；花萼筒绿白色，具三齿；花冠管漏斗形，淡黄色，喉部密生柔毛，裂片3；能育雄蕊1。

生境分布　分布于我国南方地区，如福建、广东、广西、云南、四川等地。生于向阳的林缘。现多栽培。

采收加工　冬季茎叶枯萎时采挖，洗净，煮或蒸至透心，晒干，除去须根。

性味功能　温，辛、苦。破血行气，通经止痛。

主治用法　主要用于胸胁刺痛，胸搏心痛，痛经经闭，癥瘕，风湿肩臂疼痛，跌扑肿痛。

化学成分　主要含挥发油类，如姜黄烯、莪术二酮等；姜黄素类，如姜黄素、脱甲氧基姜黄素、双脱甲氧基姜黄素等。

备　注　姜黄的块根入药称“郁金”，习称“黄丝郁金”。

Source　It is the dried rhizome of *Curcuma longa* L. (Zingiberaceae). The medicinal is called as “Jianghuang”.

Distribution　*C. longa* is distributed in southern China, e.g., Fujian, Guangdong, Guangxi, Yunnan, Sichuan. It grows on the forest edge with sun exposure. It is commonly cultivated at present.

Indications　It is used to treat stabbing pain in the chest and hypochondrium, heart pain, dysmenorrhea and amenorrhea, abdominal mass, rheumatic shoulder and arm pain due to wind–dampness, traumatic injury with painful swelling.

Chemical Constituents　It mainly contains volatile oils (e.g., curcumene, curdione, curcumins (e.g., curcumin, demethoxycurcumin, bisdemethoxycurcumin).

Note　The root is called Radix Curcumae.

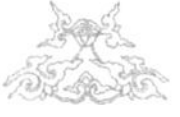

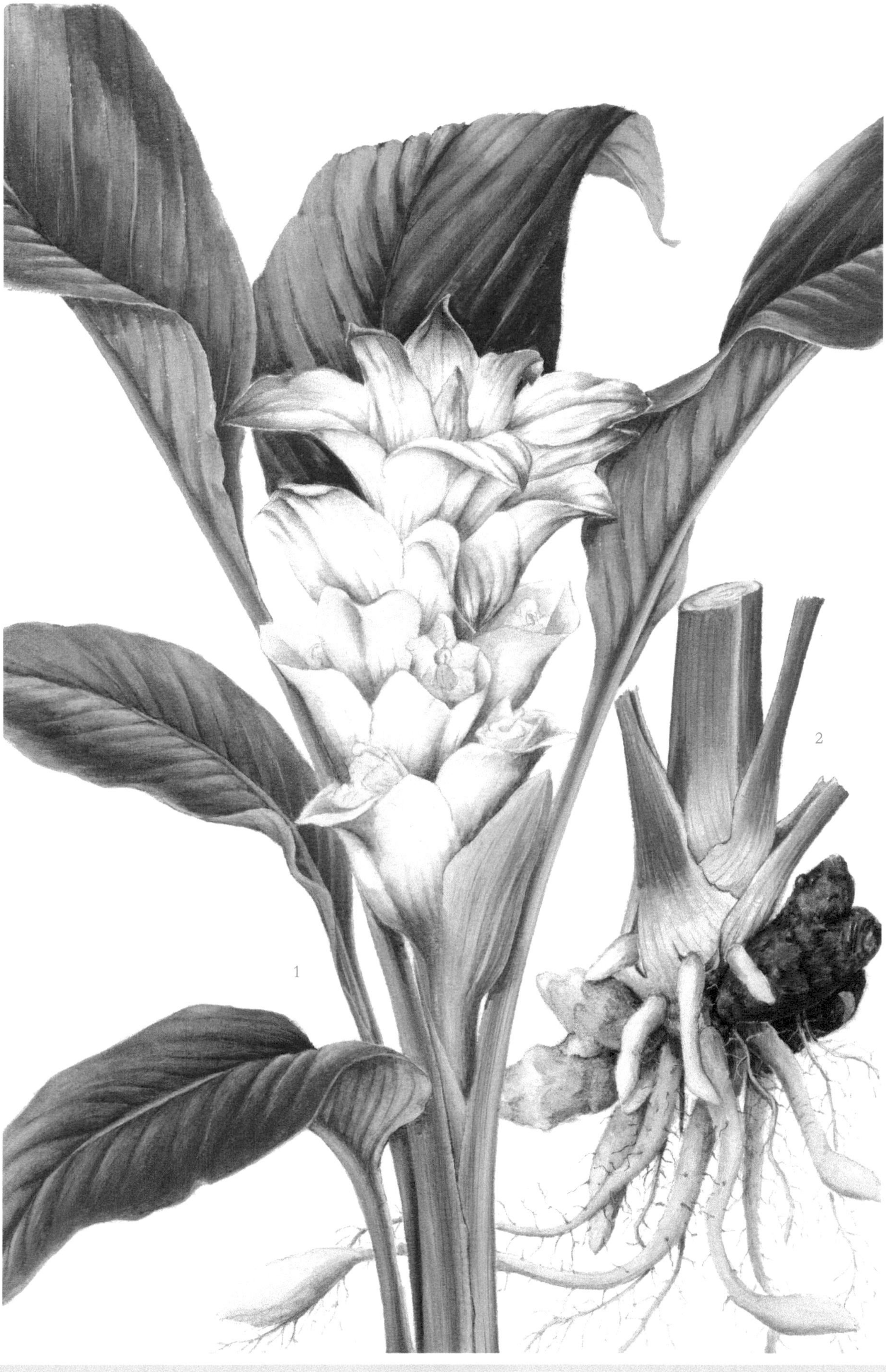

1

2

1. 花枝（flowering stem）　2. 根状茎及块根（rhizome and root tuber）

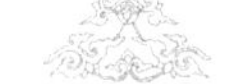

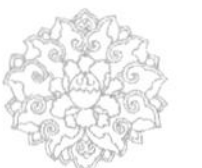

温郁金

Wenyujin

Curcuma wenyujin

基　　源　姜科 Zingiberaceae 姜黄属 *Curcuma* 植物温郁金 *Curcuma wenyujin* Y. H. Chen et C. Ling 的干燥块根。药材名为“郁金”。

形态特征　多年生草本。根茎肉质；根端膨大呈纺锤状。叶基生，叶片长圆形，顶端具细尾尖。花葶单独由根茎抽出，与叶同时发出或先叶而出，穗状花序圆柱形；花葶被疏柔毛；花冠管漏斗形，喉部被毛，裂片长圆形，白色，后方的一片较大，顶端具小尖头，被毛；侧生退化雄蕊淡黄色；唇瓣黄色，倒卵形。

生境分布　主要栽培于我国南方诸省。为著名道地药材“浙八味”之一。

采收加工　冬季茎叶枯萎后采挖，除去泥沙和细根，蒸或煮至透心，干燥。

性味功能　寒，辛、苦。活血止痛，行气解郁，清心凉血，利胆退黄。

主治用法　用于胸胁刺痛，胸痹心痛，经闭痛经，乳房胀痛，热病神昏，癫痫发狂，血热吐衄，黄疸尿赤。

化学成分　主要含有挥发油类、姜黄素类成分。

备　　注　温郁金的干燥根茎入药称“片姜黄”，具有破血行气，通经止痛的功效。

Source　It is the dried root rhizome of *Curcuma wenyujin* Y. H. Chen et C. Ling (Zingiberaceae). The medicinal material is called as “Yujin”.

Distribution　*C. wenyujin* is mainly cultivated in southern China. It is one of the famous authentic medicinal materials—“Eight Tastes of Zhejiang”.

Indications　It is used to treat stabbing pain in the chest and hypochondrium, heart pain due to chest impediment, amenorrhea and dysmenorrhea, mammary distending pain, unconsciousness due to febrile disease, epilepsy with mania, hematemesis and epistaxis due to heat in blood, jaundice with deep-colored urine.

Chemical Constituents　It mainly contains volatile oils and curcumins.

Note　The dry rhizome of *C. wenyujin* can be used as medicine and called Rhizoma Wenyujin Concisum, which has the function of breaking blood and circulating qi, and unblocking the meridian to relieve dysmenorrhea.

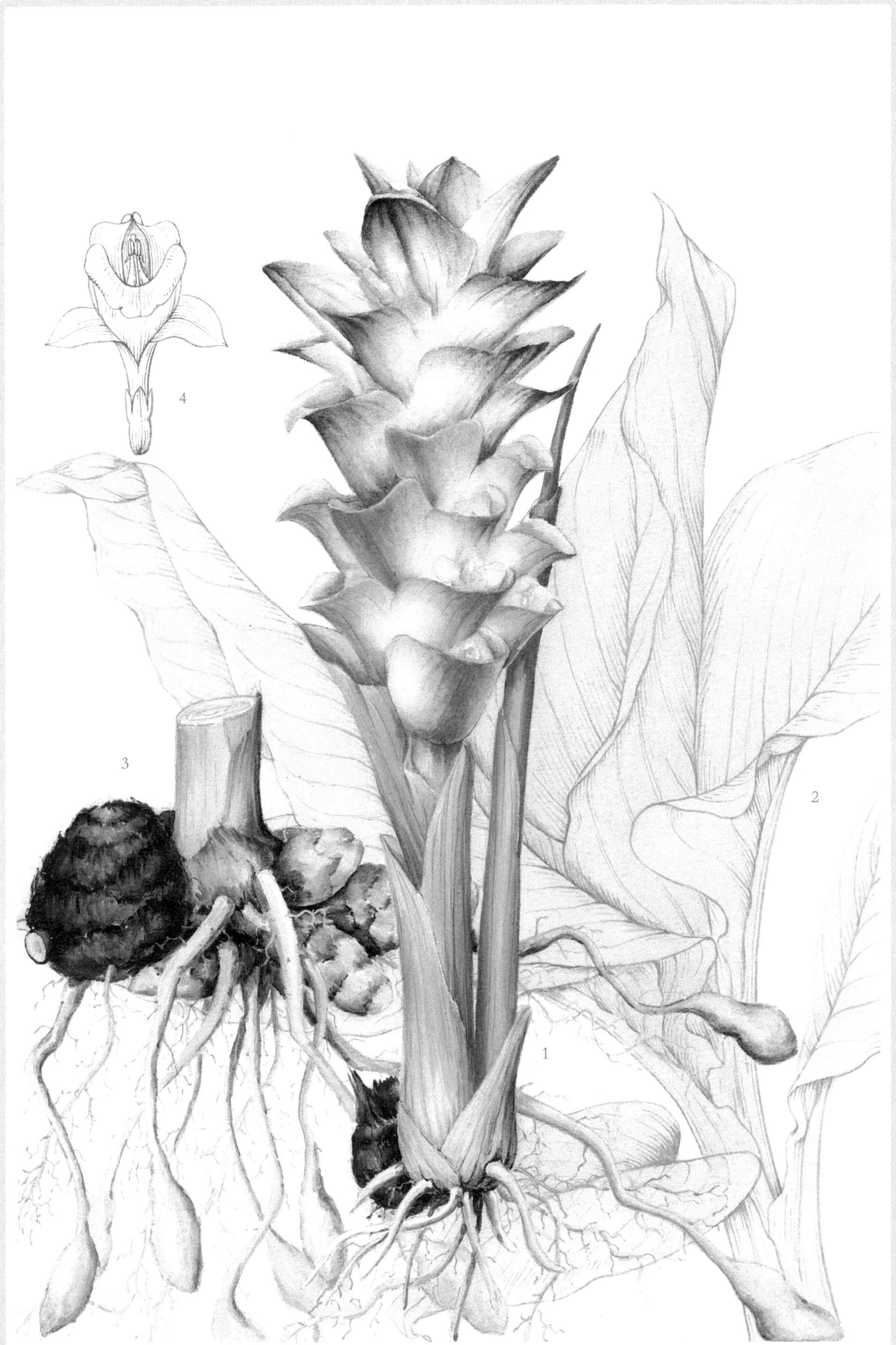

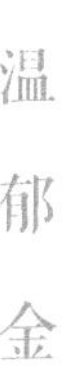
温郁金

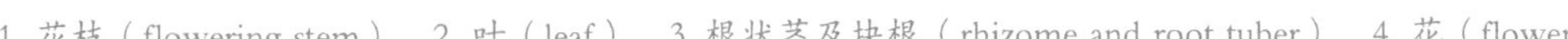
1. 花枝（flowering stem） 2. 叶（leaf） 3. 根状茎及块根（rhizome and root tuber） 4. 花（flower）

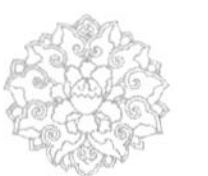

蓬莪术

Pengezhu

Curcuma phaeocaulis

基　　源　姜科 Zingiberaceae 姜黄属 *Curcuma* 植物蓬莪术 *Curcuma phaeocaulis* Val. 的干燥根茎。药材名为"莪术"。

形态特征　多年生草本。根状茎圆柱形，肉质；根细长或末端膨大成块根。叶直立，椭圆状长圆形至长圆状披针形，中部常有紫斑；叶柄较叶片为长。花葶由根状茎单独发出，常先叶而生；穗状花序阔椭圆形；花萼白色，顶端三裂；花冠裂片长圆形，黄色，后方的 1 片较大；唇瓣黄色，近倒卵形，顶端微缺。

生境分布　分布于我国福建、江西、广东、广西、四川、云南和台湾等地；栽培或野生于林荫下。

采收加工　冬季茎叶枯萎后采挖，洗净，蒸或煮至透心，晒干或低温干燥后除去须根和杂质。

性味功能　温，辛、苦。行气破血，消积止痛。

主治用法　用于癥瘕痞块，瘀血经闭，胸痹心痛，食积胀痛。

化学成分　主要含有挥发油类成分，如姜黄烯、莪术酮、姜黄酮等；另还含有姜黄素类成分。

Source　It is the dried root rhizome of *C. phaeocaulis* Val. (Zingiberaceae). The medicinal material is called as "Ezhu".

Distribution　*C. phaeocaulis* is distributed in Fujian, Jiangxi, Guangdong, Guangxi, Sichuan, Yunnan, Chinese Taiwan and other provinces. It is cultivated or grows under the shade of trees in the wild.

Indications　It is used to treat abdominal mass, static blood and amenorrhea, heart pain due to chest impediment, food accumulation and distending pain.

Chemical Constituents　It mainly contains volatile oils, e.g., curcumene, curzerenone, turmerone. It also contains curcumins.

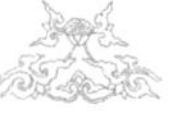

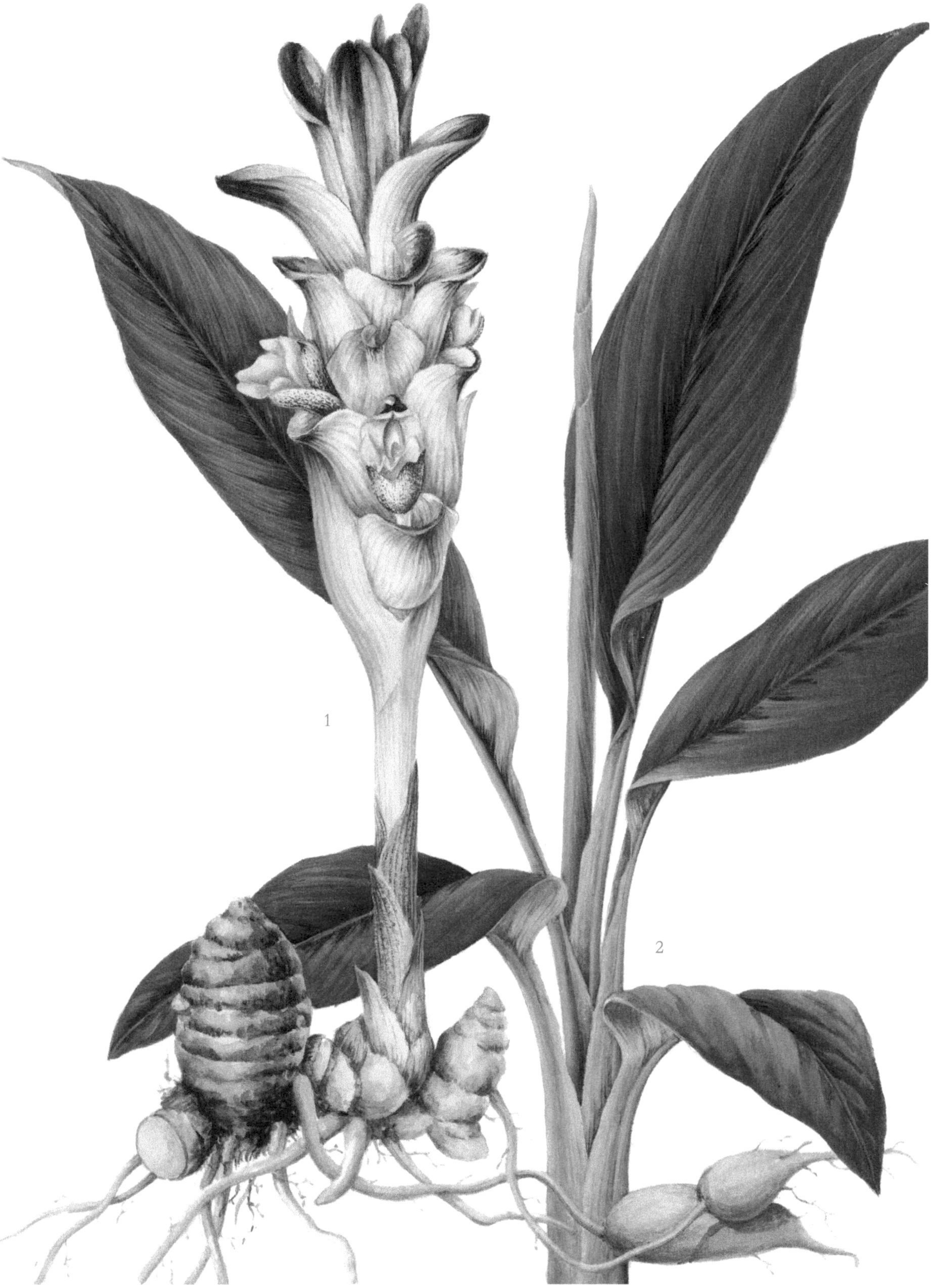

1. 植株（plant）　2. 叶（leaf）

姜

Jiang

Zingiber officinale

基　　源　姜科Zingiberaceae姜属*Zingiber*植物姜*Zingiber officinale* Rosc.的干燥根茎。药材名为“干姜”。

形态特征　多年生草本。根茎肥厚，辛辣。叶互生，排成2列，无柄，几抱茎；叶片披针形，先端渐尖，基部狭，鞘状抱茎。花葶自根茎抽出；穗状花序椭圆形；苞片卵形，淡绿色；花冠黄绿色，唇瓣中裂片有紫色条纹和淡黄色斑点，两侧裂片卵形，黄绿色，具紫色边缘；雄蕊1枚，暗紫色。蒴果。种子多数，黑色。

生境分布　我国中部、东南部至西南部各省区广为栽培。

采收加工　冬季采挖，除去须根及泥沙，晒干或低温干燥。

性味功能　热，辛。温中散寒，回阳通脉，温肺化饮。

主治用法　用于脘腹冷痛，呕吐泄泻，肢冷脉微，寒饮喘咳。

化学成分　主要含有挥发油类，如6-姜辣素、β-甜没药烯、α-姜烯、牻牛儿醇等。

备　　注　鲜品为生姜，可解表散寒，温中止呕，化痰止咳，解鱼蟹毒。干姜经砂烫至鼓起称“炮姜”，具有温经止血，温中止痛的功效。

Source　It is the dried rhizome of *Zingiber officinale* Rosc. (Zingiberaceae). The medicinal material is called as “Ganjiang”.

Distribution　*Z. officinale* is widely cultivated in the central, southeastern, and southwestern China.

Indications　It is used to treat cold pain in the stomach and abdomen, vomiting and diarrhea, cold limbs with faint pulse, cold-fluid retention, panting with coughing.

Chemical Constituents　It mainly contains volatile oils, e.g., 6-gingerol, β-bisabolene, α-zingiberene, and geraniol.

Note　The fresh product of *Z. officinale* is known as Rhizoma Zingiberis Recens. It can be used to release exterior and dissipate cold, warm middle and arrest vomiting, resolve phlegm and relieve cough, and resolve the toxin of fish and crabs. Rhizoma Zingiberis can be burnt until it is bulging, which is called Rhizoma Zingiberis Praeparatum and has the function of warming meridians to stop hemorrhage and warming the middle jiao to kill pain.

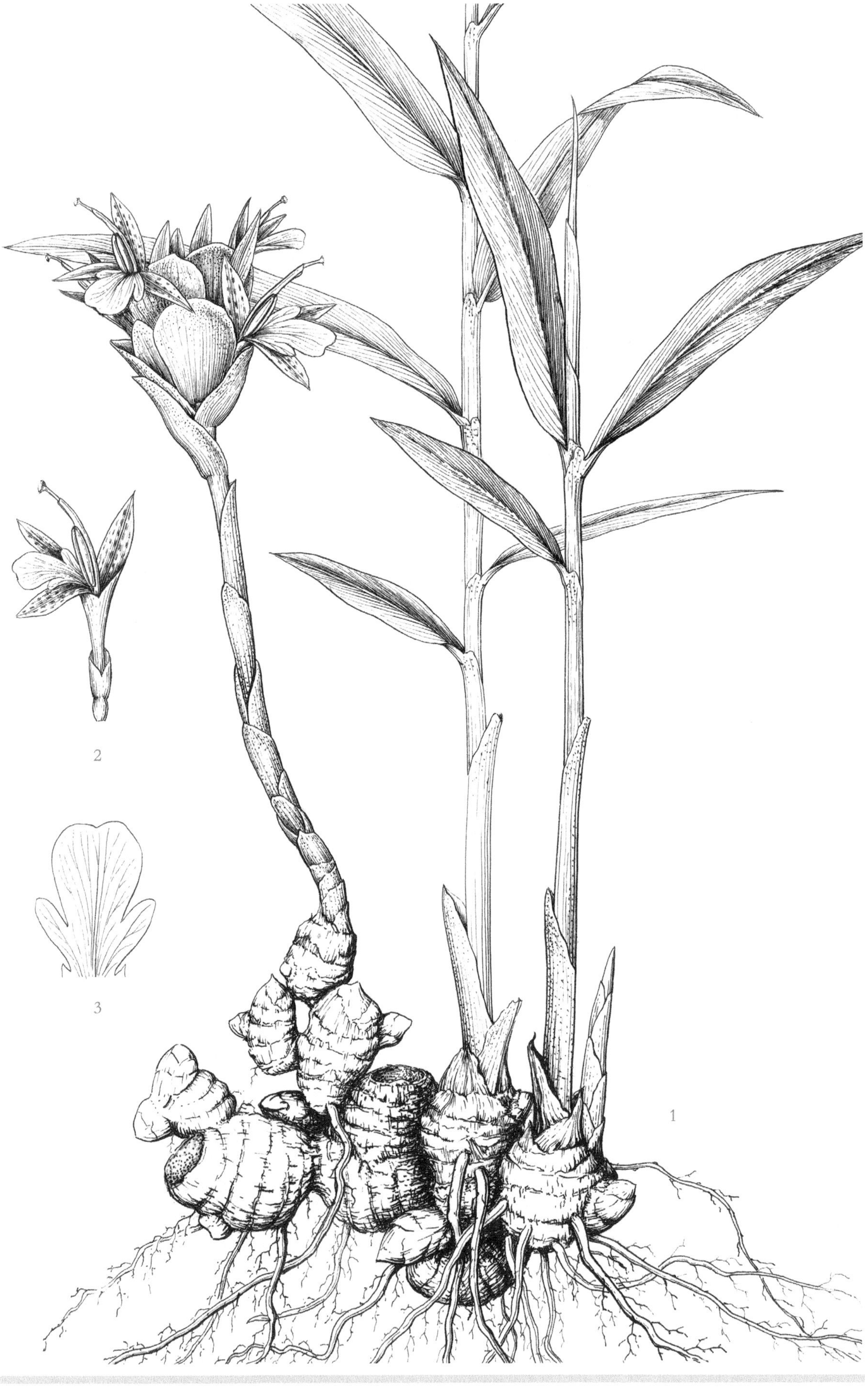

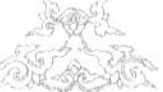

1. 植株（plant）　2. 花（flower）　3. 唇瓣（labellum）

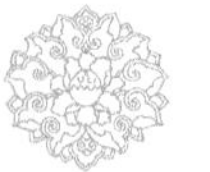

桔梗

Jiegeng

Platycodon grandiflorus

基　源　桔梗科 Campanulaceae 桔梗属 *Platycodon* 植物桔梗 *Platycodon grandiflorus* (Jacq.) A. DC. 的干燥根。药材名为“桔梗”。

形态特征　多年生草本。茎上部偶有分枝。叶序全部轮生至全部互生；叶片卵形至披针形，顶端急尖，上面绿色，下面被白粉，有时脉上有短毛，边缘具细锯齿。花单朵顶生，或数朵集成假总状花序，或有花序分枝而集成圆锥花序；花萼筒部半圆球状，被白粉；花冠大，蓝紫色。蒴果球状。种子多数。

生境分布　分布于我国东北、华北、华东、华中各省。常生于海拔 2000 m 以下的向阳处草丛、灌丛中。

采收加工　春、秋二季采挖，洗净，除去须根，趁鲜剥去外皮或不去外皮，干燥。

性味功能　平，苦、辛。宣肺，利咽，祛痰，排脓。

主治用法　主要用于咳嗽痰多，胸闷不畅，咽痛音哑，肺痈吐脓。

化学成分　主要含有皂苷类成分，如桔梗皂苷 A、桔梗皂苷 D、远志皂苷等；另还含有脂肪酸、多聚糖、维生素、蛋白质等。

备　注　我国东北以及朝韩半岛常将桔梗腌制成泡菜，供食用。

Source　It is the dried root of *Platycodon grandiflorus* (Jacq.) A. DC. (Campanulaceae). The medicinal material is called as “Jiegeng”.

Distribution　*P. grandiflorus* is distributed in the provinces of Northeast China, North China, East China and Central China. It commonly grows in underbrushes exposing to sun and shrubs below 2000 m above sea level.

Indications　It is used to treat cough with profuse sputum, stuffiness in the chest, throat pain and hoarseness, lung abscess and pyemesis.

Chemical Constituents　It mainly contains saponins, e.g., platycodin A, platycodin D, polygalacin. It also contains fatty acids, polysaccharides, vitamins, proteins, etc.

Note　In northeastern China and the Korean Peninsula, Radix Platycodonis is often used to make kimchi.

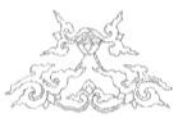

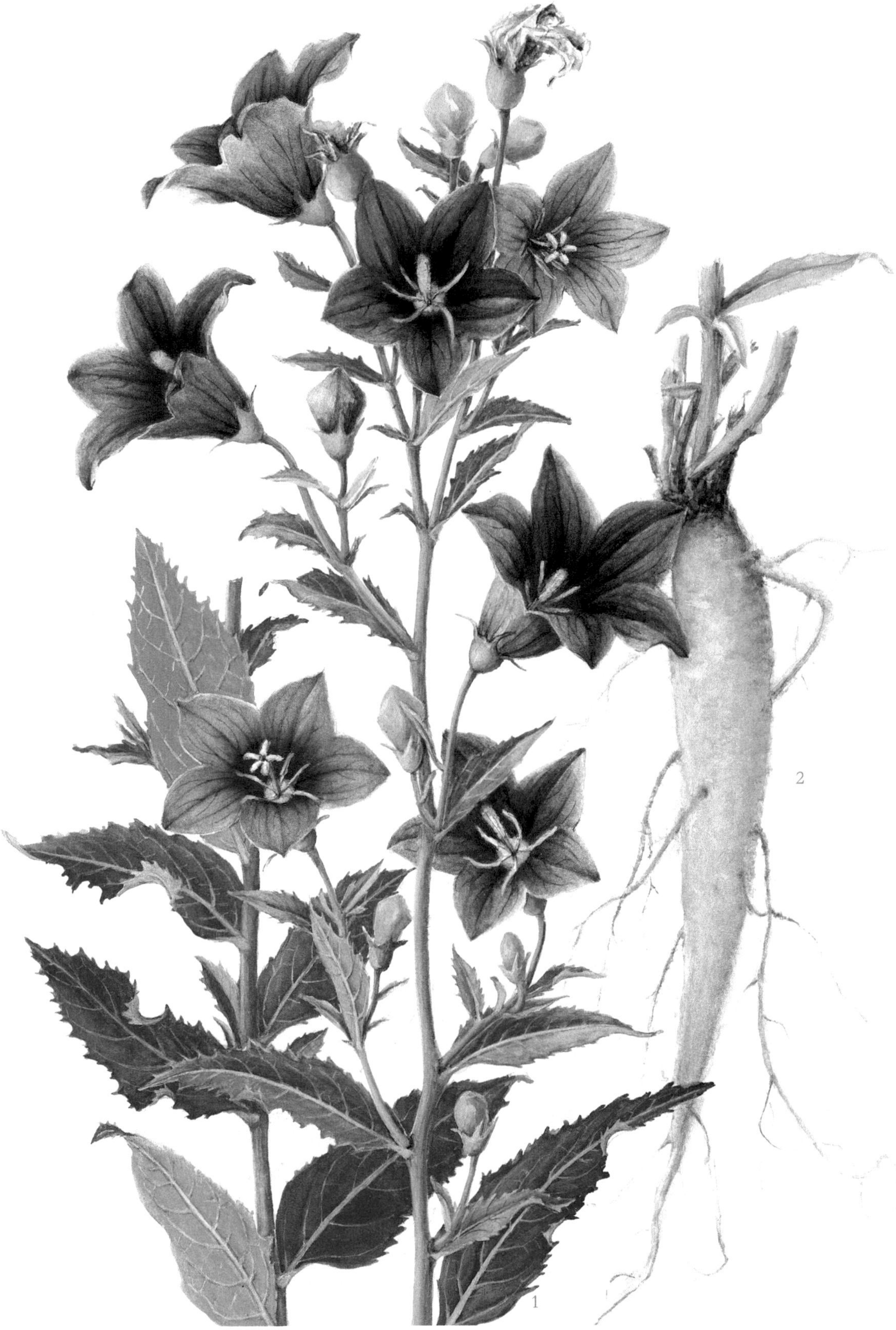

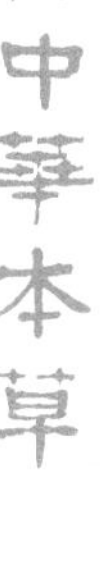

1. 花枝（flowering stem） 2. 根（root）

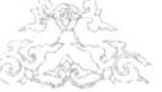

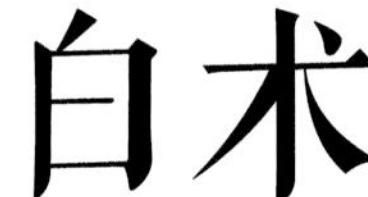

白术

Baizhu

Atractylodes macrocephala

基　　源　菊科 Asteraceae 苍术属 *Atractylodes* 植物白术 *Atractylodes macrocephala* Koidz. 的干燥根茎。药材名为“白术”。

形态特征　多年生草本。茎直立，通常自中下部长分枝。叶片通常 3-5 羽状全裂；叶薄纸质，边缘有针刺状缘毛。头状花序单生茎顶；总苞片覆瓦状排列，苞片边缘有白色蛛丝毛；小花紫红色。瘦果倒圆锥状，被稠密的白色长直毛；冠毛羽毛状。

生境分布　主要生长于我国华东等省 800 m 以上的山沟、深谷，现已极少见。浙江、安徽等地有大量栽培，浙江新昌烟山白术种植始于唐朝，为著名的道地药材“浙八味”之一。

采收加工　冬季下部叶枯黄、上部叶变脆时采挖，除去泥沙，烘干或晒干，再除去须根。

性味功能　温，苦、甘。健脾益气，燥湿利水，止汗，安胎。

主治用法　主要用于脾虚食少，腹胀泄泻，痰饮眩悸，水肿，自汗，胎动不安。

化学成分　根茎含挥发油类，如苍术酮、苍术醚等；还含有果糖、菊糖、氨基酸等。

备　　注　常用的炮制方法有土炒或麸炒，以增强功效。

Source　It is the dried rhizome of *Atractylodes macrocephala* Koidz. (Asteraceae). The medicinal material is called as “Baizhu”.

Distribution　*A. macrocephala* grows mainly in ravines and deep valleys above 800 m in East China, but now becomes rare. It is widely cultivated in Zhejiang, Anhui and other provinces. The cultivation of Rhizoma Atractylodis Macrocephalae in Yanshan Mountain of Xinchang County, Zhejiang, began in Tang Dynasty. It is one of the famous authentic medicinal materials—“Eight Tastes of Zhejiang”.

Indications　It is used to treat spleen deficiency with decreased food intake, abdominal bloating and diarrhea, dizziness and palpitation due to phlegm-fluid retention, edema, spontaneous sweating, and threatened abortion.

Chemical Constituents　The rhizome contains volatile oils, e.g., atractylone, atractyloxide. It also contains fructose, inulin and amino acids.

Note　The commonly used processing methods are stir-frying with earth or with bran, which can enhance its effects.

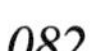

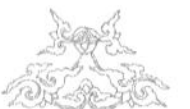

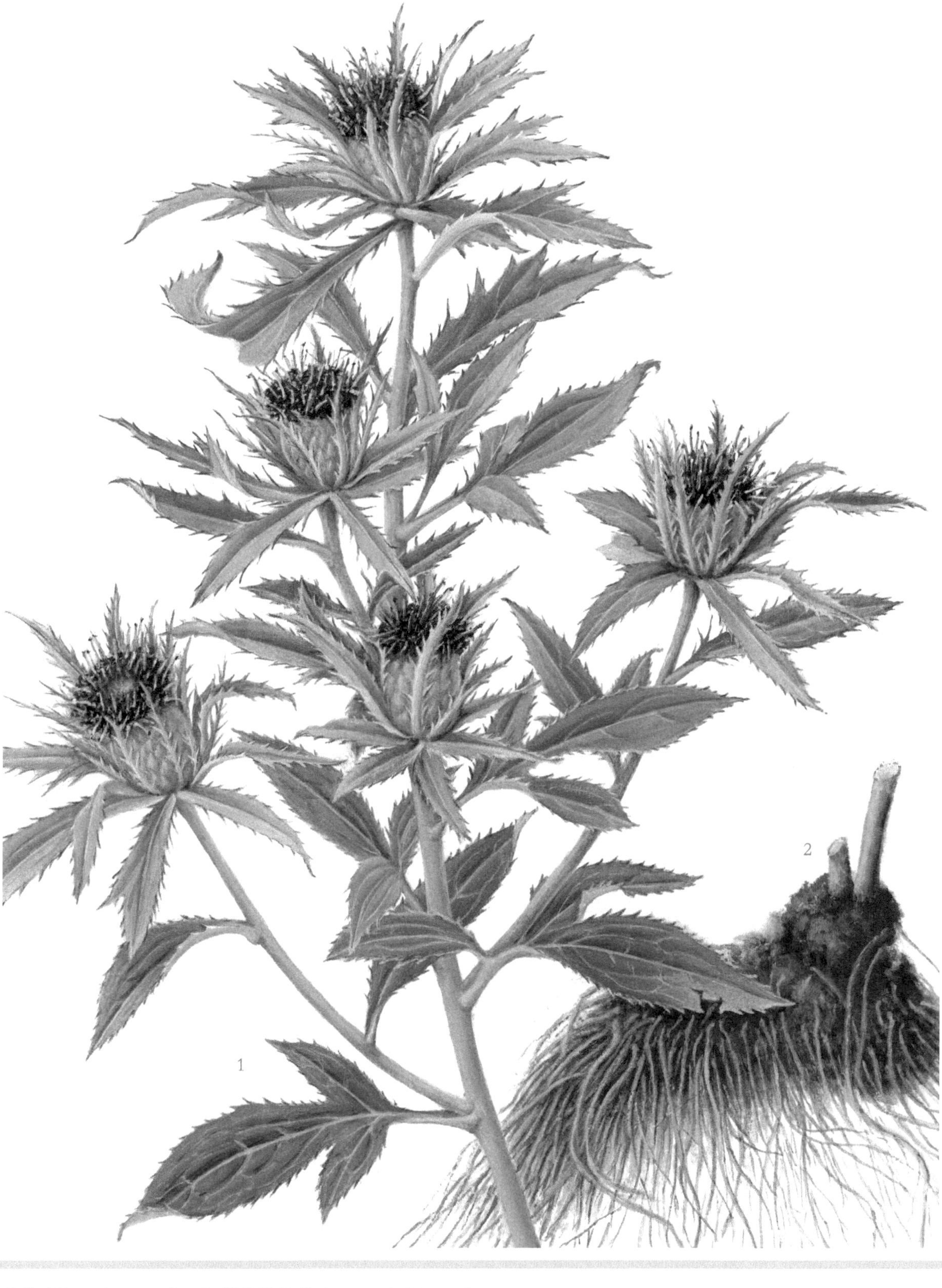

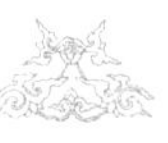

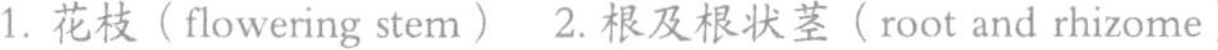

1. 花枝（flowering stem） 2. 根及根状茎（root and rhizome）

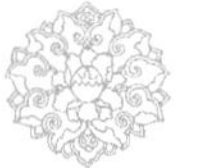

中华猕猴桃

Zhonghuamihoutao

Actinidia chinensis

基　　源　猕猴桃科 Actinidiaceae 猕猴桃属 *Actinidia* 植物中华猕猴桃 *Actinidia chinensis* Planch. 的根。药材名为“藤梨根”。

形态特征　大型落叶藤本。幼枝密被茸毛，隔年枝秃净；隔年枝皮孔长圆形；有髓，片层状。叶纸质，倒阔卵形，顶端截平，中间凹入或具突尖，基部钝圆形，叶面深绿色，散被短糙毛，背面苍绿色，密被淡褐色星状绒毛。聚伞花序；花初开白色，开后淡黄色，有香气。果近球形或椭圆形，黄褐色，被刺毛状长硬毛；宿存萼片反折。

生境分布　广泛分布于长江流域。常生于海拔 200-600 m 低山区的次生疏林中。

采收加工　一般于春、秋二季挖取，洗净，晒干，切碎用。

性味功能　凉，酸、涩。清热解毒，祛风除湿，利尿止血。

主治用法　主要用于风湿骨痛、黄疸等症。

化学成分　根含猕猴桃多糖复合物及丰富的抗坏血酸。

备　　注　中华猕猴桃的果实是一种闻名世界、富含营养的水果。

Source　It is the dried root of *Actinidia chinensis* Planch. (Actinidiaceae). The medicine material is called as “Tengligen”.

Distribution　*A. chinensis* is distributed widely in the Yangtze River Basin. It commonly grows in the secondary sparse forest in the low mountainous areas at an attitude of 200–600 m.

Indications　It is used to treat osteodynia due to wind–dampness and jaundice.

Chemical Constituents　The root contains polysaccharide complex and rich in ascorbic acid.

Note　The fruit of *A. chinensis* is a world-famous and nutritious fruit.

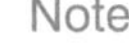

中华猕猴桃

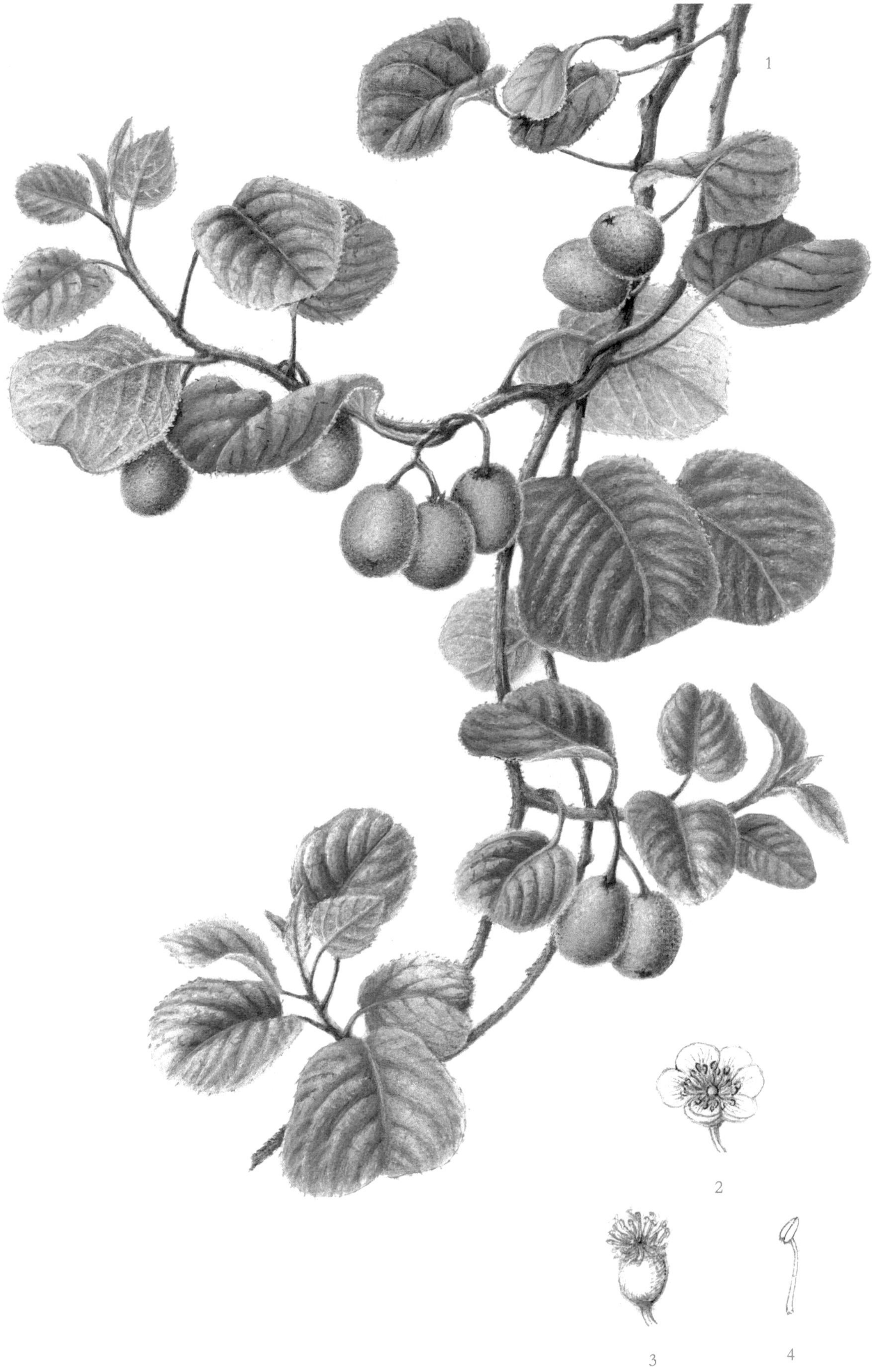

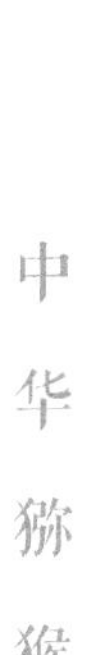

1. 果枝（fruiting stem） 2. 花（flower） 3. 雌蕊（pistil） 4. 雄蕊（stamen）

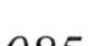

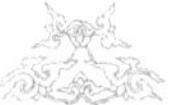

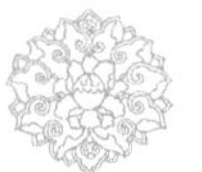

雪胆

Xuedan

Hemsleya chinensis

基　源　葫芦科 Cucurbitaceae 雪胆属 *Hemsleya* 植物雪胆 *Hemsleya chinensis* Cogn. ex Forbes et Hemsl. 的干燥块根。药材名为“雪胆”。

形态特征　多年生攀援草本。卷须线形，先端 2 歧。趾状复叶由 5-9 小叶组成；小叶片卵状披针形至宽披针形，膜质，中央小叶较大，两侧较小，外侧的略歪斜。花雌雄异株；雄花呈疏散的聚伞总状花序或圆锥花序；花萼裂片 5，卵形，反折；花冠橙红色；雌花呈稀疏的总状花序，花较大。果实矩圆状椭圆形，单生。种子黑褐色，近圆形，周生狭窄木栓质翅。

生境分布　分布于湖北、四川、江西。常见生于海拔 1200-2100 m 的杂木林下或林缘沟边。

采收加工　常年可采，洗净，切片晒干。

性味功能　寒，苦；有小毒。清热解毒，健胃止痛。

主治用法　用于胃痛，溃疡病，上呼吸道感染，支气管炎，肺炎，细菌性痢疾，肠炎，泌尿系感染，败血症及其他多种感染。

化学成分　块茎含有雪胆甲素、雪胆乙素、齐墩果酸等。

Source　It is the dried root rhizome of *Hemsleya chinensis* Cogn. ex Forbes et Hemsl. (Cucurbitaceae). The medicinal material is called as “Xuedan”.

Distribution　*H. chinensis* is distributed in Hubei, Sichuan and Jiangxi. It commonly grows under mixed wood forests or at the edge of the forest ditches at an altitude of 1200–2100 m.

Indications　It is used to treat stomach pain, ulcers, upper respiratory tract infections, bronchitis, pneumonia, bacterial dysentery, enteritis, urinary infections, septicemia and many other infections.

Chemical Constituents　The rhizome contains Curcurbitacin IIa, cucurbitacin IIb and oleanolic acid.

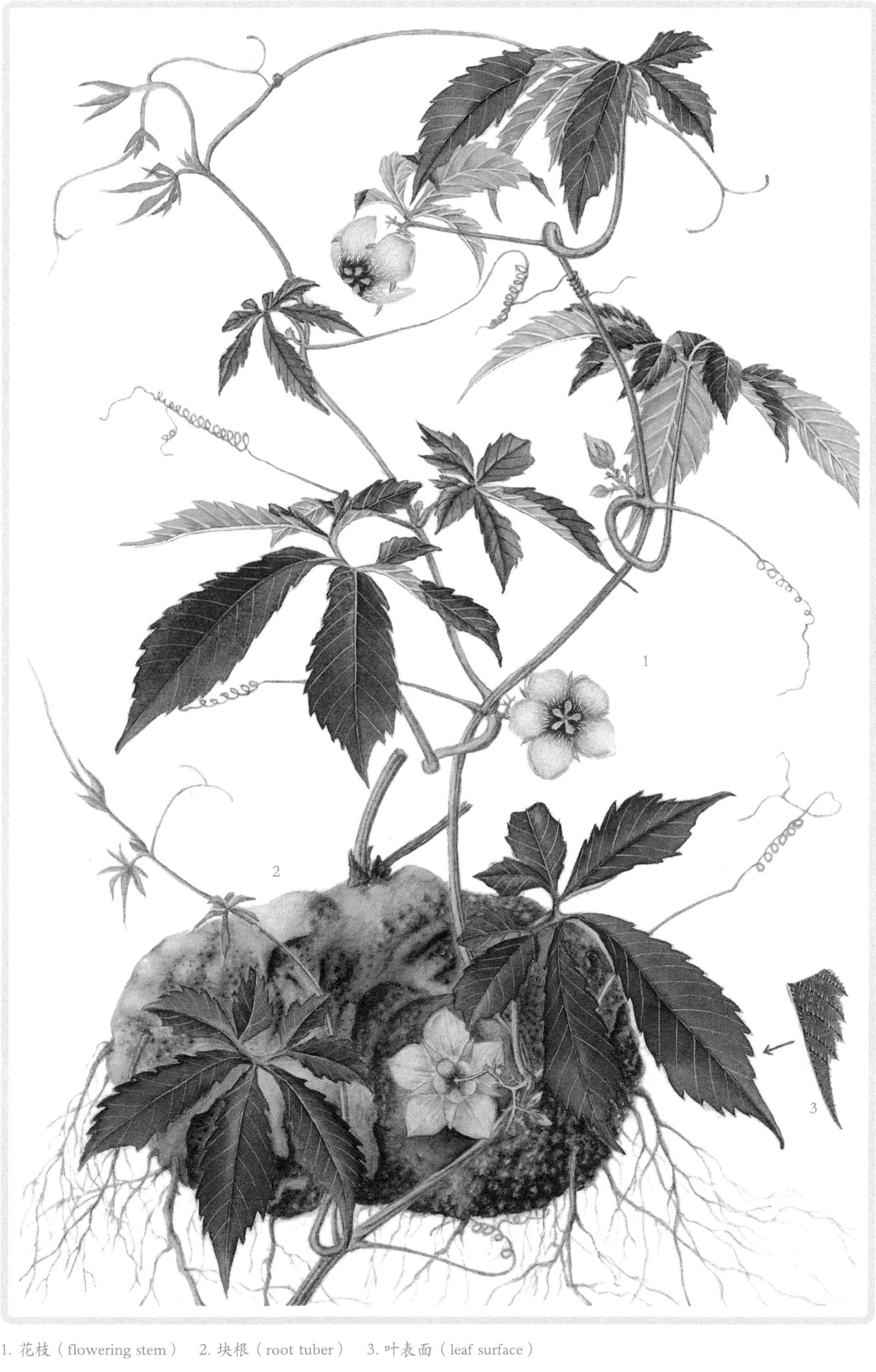

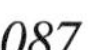

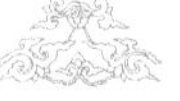

1. 花枝（flowering stem） 2. 块根（root tuber） 3. 叶表面（leaf surface）

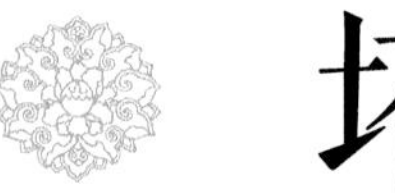

塔黄

Tahuang

Rheum nobile

基　源　蓼科 Polygonaceae 大黄属 *Rheum* 植物塔黄 *Rheum nobile* Hook. f. et Thoms. 的根茎。药材名为“塔黄”。

形态特征　多年生高大草本。茎单生不分枝，粗壮挺直。基生叶数片，呈莲座状，具多数茎生叶，近革质，顶端圆或极阔钝尖形；托叶鞘宽大，阔披针形，玫瑰红色；上部叶及叶状苞片向上渐小近圆形，苞片淡黄色。花序分枝腋生，总状；花 5-9 朵簇生。果实宽卵形或卵形，翅窄，深褐色。种子心状卵形，黑褐色。

生境分布　分布于喜马拉雅山麓及四川、青海、云南高原地带。一般生长于海拔 4000-4800 m 的高山流石滩或潮湿草地灌丛中。

采收加工　9-10 月采挖根茎，除去泥土和杂质，切片，阴干备用。

性味功能　寒，苦。导滞，散瘀，消肿。

主治用法　主要用于实热便秘，谵语发狂，食积痞滞，痢疾，湿热发黄，目赤头痛，闭经，癥瘕，痈肿疔毒。

化学成分　根及根茎中含有蒽醌类成分，主要为大黄素、大黄素甲醚和大黄酚为苷元的结合型蒽醌，还含有大量的鞣质。

备　注　塔黄为藏药常用药。

Source　It is the rhizome of *Rheum nobile* Hook. f. et Thoms. (Polygonaceae). The medicinal material is called as “Tahuang”.

Distribution　*R. nobile* is distributed in the Himalaya foothills, and the plateau area of Sichuan, Qinghai, and Yunnan. It generally grows on alpine rocky beaches or in shrubs of wet grassland at an altitude of 4000–4800 m.

Indications　It is used to treat constipation due to excessive heat, delirious speech and mania, food accumulation, dysentery, dampness–heat jaundice, red eyes and headache, amenorrhea, abdominal mass, swollen abscess and boil.

Chemical Constituents　The rhizome mainly contains bound anthraquinones,whose aglycones are emodin, physcione, chrysophanol and much tannin.

Note　It is commonly used in Tibetan medicine.

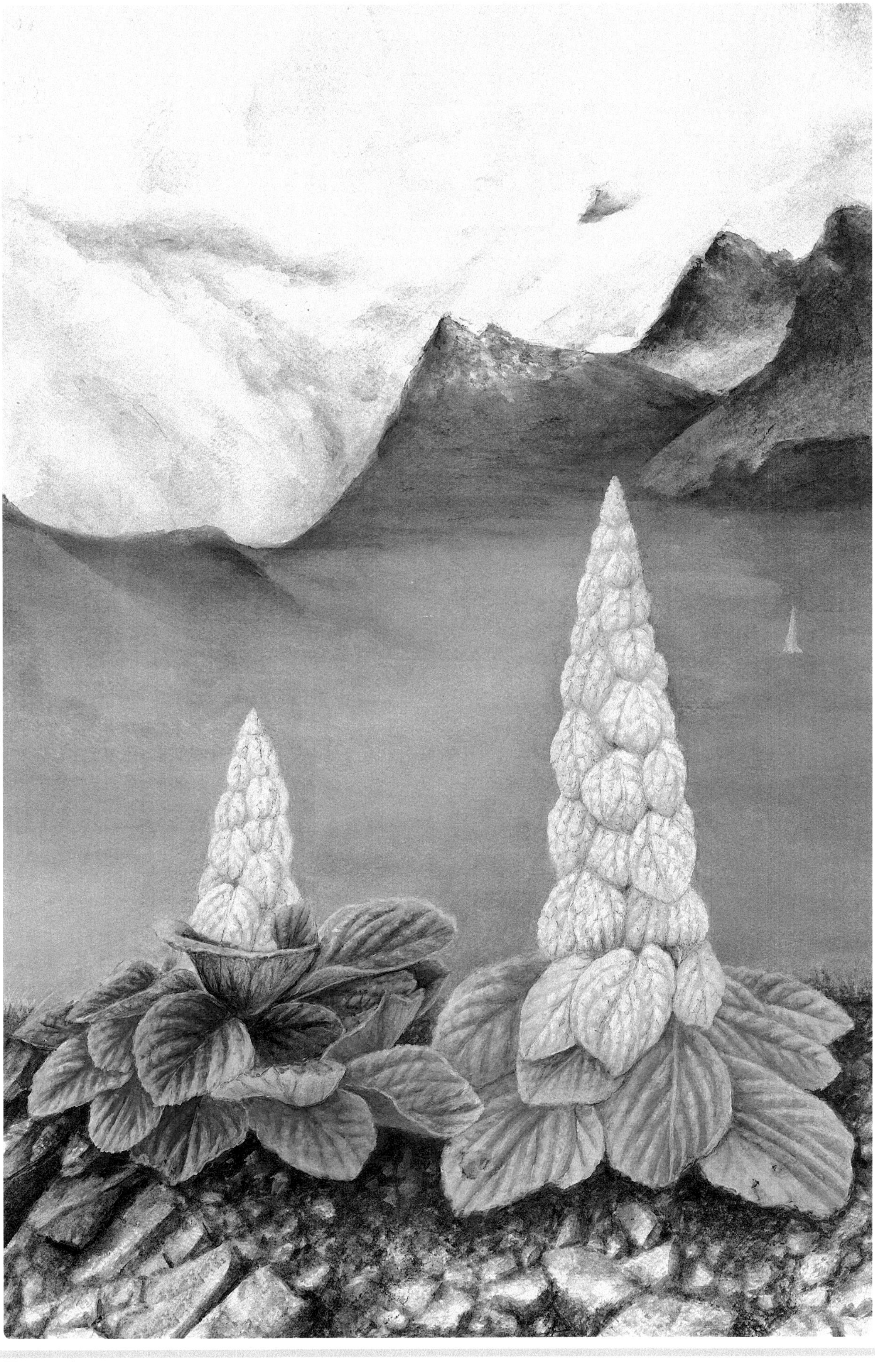

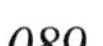

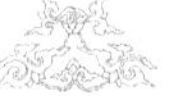

植株及生境（plant and habitat）

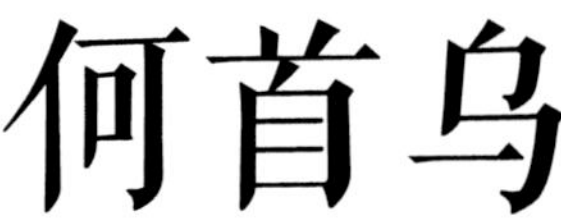

何首乌

Heshouwu

Polygonum multiflorum

基　　源　蓼科 Polygonaceae 蓼属 *Polygonum* 植物何首乌 *Polygonum multiflorum* Thunb. 的干燥块根。药材名为“何首乌”。

形态特征　多年生草本。块根肥厚，外皮紫褐色。茎缠绕，多分枝，下部木质化。叶卵形，顶端渐尖，基部心形，全缘；托叶鞘膜质。花序圆锥状，顶生或腋生；花小，花被白色或淡绿色。瘦果卵形，具三棱，黑褐色，包于宿存花被内。

生境分布　主要分布于我国华中、华东、西南各地。生于山坡路旁、林下等环境。

采收加工　秋、冬二季叶枯萎时采挖，削去两端，洗净，个大的切成块，干燥。

性味功能　微温，苦、甘、涩。解毒，消痈，截疟，润肠通便。

主治用法　用于疮痈，瘰疬，风疹瘙痒，久疟体虚，肠燥便秘。不宜长期超量服用，避免与肝毒性药物同时使用，注意监测肝功能。

化学成分　块根主要含有蒽醌类化合物，如大黄素、大黄酚、大黄素甲醚等；还含有穆坪马兜铃酰胺、二苯乙烯苷、没食子酸、磷脂等。

备　　注　何首乌的茎藤入药称“夜交藤”，用于养心安神。现代植物分类学研究认为，何首乌应属于何首乌属，学名修订为 *Fallopia multiflora* (Thunb.) Harald.。

Source　It is the dried root rhizome of *Polygonum multiflorum* Thunb. (Polygonaceae). The medicinal material is called as “Heshouwu”.

Distribution　*P. multiflorum* is mainly distributed in Central East and Southwest China. It commonly grows by the roadside of hills and under forests.

Indications　It is used to treat sore and abscess, scrofula, itch due to rubella, protracted malaria and weakness, and intestinal dryness with constipation. It is not advisable to take large doses for prolonged periods. Hepatotoxic drugs are not allowed to take with it and liver function should be monitored.

Chemical Constituents　The root tuber mainly contains anthraquinones, e.g., emodin, chrysophanol, physcione. It also contains moupinamide, diphenylethylene-2-O-glucoside, gallic acid, phospholipids, etc.

Note　The stem and vine are called Caulis Polygoni Multiflori, which can be used as medicine to nourish the heat and calm the mind. Modern plant taxonomy studies suggest that the plant should be classified into the genus *Fallopia*. The scientific name has been revised to *F. multiflora* (Thunb.) Harald.

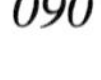

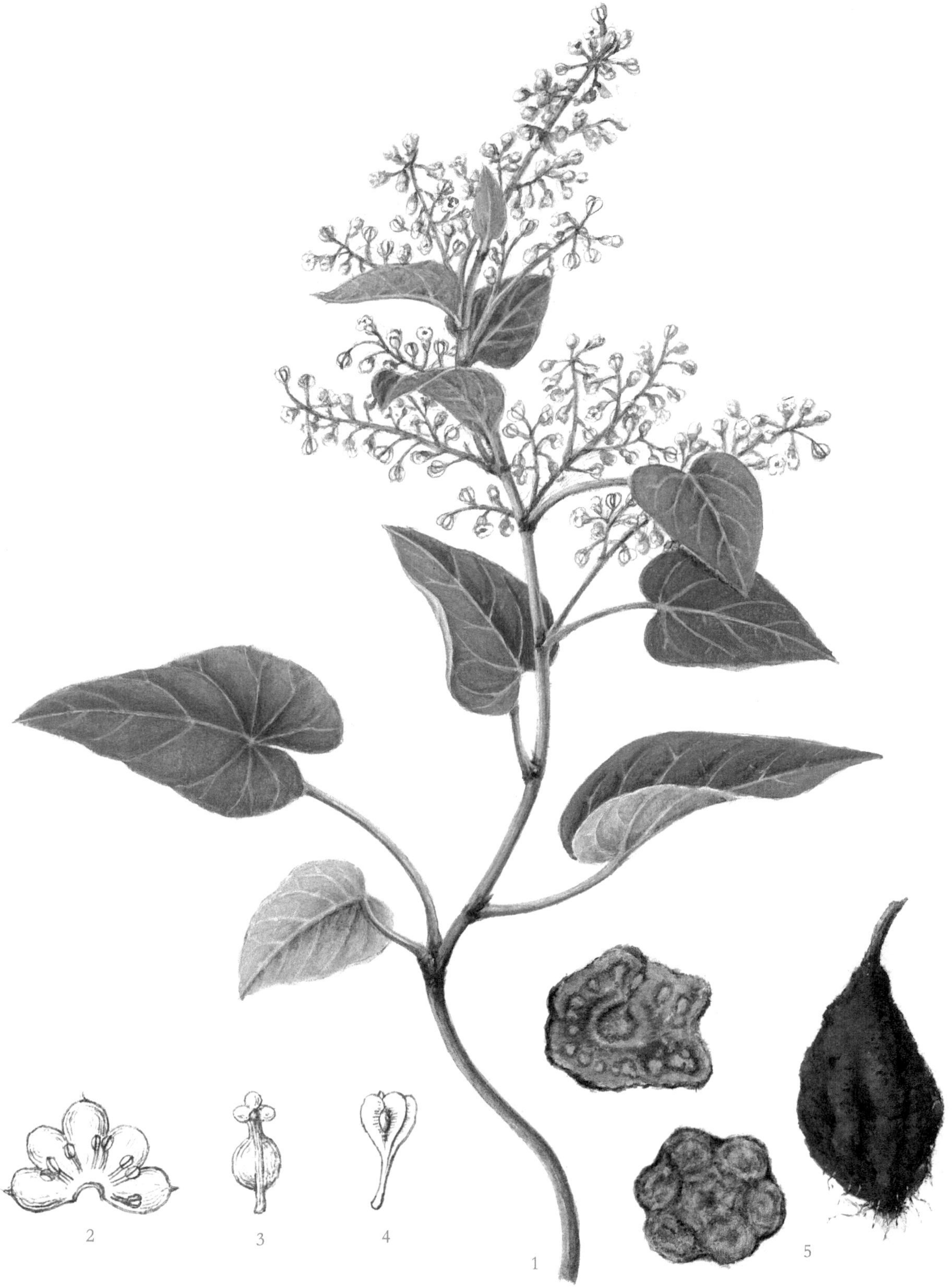

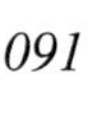

1. 花枝（flowering stem） 2. 花内面（inner flower） 3. 雌蕊（pistil） 4. 果实（fruit） 5. 块根及横切面（root tuber and transection）

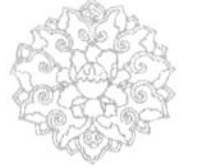

伏生紫堇

Fushengzijin

Corydalis decumbens

基　　源　罂粟科 Papaveraceae 紫堇属 *Corydalis* 植物伏生紫堇（夏天无）*Corydalis decumbens* (Thunb.) Pers. 的干燥块茎。药材名为“夏天无”。

形态特征　多年生草本。块茎小，形状不规则；茎柔弱，细长，不分枝。叶二回三出；小叶片倒卵圆形，全缘。总状花序；花近白色至淡粉红色或淡蓝色；萼片早落；外花瓣顶端下凹；上花瓣瓣片和距微上弯；下花瓣宽匙形；内花瓣具超出顶端的宽而圆的鸡冠状突起。蒴果线形，多少扭曲。

生境分布　分布于我国中部、东部部分省区；日本南部也有分布。常生于海拔 300 m 以下的疏林下和路边。

采收加工　春季或初夏出苗后采挖，除去茎、叶及须根，洗净，干燥。

性味功能　温，苦、微辛。活血通络，行气止痛。

主治用法　主要用于中风偏瘫，跌扑损伤，风湿性关节炎，坐骨神经痛。

化学成分　块茎主要含有生物碱类成分，如原阿片碱、巴马汀、夏天无碱等；另还含有甾酸、棕榈酸、阿魏酸等。

Source　It is the dried rhizome of *Corydalis decumbens* (Thunb.) Pers. (Papaveraceae). The medicinal material is called as “Xiatianwu”.

Distribution　*C. decumbens* is distributed in central and eastern parts of China and south Japan. It commonly grows in sparse forest and by the roadside below the altitude of 300 m.

Indications　It is used to treat stroke marked by hemiplegia, traumatic injury, rheumarthritis, and sciatica.

Chemical Constituents　The stem tuber mainly contains alkaloids, e.g., protopine, palmatine, decumbenine. It also contains steroidal acid, palmitic acid, ferulic acid, etc.

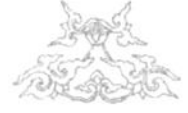

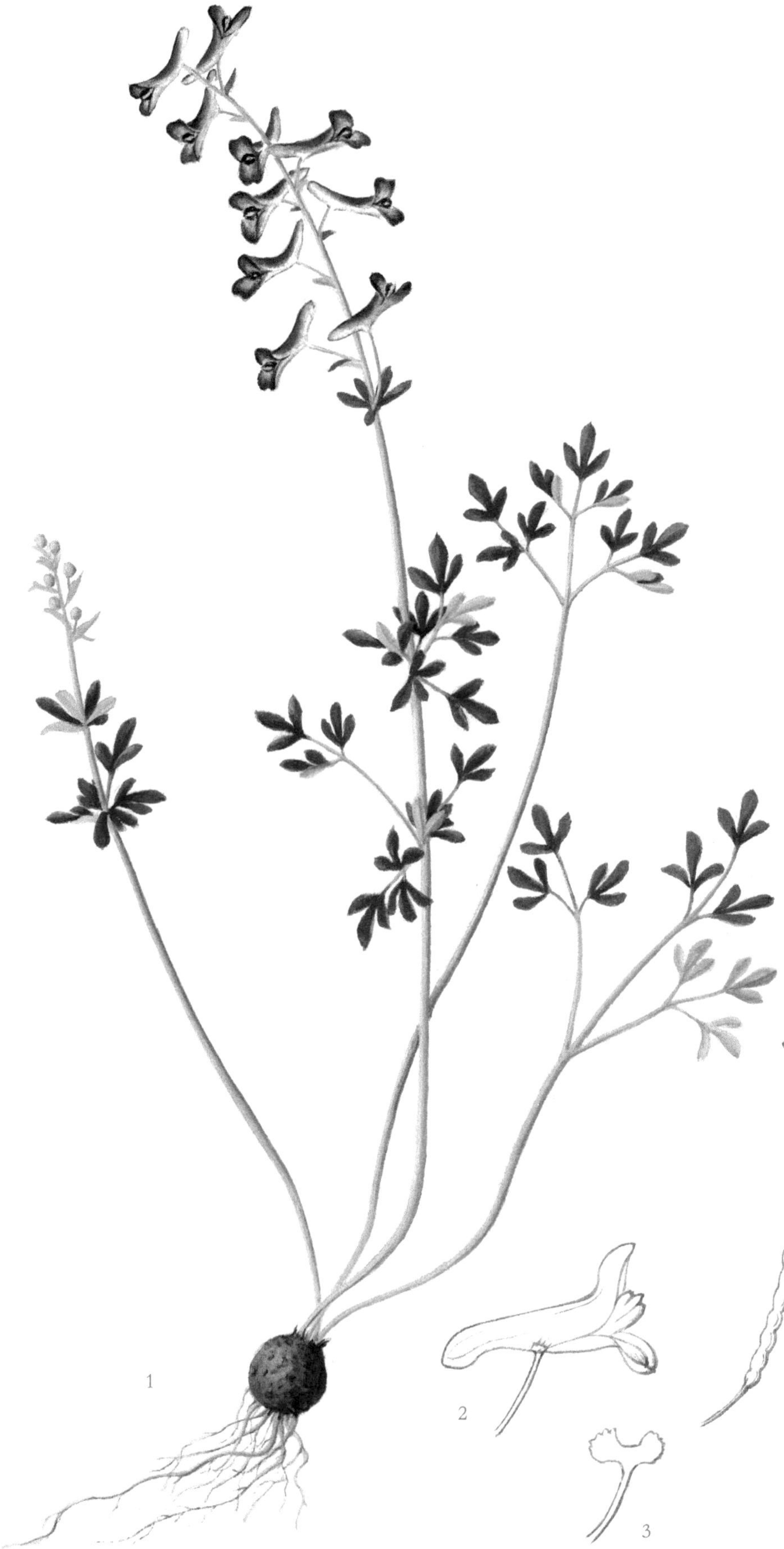

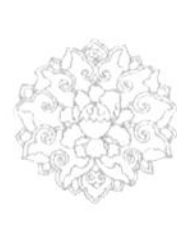

伏生紫堇

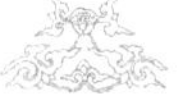

1. 植株（plant） 2. 花（flower） 3. 柱头（stigma） 4. 果实（fruit）

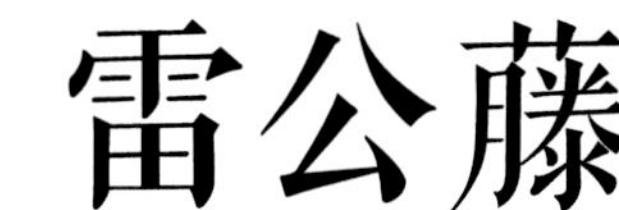

雷公藤

Leigongteng

Tripterygium wilfordii

基　　源　卫矛科 Celastraceae 雷公藤属 *Tripterygium* 植物雷公藤 *Tripterygium wilfordii* Hook. f. 根的木质部。药材名为“雷公藤”。

形态特征　藤本灌木。小枝棕红色，具四细棱，密被毛及细密皮孔。叶椭圆形或卵形，先端急尖，基部阔楔形，边缘有细锯齿；叶柄密被锈色毛。圆锥聚伞花序较窄小，通常有 3-5 分枝，花序、分枝及小花梗均被锈色毛；花白色。翅果长圆形。种子细柱状。

生境分布　分布于长江流域以南各地及西南地区；朝鲜、日本也有分布。生于山地林内阴湿处。

采收加工　秋季挖取根部，抖净泥土，晒干，或去皮晒干。

性味功能　凉，苦、辛。有大毒。祛风除湿、活血通络、消肿止痛、杀虫解毒。

主治用法　主要用于治疗类风湿性关节炎，风湿性关节炎，肾小球肾炎，肾病综合征，红斑狼疮，疥疮，顽癣等。煎汤内服需久煎，也可制成糖浆，外用可制成酊剂、软膏涂擦。凡疮痒出血者慎用。

化学成分　根木质部含雷公藤三萜内酯 A、南蛇藤素、雷公藤三萜酸 A、直楔草酸、雷公藤酮、雷公藤内酯三醇、亚麻酸等；根皮含雷公藤碱、雷公藤内酯酮、雷公藤内酯二醇、山海棠素、雷公藤素、美登木酸等。

备　　注　雷公藤毒性剧烈，现主要制成制剂，用于治疗自身免疫性疾病。

Source　It is the xylem of root of *Tripterygium wilfordii* Hook. f. (Celastraceae). The medicinal material is called as “Leigongteng”.

Distribution　*T. wilfordii* is distributed in the southern regions of the Yangtze River Basin and Southwest China. It is also found the in Democratic People’s Republic of Korea and Japan. It grows in shady and damp mountain forests.

Indications　It is used to treat rheumatoid arthritis, rheumatic arthritis, glomerulonephritis, nephrotic syndrome, lupus erythematosus, scabies, tinea, etc. For internal use, it should be decocted for extended periods of time or made into syrup. It can be used as a tincture or ointment for external application. Those who have itchy and bleeding sore should use it with caution.

Chemical Constituents　The xylem of the root contains triptoterpenoid lactone A, celasterol, triptotriterpenic acid A, orthosphenic acid, tripterygone, triptriolide, linolenic acid, etc. The root bark contains wilfordine, triptonide, tripdiolide, hypolide, wilforonide, maytenonic acid, etc.

Note　It is highly toxic and is now mainly made into preparations for the treatment of autoimmune diseases.

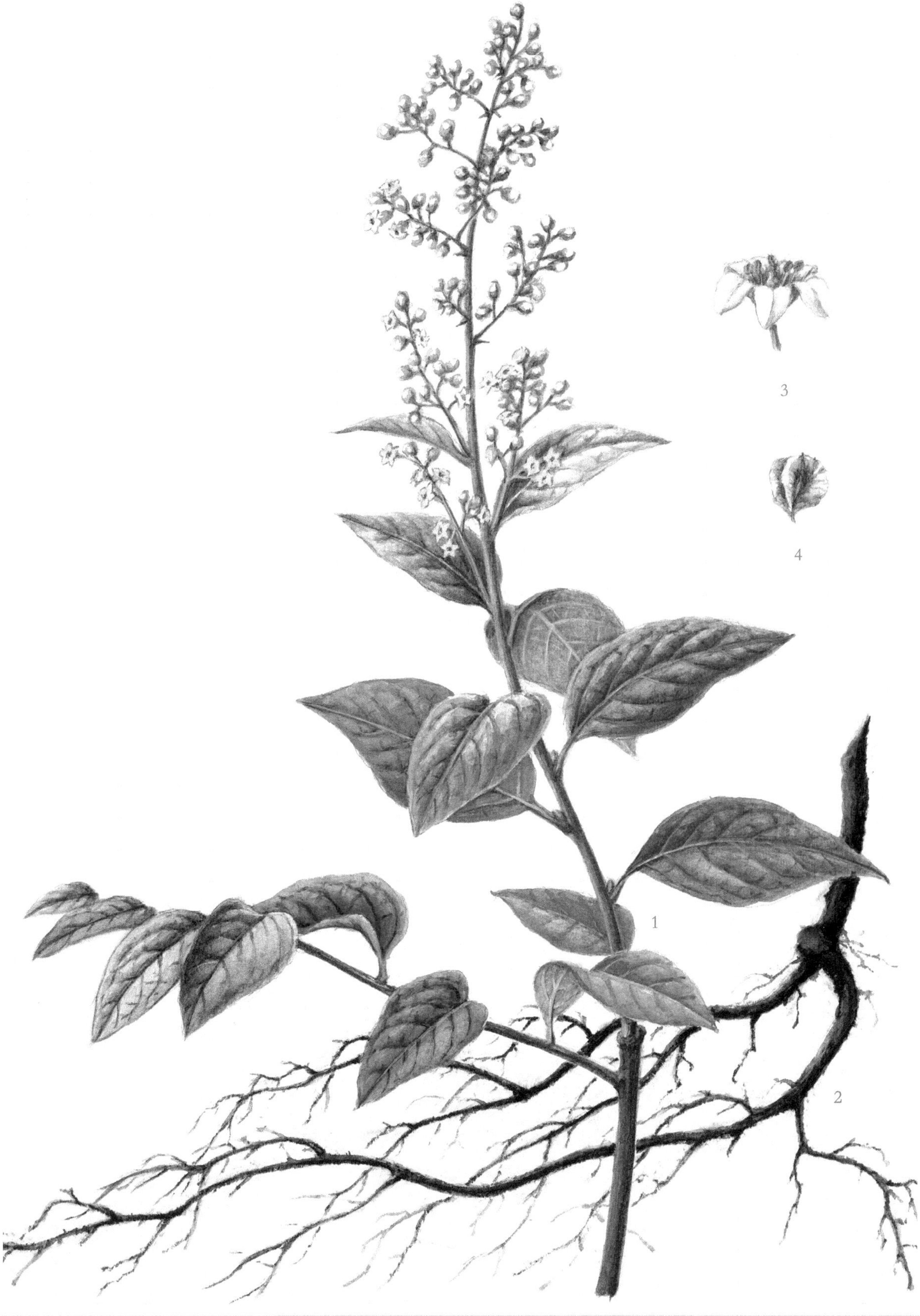

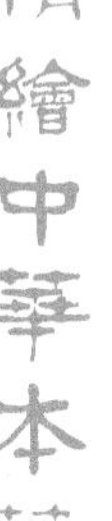

1. 花枝（flowering stem） 2. 根（root） 3. 花（flower） 4. 果实（fruit）

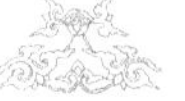

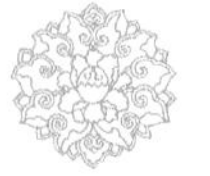

大血藤

Daxueteng

Sargentodoxa cuneata

基　源　木通科 Lardizabalaceae 大血藤属 *Sargentodoxa* 植物大血藤 *Sargentodoxa cuneata* (Oliv.) Rehd. et Wils. 的干燥藤茎。药材名为“大血藤”。

形态特征　落叶木质藤本。全株无毛；当年枝条暗红色。三出复叶；小叶革质，顶生小叶近倒卵圆形，全缘，侧生小叶斜卵形，上面绿色，下面淡绿色，干时常变为红褐色，无小叶柄。总状花序；雄花与雌花同序或异序；萼片 6，花瓣状，长圆形；花瓣 6。浆果近球形，成熟时黑蓝色。

生境分布　分布于我国南方大部分省区。生于土壤肥沃的深山疏林中。

采收加工　秋、冬二季采收，除去侧枝，截段，干燥。

性味功能　平，苦。清热解毒，活血，祛风止痛。

主治用法　用于肠痈腹痛，热毒疮疡，经闭，痛经，跌扑肿痛，风湿痹痛。

化学成分　茎藤中主要含有蒽醌类成分，如大黄素、大黄素甲醚、大黄酚等；另还含有 β-谷甾醇、胡萝卜甙、硬脂酸、毛柳甙、香草酸和原儿茶酸等。

Source　It is the dried cane of *Sargentodoxa cuneata* (Oliv.) Rehd.et Wils. (Lardizabalaceae). The medicinal material is called as “Daxueteng”.

Distribution　*S. cuneata* is distributed in most provinces of southern China. It grows in sparse fertile forests in deep mountains.

Indications　It is used to treat intestinal abscess and abdominal pain, sore and ulcer due to heat toxin, amenorrhea, dysmenorrhea, traumatic injury with pain and swelling, wind–dampness impediment pain.

Chemical Constituents　The stem and vine mainly contain anthraquinones (e.g., emodin, physcion, chrysophanol), β-sitosterol, daucosterol, stearic acid, salidroside, vanillic acid, protocatechuic acid, etc.

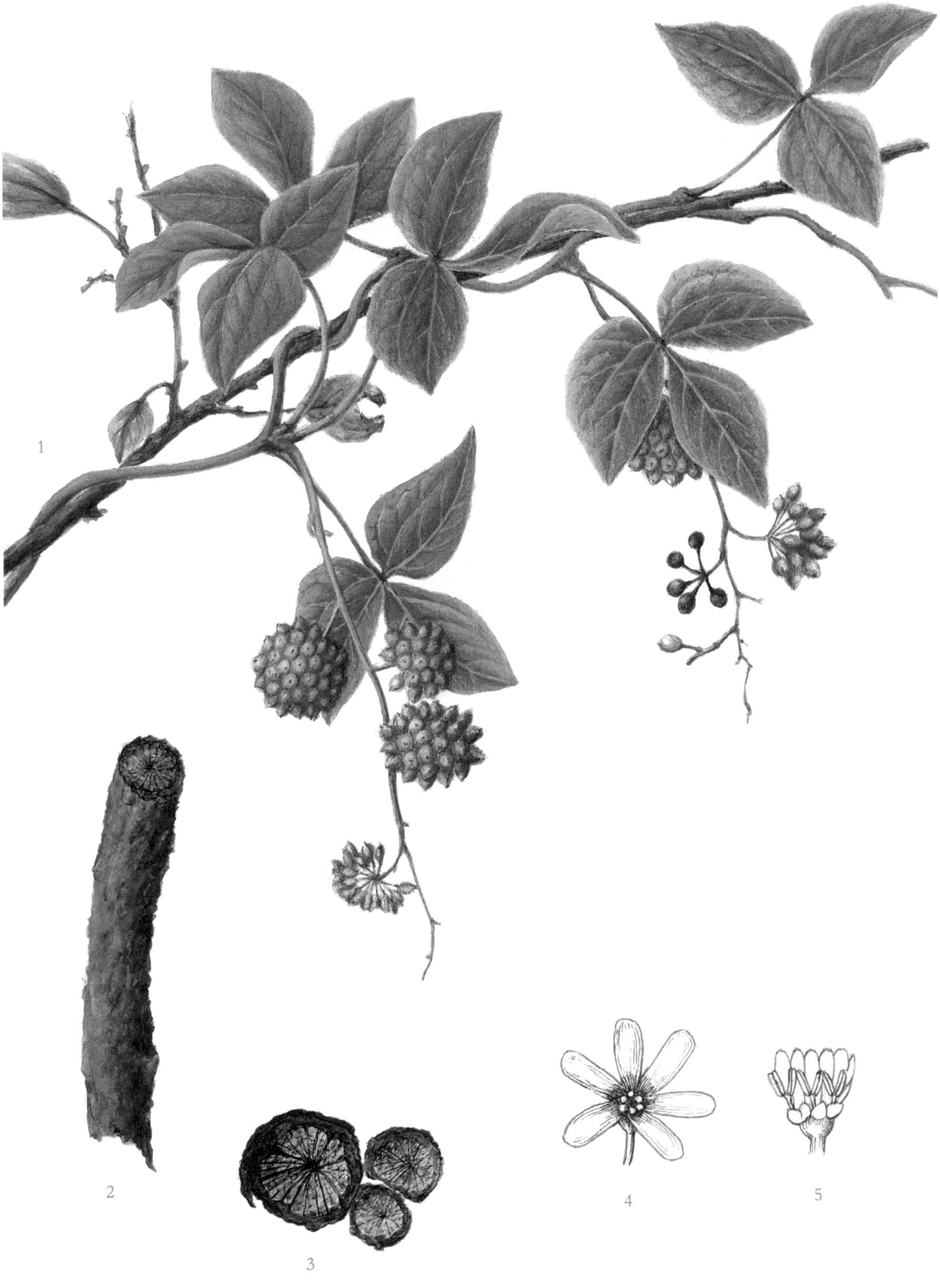

1. 果枝（fruiting stem） 2. 茎（stem） 3. 茎横切面（transection of stem） 4. 花（flower） 5. 雄蕊（stamen）

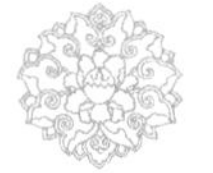

三叶木通

Sanyemutong

Akebia trifoliata

基　源　木通科 Lardizabalaceae 木通属 *Akebia* 植物三叶木通 *Akebia trifoliata* (Thunb.) Koidz. 的干燥藤茎。药材名为“木通”。

形态特征　落叶木质藤本。掌状复叶互生或在短枝上的簇生；小叶 3 片，纸质或薄革质，卵形至阔卵形，边缘具波状齿或浅裂。总状花序自短枝上簇生叶中抽出，下部有 1-2 朵雌花，以上约有 15-30 朵雄花。雄花萼片 3，淡紫色。雌花萼片 3，紫褐色；心皮 3-9 枚，离生。果长圆形，成熟时近灰白色；种子多数，扁卵形，种皮褐色，稍有光泽。

生境分布　分布于我国华北和长江流域各省区。常生于海拔 250-2000 m 的山谷疏林或丘陵灌丛中。

采收加工　秋季采收，截取茎部，除去细枝，阴干。

性味功能　寒，苦。利尿通淋，清心除烦，通经下乳。

主治用法　用于淋证，水肿，心烦尿赤，口舌生疮，经闭乳少，湿热痹痛。

化学成分　主要含有萜类，如白桦脂醇、齐墩果酸；皂苷类，如木通皂苷等；另还含有豆甾醇、胡萝卜苷等。

备　注　三叶木通干燥近成熟果实亦可入药，称“预知子”，具有疏肝理气、活血止痛、散结、利尿的功效。

Source　It is the dried cane of *Akebia trifoliata* (Thunb.) Koidz. (Lardizabalaceae). The medicinal material is called as “Mutong”.

Distribution　*A. trifoliata* is distributed in North China and the Yangtze River Basin. It commonly commonly grows in sparse forests or shrubs of valleys at an altitude of 250–2000 m.

Indications　It is used to treat strangury, edema, vexation and deep-colored urine, mouth and tongue sore, amenorrhea with scant breast milk, damp–heat impediment.

Chemical Constituents　It mainly contains terpenes (e.g., betulin, oleanolic acid) and saponins (e.g., akeboside). It also contains stigmasterol, daucosterol, etc.

Note　The dried near-ripe fruits can also be used as medicine, which is known as Fructus Akebiae. It has the function of soothing liver and regulating qi, activating blood circulation to relieve pain, and dispersing masses.It is also used as a diuretic.

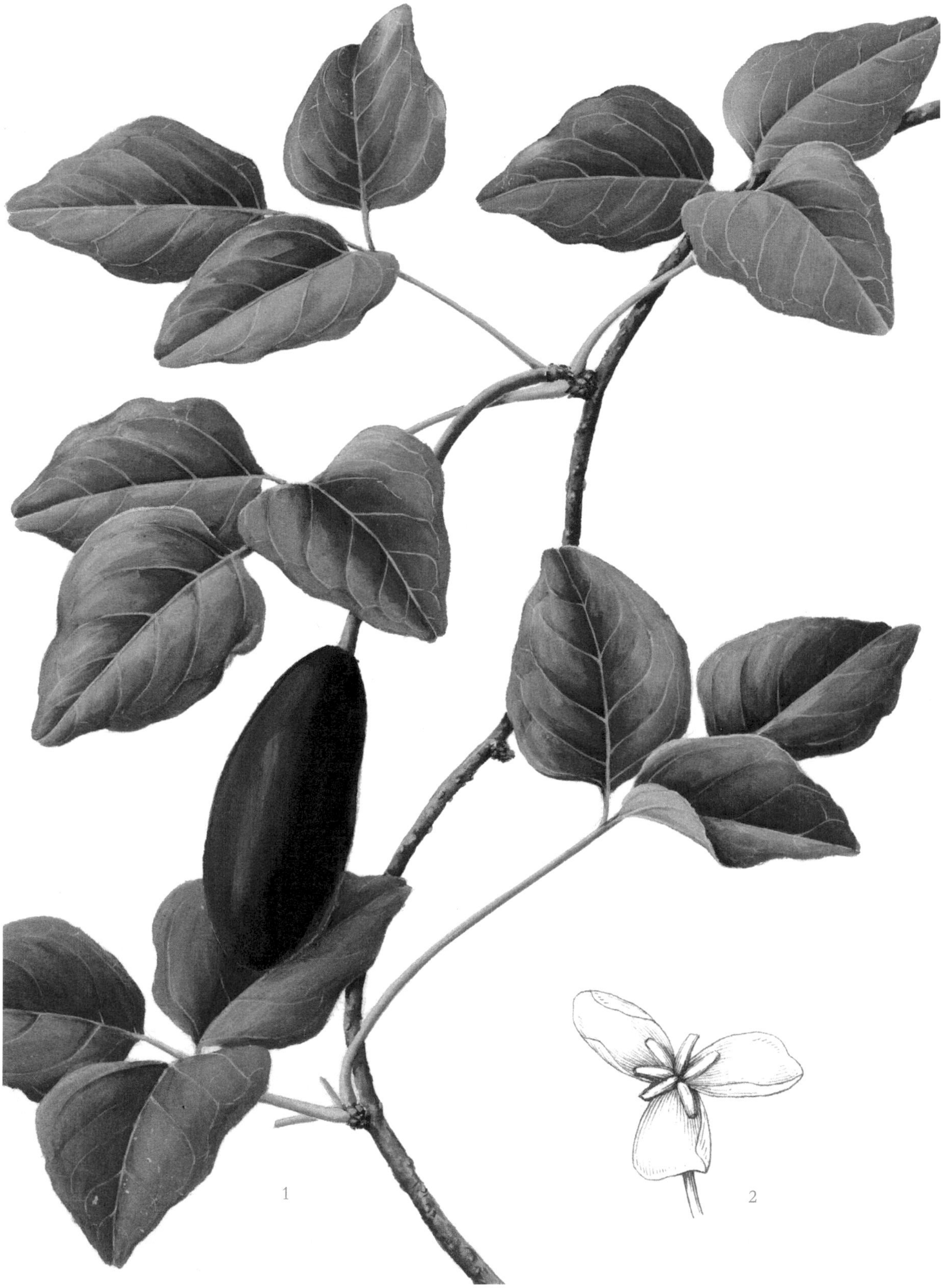

1

2

1. 果枝（fruiting stem） 2. 雌花（female flower）

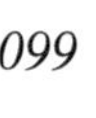

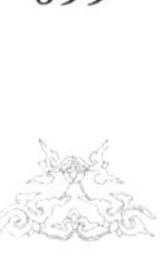

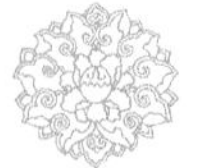

金钗石斛

Jinchaishihu

Dendrobium nobile

基　　源　兰科 Orchidaceae 石斛属 *Dendrobium* 植物金钗石斛 *Dendrobium nobile* Lindl. 的新鲜或干燥茎。药材名为“石斛”。

形态特征　多年生草本。茎直立，肉质状肥厚，稍扁的圆柱形，上部多少回折状弯曲，基部明显收狭，不分枝，具多节。叶革质，长圆形，先端钝并且不等侧二裂，基部具抱茎的鞘。总状花序从具叶或落了叶的老茎中部以上部分发出；花大，多为白色，先端淡紫色；唇瓣宽卵形，先端钝，唇盘中央具 1 个紫红色大斑块。

生境分布　分布于我国南方的部分省区。附生于海拔数百米的林中树干或岩石上。

采收加工　全年均可采收，鲜用者除去根和泥沙；干用者采收后，除去杂质，用开水略烫或烘软，再边搓边烘晒，至叶鞘搓净，干燥。

性味功能　微寒，甘。益胃生津，滋阴清热。

主治用法　主要用于热病津伤，口干烦渴，胃阴不足，食少干呕，病后虚热不退，阴虚火旺，骨蒸劳热，目暗不明，筋骨痿软。

化学成分　茎中主要含有生物碱类成分，如石斛碱、石斛次碱等。

备　　注　金钗石斛花大而美丽，可栽培用于观赏。

Source　It is the fresh or dried stem of *Dendrobium nobile* Lindl. (Orchidaceae). The medicinal material is called as “Shihu”.

Distribution　*D. nobile* is distributed in some provinces of southern China. It commonly grows on tree trunks or rocks in the forests at an altitude of hundreds of meters.

Indications　It is mainly used to treat febrile disease and fluid damaging, dry mouth and extreme thirst, insufficiency of stomach yin, low food intake and retching, heat deficiency condition after illness, yin deficiency with effulgent fire, bone-steaming with hectic fever, dim vision, and flaccidity of sinews and bones.

Chemical Constituents　The stem mainly contains alkaloids, e.g., dendrobine and nobilonine.

Note　The flowers are large and beautiful, and it can be cultivated for viewing.

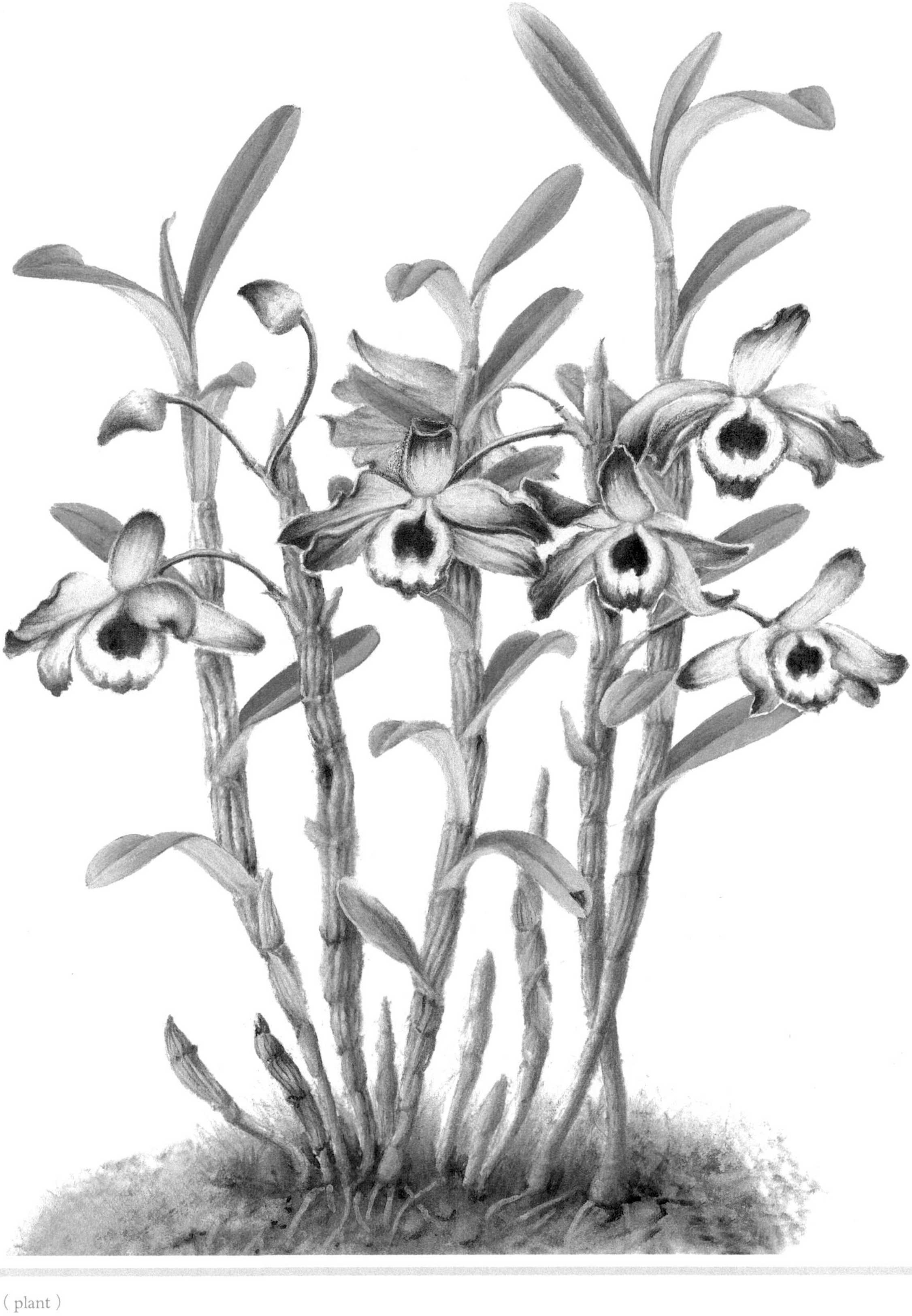

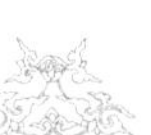

植株（plant）

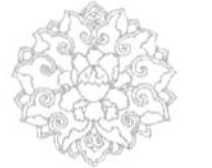

铁皮石斛

Tiepishihu

Dendrobium officinale

基　源　兰科 Orchidaceae 石斛属 *Dendrobium* 植物铁皮石斛 *Dendrobium officinale* Kimura et Migo 的干燥茎。药材名为“铁皮石斛”。

形态特征　附生草本。茎直立，圆柱形，不分枝，具多节，常在中部以上互生 3-5 枚叶；叶二列，纸质，长圆状披针形，基部下延为抱茎的鞘；叶鞘常具紫斑。总状花序常从落了叶的老茎上部发出，具 2-3 朵花；萼片和花瓣黄绿色；唇瓣白色；唇盘密布细乳突状的毛，并且在中部以上具 1 个紫红色斑块。

生境分布　分布于我国华东、华南部分省区以及云南。多附生于半阴湿的山崖或大树上。现多栽培。

采收加工　11 月至翌年 3 月采收，除去杂质，剪去部分须根，边加热边扭成螺旋形或弹簧状，烘干；或切成段，干燥或低温烘干。前者习称“铁皮枫斗”（耳环石斛）；后者习称“铁皮石斛”。

性味功能　微寒，甘。益胃生津，滋阴清热。

主治用法　主要用于热病津伤，口干烦渴，胃阴不足，食少干呕，病后虚热不退，阴虚火旺，骨蒸劳热，目暗不明，筋骨痿软。

化学成分　铁皮石斛主要含有生物碱类，如石斛碱、石斛胺碱等；另含有多糖类、氨基酸类和菲类等成分。

Source　It is the dried stem of *Dendrobium officinale* Kimura et Migo. (Orchidaceae). The medicinal material is called as “Tiepishihu”.

Distribution　*D. officinale* is distributed in some regions in East and South China as well as Yunnan province. It commonly grows on semi-damp and shady cliffs or trees. Nowadays, it is commonly cultivated.

Indications　It is used to treat febrile disease and fluid damaging, dry mouth and extreme thirst, insufficiency of stomach yin, low food intake and retching, heat deficiency condition after illness, yin deficiency with effulgent fire, bone-steaming with hectic fever, dim vision, and flaccidity of sinews and bones.

Chemical Constituents　It mainly contains alkaloids (e.g., dendrobine, dendramine). It also contains polysaccharides, amino acids, phenanthrenes, etc.

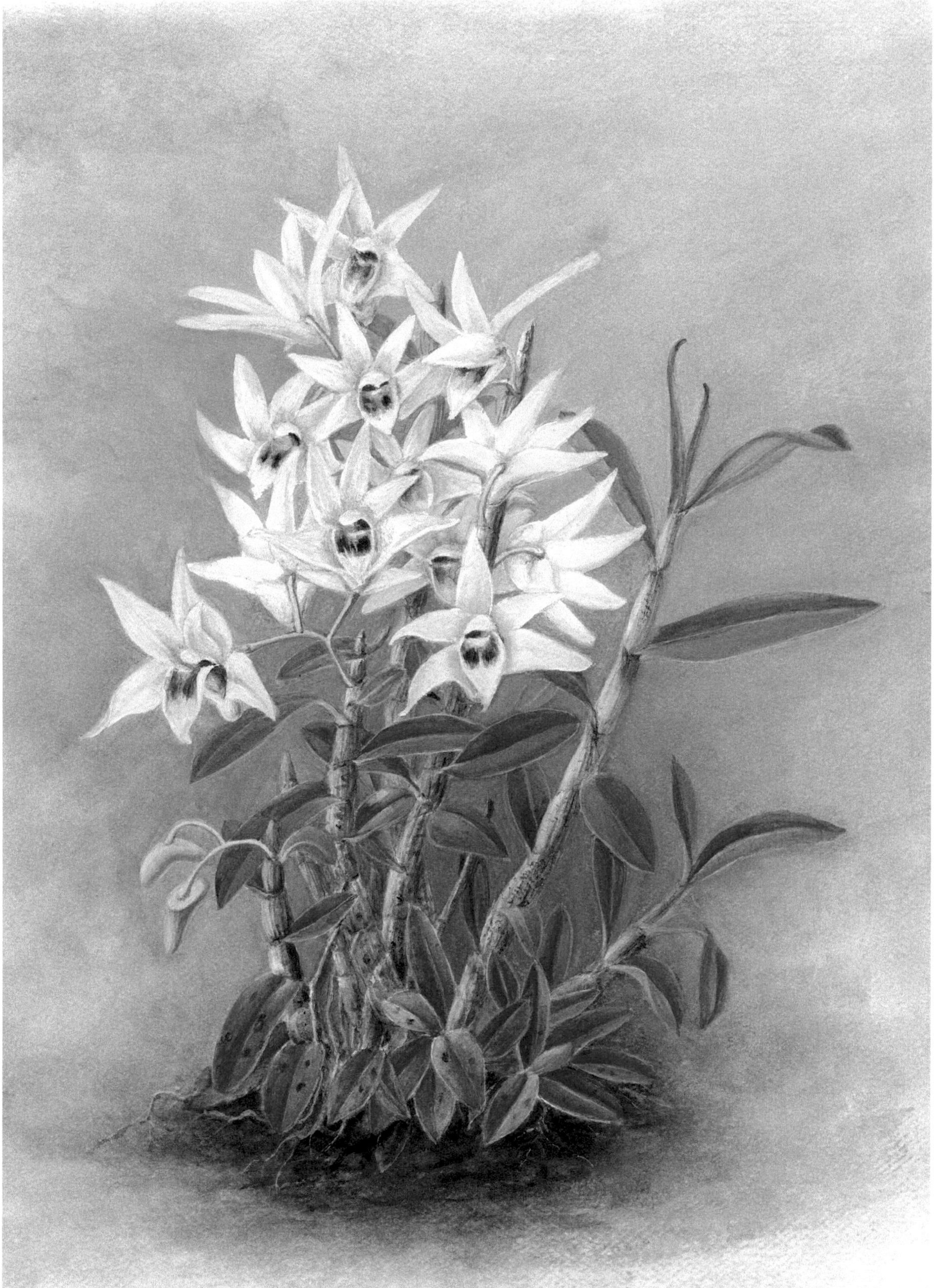

植株（plant）

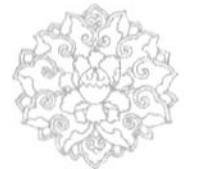

霍山石斛

Huoshanshihu

Dendrobium huoshanense

基　源　兰科 Orchidaceae 石斛属 *Dendrobium* 植物霍山石斛 *Dendrobium huoshanense* C. Z. Tang et S. J. Cheng 的新鲜或干燥茎。药材名为“石斛”，习称“米斛”。

形态特征　多年生草本。茎直立，肉质，不分枝，具3-7节，淡黄绿色，有时带淡紫红色斑点。叶革质，2-3枚互生于茎的上部，斜出，舌状长圆形。总状花序1-3个，从落了叶的老茎上部发出，具1-2朵花；花淡黄绿色，开展；花瓣卵状长圆形，先端钝，具5条脉；唇瓣近菱形，长和宽约相等。

生境分布　分布于安徽大别山区。生于云雾缭绕的悬崖峭壁崖石缝隙间。现多栽培。

采收加工　11月至翌年3月采收，除去杂质，剪去部分须根，边加热边扭成螺旋形或弹簧状，烘干。

性味功能　微寒，甘。益胃生津，滋阴清热。

主治用法　主要用于热病津伤，口干烦渴，胃阴不足，食少干呕，病后虚热不退，阴虚火旺，骨蒸劳热，目暗不明，筋骨痿软。

化学成分　霍山石斛的茎中主要含有多糖类、生物碱类以及果糖等成分。

备　注　霍山石斛以形似蚱蜢髀，色青黄，味甘，黏性足，无渣为佳。“米斛”为安徽霍山地理标志产品，加工成的枫斗具有“龙头凤尾”的特征。有专家考证，“斛”为“觓”之误，形如病羊之角，为历史传承中印刷错误所致。

Source　It is the fresh or dried stem of *Dendrobium huoshanense* C. Z. Tang et S. J. Cheng (Orchidaceae). The medicinal is called as “Shihu”.

Distribution　*D. huoshanense* is distributed in Dabie Mountains in Anhui Province. It grows between the cliffs and rocks surrounded by clouds and mist. It is commonly cultivated at present.

Indications　It is mainly used to treat febrile disease and fluid damaging, dry mouth and extreme thirst, insufficiency of stomach yin, low food intake and retching, heat deficiency after illness, yin deficiency with effulgent fire, bone-steaming with hectic fever, dim vision, flaccidity of sinews and bones.

Chemical Constituents　The stem mainly contains polysaccharides, alkaloids, fructose, etc.

Note　The best Herba Dendrobii Huoshanensis is characterized by the shape of grasshopper’s thigh, bluish yellow color, sweet flavor, high viscosity, and no slags. Herba Dendrobii Huoshanensis is the geographically representative product of Huoshan County, Anhui Province. The processed product is characterized by “dragon head and phoenix tail”. Some experts have researched that the “Hu” is the mistake of “Qiu”. It means that the shape is like the horn of a sick sheep, which is caused by a typographical error in historical inheritance.

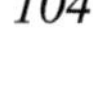

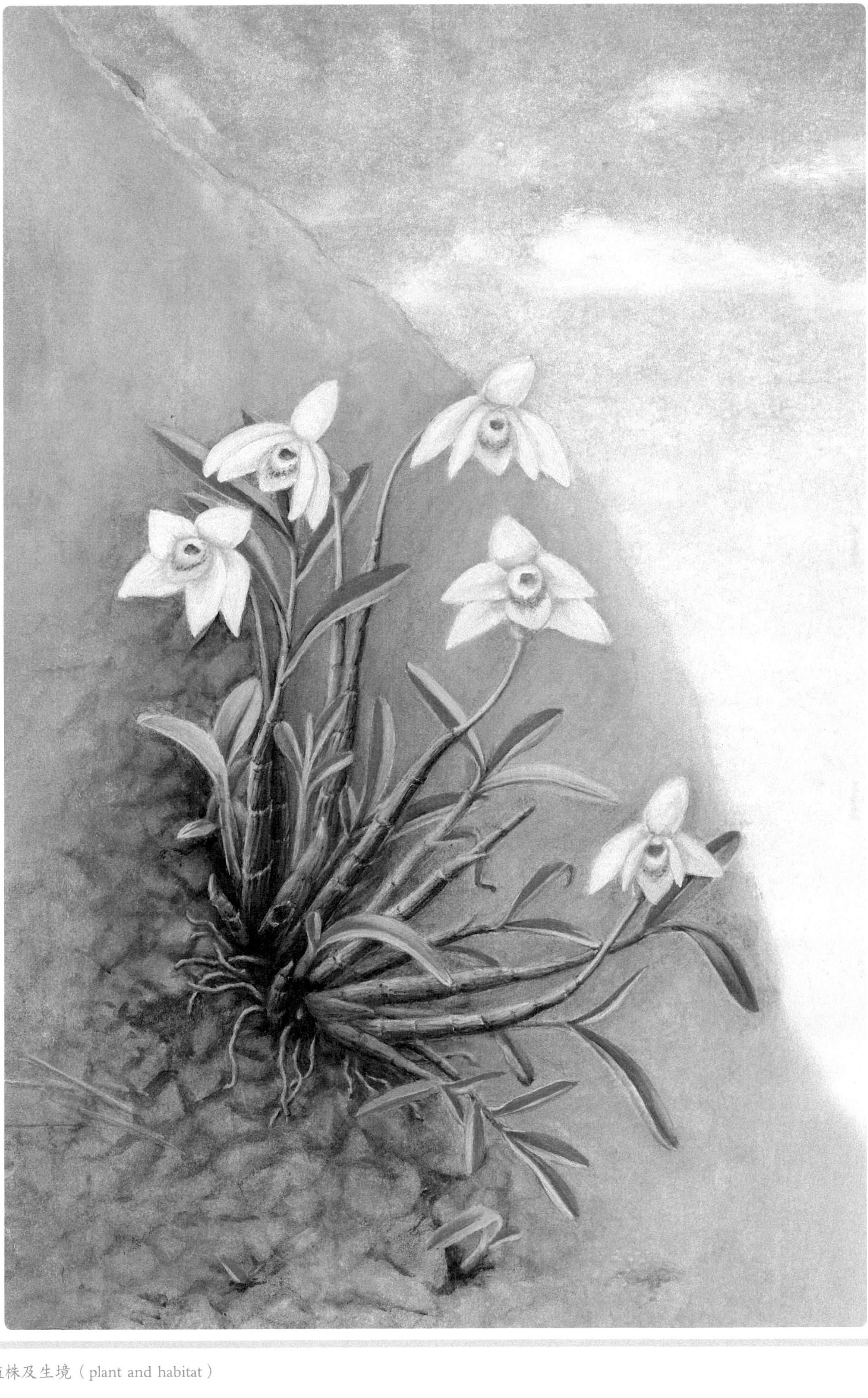

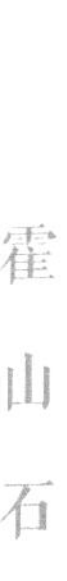
霍山石斛

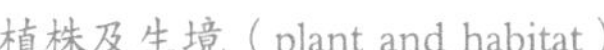
植株及生境（plant and habitat）

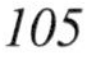

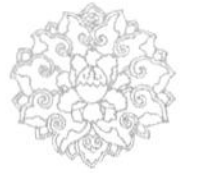

白木香

Baimuxiang

Aquilaria sinensis

基　源　瑞香科 Thymelaeaceae 沉香属 *Aquilaria* 植物白木香 *Aquilaria sinensis* (Lour.) Spreng. 含有树脂的木材。药材名为“沉香”。

形态特征　乔木。树皮暗灰色。叶革质，圆形至长圆形，先端锐尖具短尖头，基部宽楔形，上面暗绿色，光亮，下面淡绿色，两面无毛；叶柄被毛。花芳香，黄绿色，伞形花序；萼筒浅钟状，五裂；花瓣 10，鳞片状，着生于花萼筒喉部，密被毛。蒴果，卵球形，二瓣裂，2 室，每室具有 1 粒种子，种子褐色，卵球形，基部有附属体。

生境分布　主要分布于福建、广东、广西、海南、台湾。生于低海拔的山地、丘陵以及路边向阳处的疏林中，现多栽培。

采收加工　全年均可采收，割取含树脂的木材，除去不含树脂的部分，阴干。

性味功能　微温，辛、苦。行气止痛，温中止呕，纳气平喘。入煎剂后下。

主治用法　用于胸腹胀闷疼痛，胃寒呕吐呃逆，肾虚气逆喘急。如汤剂宜后下。

化学成分　药材沉香主要含有倍半萜类和色原酮类成分。白木香原植物主要含有黄酮类、二苯甲酮类、木脂素类、简单酚类化合物、萜类、甾类和生物碱类等。

备　注　白木香为保持水土的优良树种。天然沉香产量稀少，结香多为意外受损或虫蚁咬噬，历史上进口沉香为瑞香科植物沉香 *Aquilaria agallocha* (Lour.) Roxb. 含有树脂的木材，商品规格分大帽盔和小帽盔，并印有火漆。现在栽培白木香使其结香的方法多为刀砍、斧劈、钻孔，俗称“开香门”，历经数年，方可采收。

Source　It is the *Aquilaria sinensis* (Lour.) Roxb. (Thymelaeaceae). The medicinal material is called as “Chenxiang”.

Distribution　*A. sinensis* is mainly distributed in Fujian, Guangdong, Guangxi, Hainan and Chinese Taiwan. It commonly grows in mountains, hills and sparse forests exposed to the sun and roadside at low altitude.It is often cultivated nowadays.

Indications　It is used to treat distention, and oppression and pain in the chest and abdomen, vomiting with hiccup due to stomach cold, qi counterflow and rapid panting with kidney deficiency. It should be decocted later.

Chemical Constituents　It mainly contains sesquiterpenes and chromones. *A. sinensis* mainly contains flavonoids, benzophenones, lignans, simple phenolic compounds, terpenoids, steroids, alkaloids, etc.

Note　*A. sinensis* is an excellent species for soil and water conservation. The yield of natural *A. sinensis* is scarce. Most of them is produced due to accidental damage or bites by insects and ants. Historically, the imported Lignum Aquilariae Resinatum is the resin-containing wood of Aquilaria sinensis (Lour.) Gilg. The product is divided by specification into large helmet and small helmet and printed with sealing wax. At present, the methods of cultivating *A. sinensis* are mostly cutting, chopping, and drilling hole. It can only be harvested after several years.

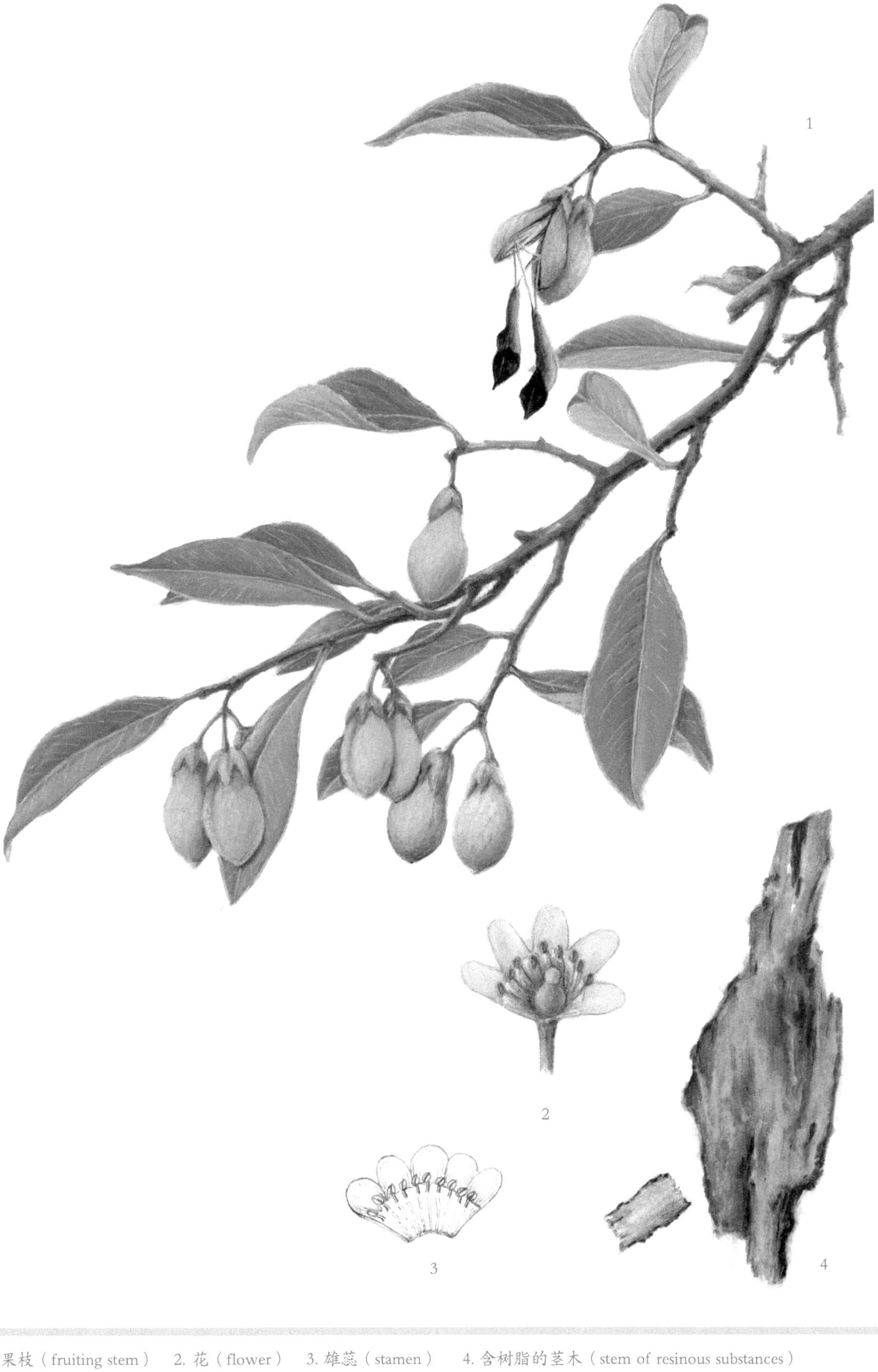

1

2

3

4

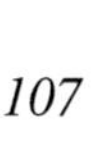

1. 果枝（fruiting stem） 2. 花（flower） 3. 雄蕊（stamen） 4. 含树脂的茎木（stem of resinous substances）

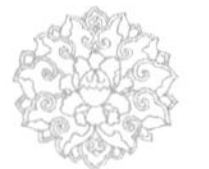

异果小檗

Yiguoxiaobo

Berberis heteropoda

基　　源　小檗科 Berberidaceae 小檗属 *Berberis* 植物异果小檗 *Berberis heteropoda* Schrenk. 的根皮和茎皮。药材名为“黑果小檗”。

形态特征　落叶灌木。茎直立，基部多分枝，嫩枝褐色，老枝灰色，刺单一或 3 分叉，暗褐色。叶簇生，革质；叶片卵圆形，全缘或具疏齿，上面绿色，下面黄绿色，叶脉不清晰。总状花序具 3-9 花；花黄色；萼片宽卵形，淡红色；花瓣 6，基部具 2 个圆形腺体。浆果球形，紫黑色，被 1 层灰粉。种子 5-6 粒，多皱纹。

生境分布　分布于新疆。常生于石质山坡、河滩地、疏林或云杉林下、灌丛中或干旱荒漠。海拔区间一般为 950-3200 m。

采收加工　春、秋季采收，除去枝叶、须根，剥取皮部，晒干。

性味功能　寒，苦。清湿热，泻火解毒。

主治用法　用于湿热痢疾，泄泻，目赤肿痛，咽喉肿痛，口疮，湿疹。

化学成分　茎皮含有小檗碱、小檗胺、掌叶防已碱、药根碱等。

Source　The root bark and stem bark of *Berberis heteropoda* Schrenk. (Berberidaceae). The medicinal material is called as “Heiguoxiaobo”.

Distribution　*B. heteropoda* is distributed in Xinjiang. It commonly grows on rocky hillsides, river flats, sparse or spruce forests, shrubs or dry deserts at an altitude of 950–3200 m generally.

Indications　It is used to treat dysentery due to dampness–heat, diarrhea, red eyes with pain and swelling, sore swollen throat, aphtha, and eczema.

Chemical Constituents　The stem bark contains berberine, berbamine, palmatine, jatrorrhizine, etc.

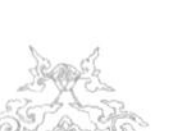

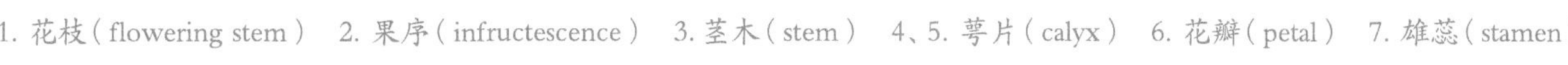

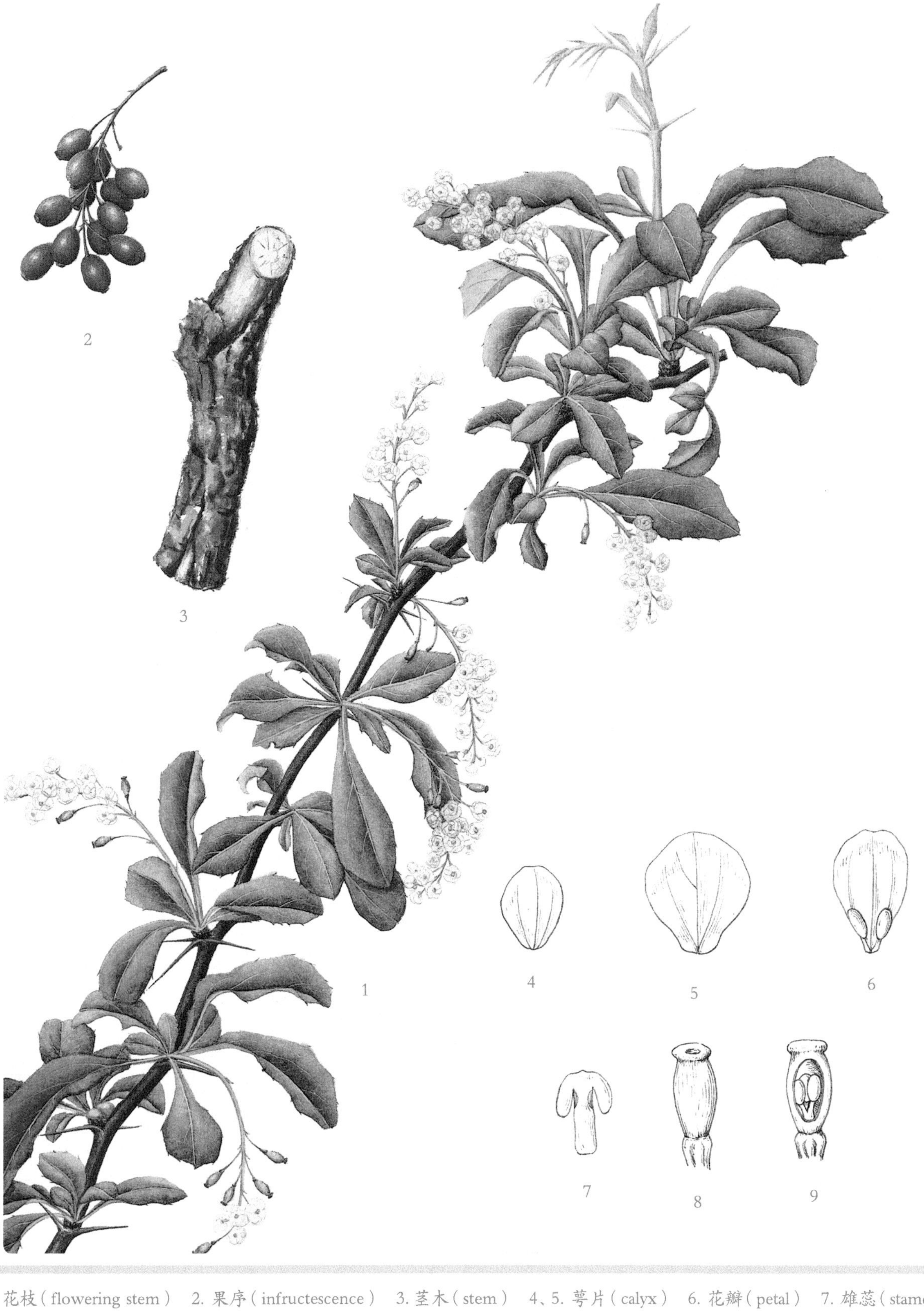

1. 花枝（flowering stem） 2. 果序（infructescence） 3. 茎木（stem） 4、5. 萼片（calyx） 6. 花瓣（petal） 7. 雄蕊（stamen） 8. 雌蕊（pistil） 9. 子房纵切面（vertical section of ovary）

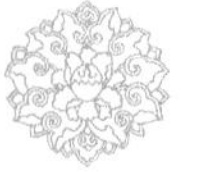

厚朴

Houpo
Magnolia officinalis

基　　源　木兰科 Magnoliaceae 木兰属 *Magnolia* 植物厚朴 *Magnolia officinalis* Rehd. et Wils. 的干燥干皮、根皮及枝皮。药材名为“厚朴”。

形态特征　落叶乔木。树皮褐色。叶大，近革质，7-9 片聚生于枝端，长圆状倒卵形，全缘而微波状。花叶同放，单生枝顶，杯状，白色，芳香；花被片 9-12，厚肉质，外轮 3 片盛开时反卷，内两轮白色，倒卵状匙形。聚合果长椭圆状卵形，心皮排列紧密，成熟时木质，顶端有弯尖头。种子三角状倒卵形，外种皮红色。

生境分布　主要分布于湖北西部、四川中部和东部。生于海拔 300-1500 m 的山地林间。现多栽培。为四川道地药材，习称“川朴”。

采收加工　4-6 月剥取根皮和枝皮直接阴干；干皮置沸水中微煮后，堆置阴湿处，“发汗”至内表面变紫褐色或棕褐色时，蒸软，取出，卷成筒状，干燥。

性味功能　温，苦、辛。燥湿消痰，下气除满。

主治用法　主要用于湿滞伤中，脘痞吐泻，食积气滞，腹胀便秘，痰饮喘咳。

化学成分　皮中主要含有木脂素类，如厚朴酚、和厚朴酚、四氢厚朴酚、异厚朴酚、厚朴三醇 B、厚朴木脂素 F、辣薄荷基厚朴酚等；另还含有桉叶油醇、对聚伞花烯、木兰箭毒碱等。

备　　注　干皮习称“筒朴”；近根部的干皮一端展开如喇叭口，习称“靴筒朴”；根皮习称“鸡肠朴”。厚朴花亦可入药。现代植物分类学研究已将厚朴学名修订为 *Houpoea officinalis* (Rehder et E. H. Wilson) N. H. Xia et C. Y. Wu。

Source　It is the dried trunk bark, root bark and branch bark of *Magnolia officinalis* Rehd. et Wils. (Magnoliaceae). The medicinal material is called as “Houpo”.

Distribution　*M. officinalis* is mainly distributed in the western Hubei and central and eastern Sichuan. It grows in the mountain forest at an altitude of 300–1500 m and is commonly cultivated at present. It is an authentic medicinal material in Sichuan called “Chuanpo”.

Indications　It is used to treat dampness damaging middle qi, gastric stuffiness with vomiting and diarrhea, food accumulation and qi stagnation, abdominal bloating and constipation, phlegm-fluid retention, and panting with coughing.

Chemical Constituents　The bark mainly contains lignans (e.g., magnolol, honokiol tetrahydromagnolol, isomagnolol, magnatriol B, magnolignan F, piperitylmagnolol, etc. It also contains eudesmol, *p*-cymene, magnocurarine, etc.

Note　The dry bark is known as “Tongpo”. The dry bark with the end near the root being unfolded like a bell mouth is called as “Xuetongpo”. The root bark is commonly called “Jichangpo”. The flowers can also be used as medicine. The modern plant taxonomy study has revised its scientific name to *Houpoea officinalis* (Rehder et E. H. Wilson) N. H. Xia et C. Y. Wu.

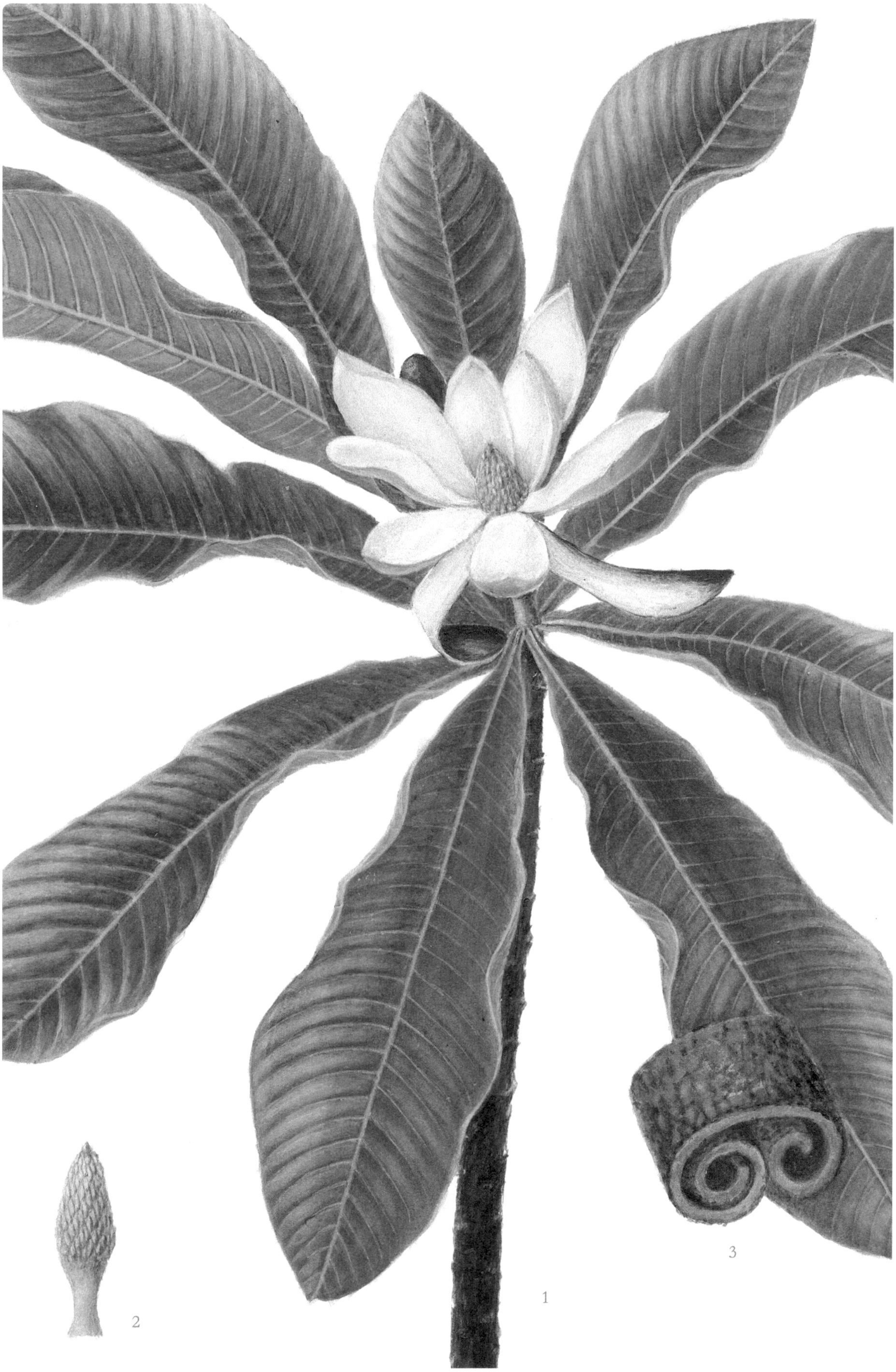

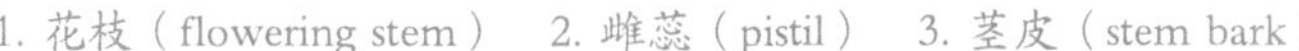

1. 花枝（flowering stem）　2. 雌蕊（pistil）　3. 茎皮（stem bark）

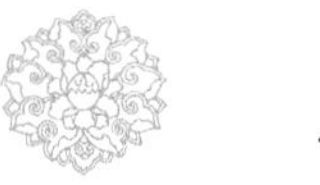

石榴

Shiliu

Punica granatum

基　　源　石榴科 Punicaceae 石榴属 *Punica* 植物石榴 *Punica granatum* L. 的干燥果皮。药材名为“石榴皮”。

形态特征　落叶灌木。枝顶常成尖锐长刺。叶对生，纸质，矩圆状披针形，顶端短尖或微凹，基部短尖，上面光亮，侧脉稍细密，叶柄短。花大，1-5 朵生枝顶；萼筒红色，裂片略外展，卵状三角形；花瓣大，红色、黄色或白色。浆果近球形，淡黄褐色，有时白色。种子多数，钝角形，红色至乳白色，肉质外种皮可食。

生境分布　原产巴尔干半岛至伊朗及其邻近地区。我国中部、南部各省均有种植。

采收加工　秋季果实成熟后收集果皮，晒干。

性味功能　温，酸、涩。涩肠止泻，止血，驱虫。

主治用法　主要用于久泻，久痢，便血，脱肛，崩漏，带下，虫积腹痛。

化学成分　主要含有鞣质，如石榴皮苦素、石榴皮鞣质和安石榴苷；有机酸类，如没食子酸、苹果酸、熊果酸等；黄酮苷类，如异槲皮苷等；生物碱类，如石榴皮碱、异石榴皮碱等。

Source　It is the dried pericarp of *Punica granatum* L. (Punicaceae). The medicinal material is called as “Shiliupi”.

Distribution　*P. granatum* is native to the region from the Balkan Peninsula to Islamic Republic of Iran and its adjacent areas. It is also cultivated in the central and southern China.

Indications　It is used to treat chronic diarrhea, enduring dysentery, bloody stool, prolapse of rectum, metrorrhagia and metrostaxis, leukorrhea, and abdominal pain due to parasitic accumulation.

Chemical Constituents　It mainly contains tannins (e.g., granatin, punicalin, and punicalagin), organic acids (e.g., gallic acid, malic acid, ursolic acid), flavonoid glycosides (e.g., isoquercetrin), and alkaloids (e.g., punicine, isopelletierine).

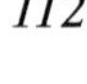

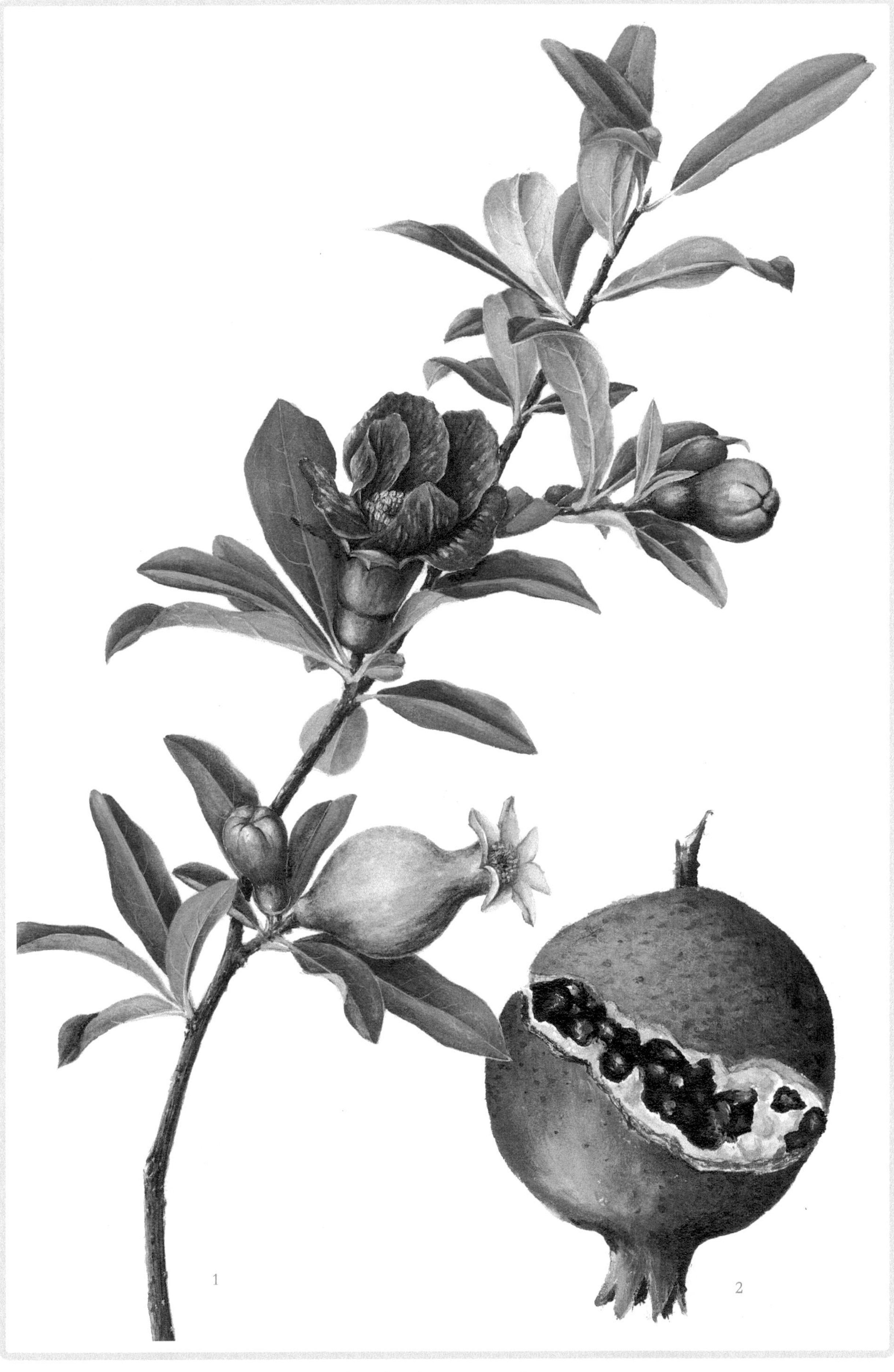

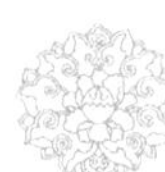

1 2

1. 花果枝（flowering and fruiting stem） 2. 果实及种子（fruit and seed）

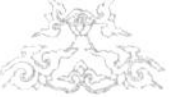

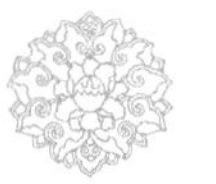

鸡蛋花

Jidanhua

Plumeria rubra

基　　源　夹竹桃科 Apocynaceae 鸡蛋花属 *Plumeria* 植物鸡蛋花 *Plumeria rubra* L. 的茎皮。药材名为"鸡蛋花"。

形态特征　小乔木。枝条具丰富乳汁。叶厚纸质，长圆状倒披针形，顶端急尖，基部狭楔形，叶面深绿色，中脉凹陷。聚伞花序顶生；总花梗 3 歧，肉质；花萼压紧花冠筒；花冠深红色，裂片狭倒卵圆形或椭圆形。蓇葖双生，广歧，长圆形，顶端急尖，淡绿色。种子长圆形，扁平；顶端具长圆形膜质的翅。

生境分布　原产墨西哥。现广泛栽培于亚洲热带和亚热带地区。常见栽培于我国南部各省的公园及路边。

采收加工　夏、秋二季采茎皮，晒干。

性味功能　凉，甘、微苦。清热，利湿，解暑。

主治用法　主要用于感冒发热，肺热咳嗽，湿热黄疸，泄泻痢疾，尿路结石，预防中暑。

化学成分　树皮中含有 α - 香树脂醇、β - 香树脂醇、β - 谷甾醇、鸡蛋花甙、东莨菪素等。根中含有环烯醚萜类化合物，如 β - 二氧鸡蛋花新酸葡萄糖酯苷、原鸡蛋花素等。

备　　注　鸡蛋花的花亦可同等入药。

Source　It is the stem bark of *Plumeria rubra* L. (Apocynaceae). The medicinal material is called as "Jidanhua".

Distribution　*P. rubra* is native to Mexico. It is widely cultivated in tropical and subtropical Asia. In China, it's commonly cultivated in parks and by the roadside in the southern provinces.

Indications　It is used to treat cold and fever, cough with lung heat, jaundice due to dampness–heat, diarrhea and dysentery, lithangiuria, and heat stroke stroke prevention.

Chemical Constituents　The bark contains α-amyrin, β-amyrin, β-sitosterol, plumieride, scopoletin, etc. The root contains iridoids, e.g., β-dihydroplumericinic acid glucosyl ester, protoplumericin.

Note　The flower of the *P. rubra* can also be used as the medicine.

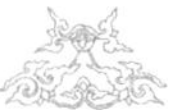

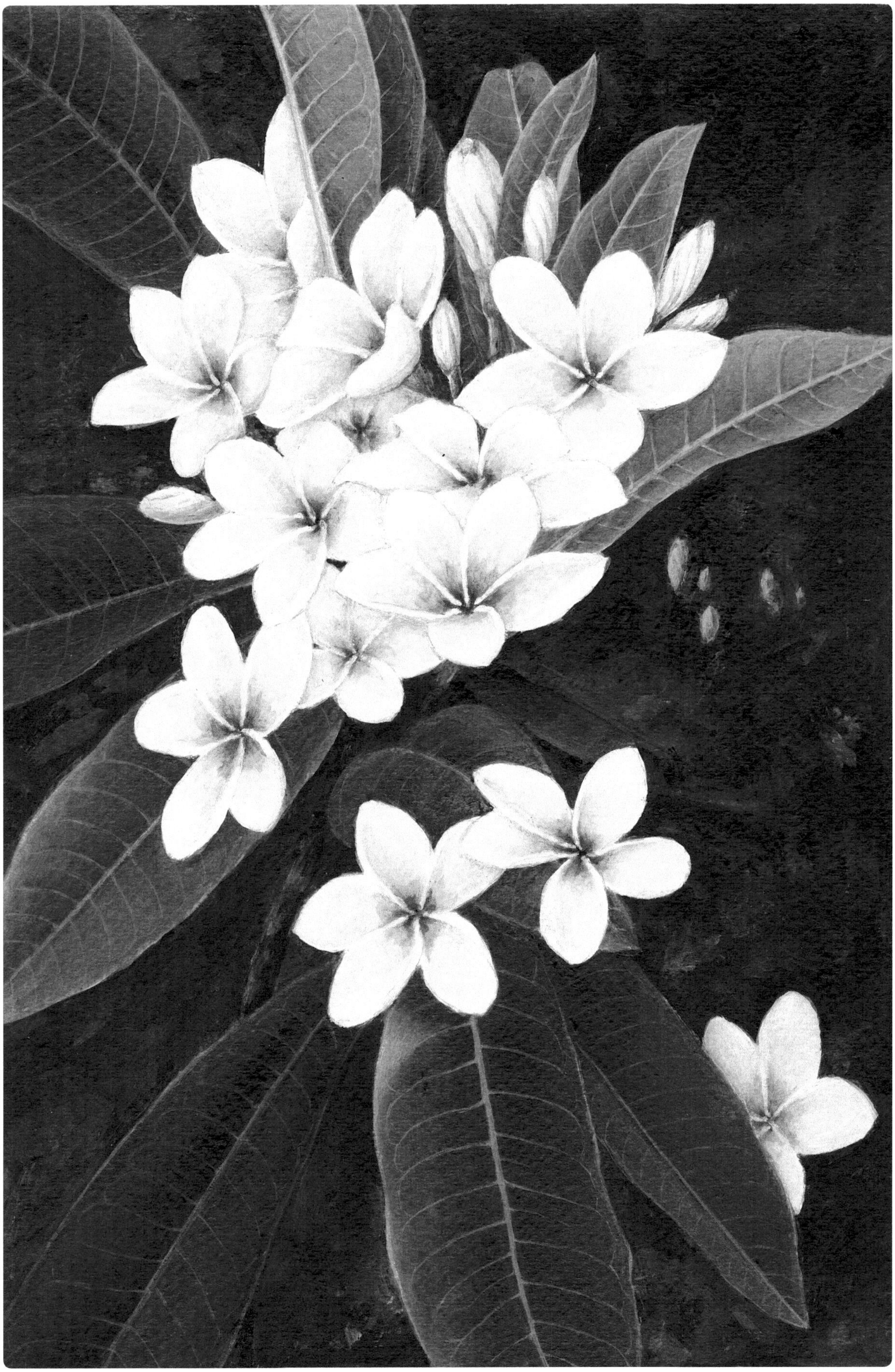

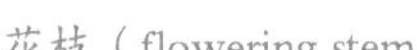

花枝（flowering stem）

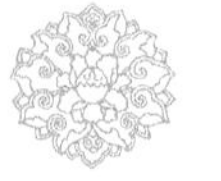

杜仲

Duzhong
Eucommia ulmoides

基　　源　杜仲科 Eucommiaceae 杜仲属 *Eucommia* 植物杜仲 *Eucommia ulmoides* Oliv. 的干燥树皮。药材名为“杜仲”。

形态特征　落叶乔木。树皮灰褐色，粗糙，内含胶丝。嫩枝有黄褐色毛，老枝有明显的皮孔。芽体卵圆形，红褐色。叶常椭圆形，薄革质；上面暗绿色，老叶略有皱纹，下面淡绿，脉上有毛。花生于当年枝基部，雄花无花被；雌花单生。翅果扁平，长椭圆形，先端二裂，周围具薄翅；坚果位于中央，稍突起。

生境分布　野生植株分布于陕西、河南、湖北、四川、云南、贵州、湖南、浙江等地。生于海拔 300-500 m 的低山、谷地、疏林中。现各地广泛栽种。

采收加工　4-6 月剥取，刮去粗皮，堆置“发汗”至内皮呈紫褐色，晒干。

性味功能　温，甘。补肝肾，强筋骨，安胎。

主治用法　用于肝肾不足，腰膝酸痛，筋骨无力，头晕目眩，妊娠漏血，胎动不安。

化学成分　主要含有木脂素类，如杜仲醇二葡萄糖苷、橄榄树脂素等；环烯醚萜类，如桃叶珊瑚苷、京尼平苷等；另还含有绿原酸、氨基酸、生物碱、杜仲丙烯醇等成分。

备　　注　杜仲为孑遗植物，也是中国特有的单属种植物；常作为绿化行道树栽培。杜仲所含的杜仲胶经硫化后改良了性能，现在用途十分广泛。

Source　It is the dried bark of *Eucommia ulmoides* Oliv. (Eucommiaceae). The medicinal material is called as “Duzhong”.

Distribution　The wild *E. ulmoides* is distributed in Shaanxi, Henan, Hubei, Sichuan, Yunnan, Guizhou, Hunan, Zhejiang and other provinces and regions. It commonly grows in low mountains, valleys or sparse forests at an altitude of 300–500 m. It is cultivated widely at present.

Indications　It is used to treat insufficiency of the liver and kidney, aching pain of lumbus and knees, weak sinews and bones, dizziness and blurred vision, hemorrhage during pregnancy, threatened abortion.

Chemical Constituents　It mainly contains lignans (e.g., eucommiol diglucoside, olivil) and iridoids (e.g., aucubin, geniposide). It also contains chlorogenic acid, amino acids, alkaloids, ulmoprenol and other components.

Note　*E. ulmoides* is a relict plant and unispecific in monotypic genus in China. It is often cultivated as a landscaping tree. The properties of gutta percha contained in Cortex Eucommiae has been improved after sulfurization and the product is now widely used.

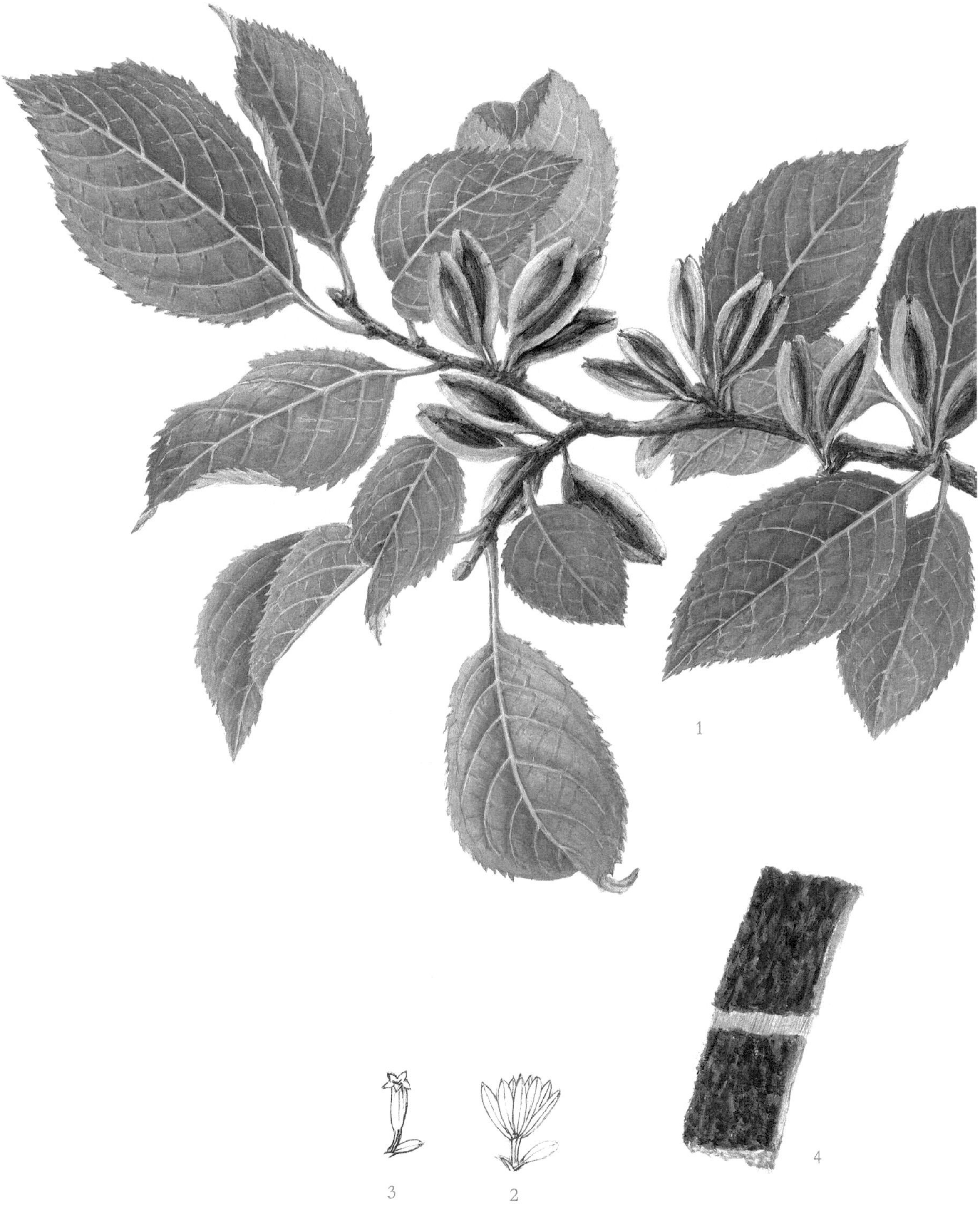

1. 果枝（fruiting stem） 2. 雄花及苞片（male flower and bract） 3. 雌花及苞片（female flower and bract） 4. 茎皮（stem bark）

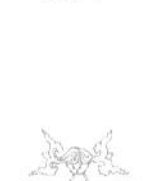

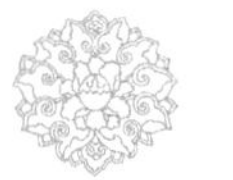

枸杞

Gouqi

Lycium chinense

基　　源　茄科 Solanaceae 枸杞属 *Lycium* 植物枸杞 *Lycium chinense* Mill. 的干燥根皮。药材名为“地骨皮”。

形态特征　多分枝灌木。枝条细弱，俯垂，有棘刺；小枝顶端锐尖成棘刺状。叶纸质，单叶互生或 2-4 枚簇生，卵形。花在长枝上单生或双生于叶腋，在短枝上则同叶簇生；花萼通常三中裂；花冠漏斗状，淡紫色，五深裂；雄蕊花丝在近基部处生绒毛；花冠筒内壁密生一圈绒毛。浆果红色，卵状。种子扁肾形，黄色。

生境分布　分布于我国大部分省区。常生于山坡、荒地、丘陵地、盐碱地、路旁及宅边。

采收加工　春初或秋后采挖根部，洗净，剥取根皮，晒干。

性味功能　寒，甘。凉血除蒸，清肺降火。

主治用法　用于阴虚潮热，骨蒸盗汗，肺热咳嗽，咯血，衄血，内热消渴。

化学成分　根皮主要含有生物碱类成分，如甜菜碱、地骨皮甲素等；有机酸类，如桂皮酸、亚油酸、亚麻酸等；另还含有大黄素、胆甾醇、芹菜素、蒙花苷等。

备　　注　枸杞子为宁夏枸杞 *Lycium barbarum* L. 的干燥果实，可滋补肝肾，益精明目。

Source　It is the dried root bark of *Lycium chinense* Mill. (Solanaceae). The medicinal material is called as “Digupi”.

Distribution　*L. chinense* is distributed in most provinces and regions in China. It commonly grows on hillsides, wasteland, hilly land, saline and alkaline land, roadside and residential area.

Indications　It is used to treat tidal fever due to yin-deficiency, steaming bone fever and night sweating, cough with lung heat, hemoptysis, epistaxis, and internal heat and wasting thirst.

Chemical Constituents　The root bark mainly contains alkaloids (e.g., betaine, kukoamine), organic acids (e.g., cinnamic acid, linoleic acid, linolenic acid). It also contains emodin, cholesterol, apigenin, linarin, etc.

Note　Fructus Lycii is the dried fruit of *L. barbarum* L., which can nourish the liver and kidney, tonify essence and improve vision.

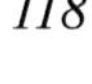

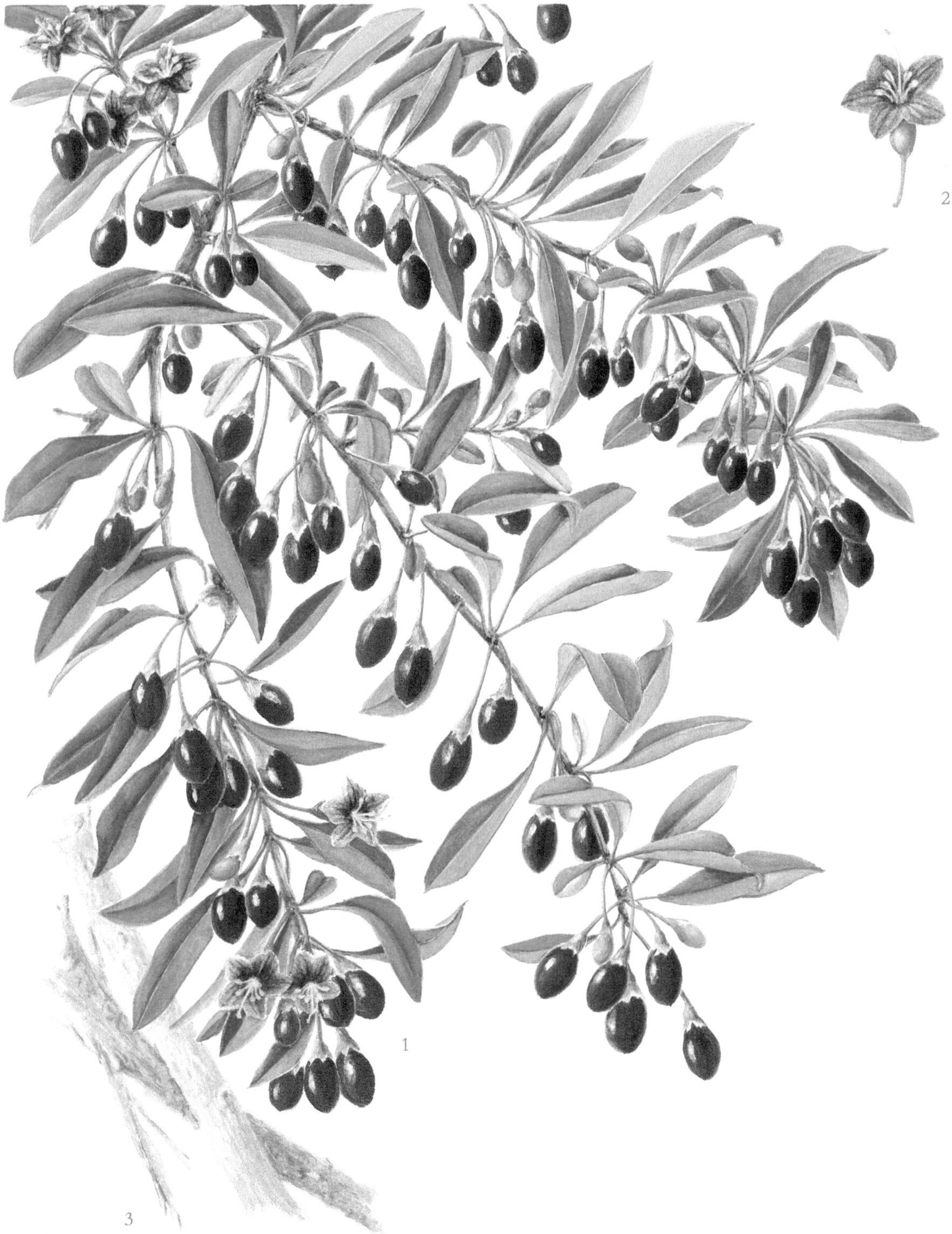

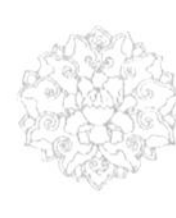

1. 果枝（fruiting stem）　2. 花（flower）　3. 根皮（root bark）

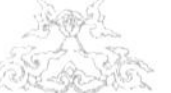

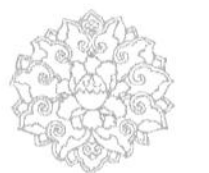

白千层

Baiqianceng
Melaleuca leucadendron

基　　源　桃金娘科 Myrtaceae 白千层属 *Melaleuca* 植物白千层 *Melaleuca leucadendron* L. 的干燥树皮。药材名为“白千层”。

形态特征　乔木。树皮灰白色，呈薄层状剥落。叶互生，革质，披针形或狭长圆形，两端尖，多油腺点，香气浓郁；叶柄极短。花白色，密集于枝顶成穗状花序，花序轴常有短毛；萼管卵形，萼齿 5，圆形；花瓣 5，卵形。蒴果近球形。

生境分布　原产澳大利亚。我国南方有作行道树栽种。

采收加工　全年均可采剥，洗净，晒干。

性味功能　平，淡。安神，解毒。

主治用法　主要用于治疗失眠多梦，神志不安，创伤化脓。

化学成分　树皮主要含木质素、黄酮类和三萜类等成分。

Source　It is the dried bark of *Melaleuca leucadendron* L. (Myrtaceae). The medicinal material is called as “Baiqianceng”.

Distribution　*M. leucadendron* is native to Australia. It is cultivated along roadside in southern China.

Indications　It is used to treat insomnia and dream-disturbed sleep, mind-wandering, and trauma with suppuration.

Chemical Constituents　The bark mainly contains lignin, flavonoids, triterpenoids, etc.

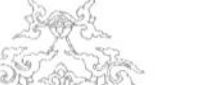
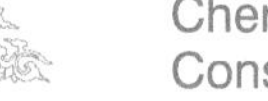

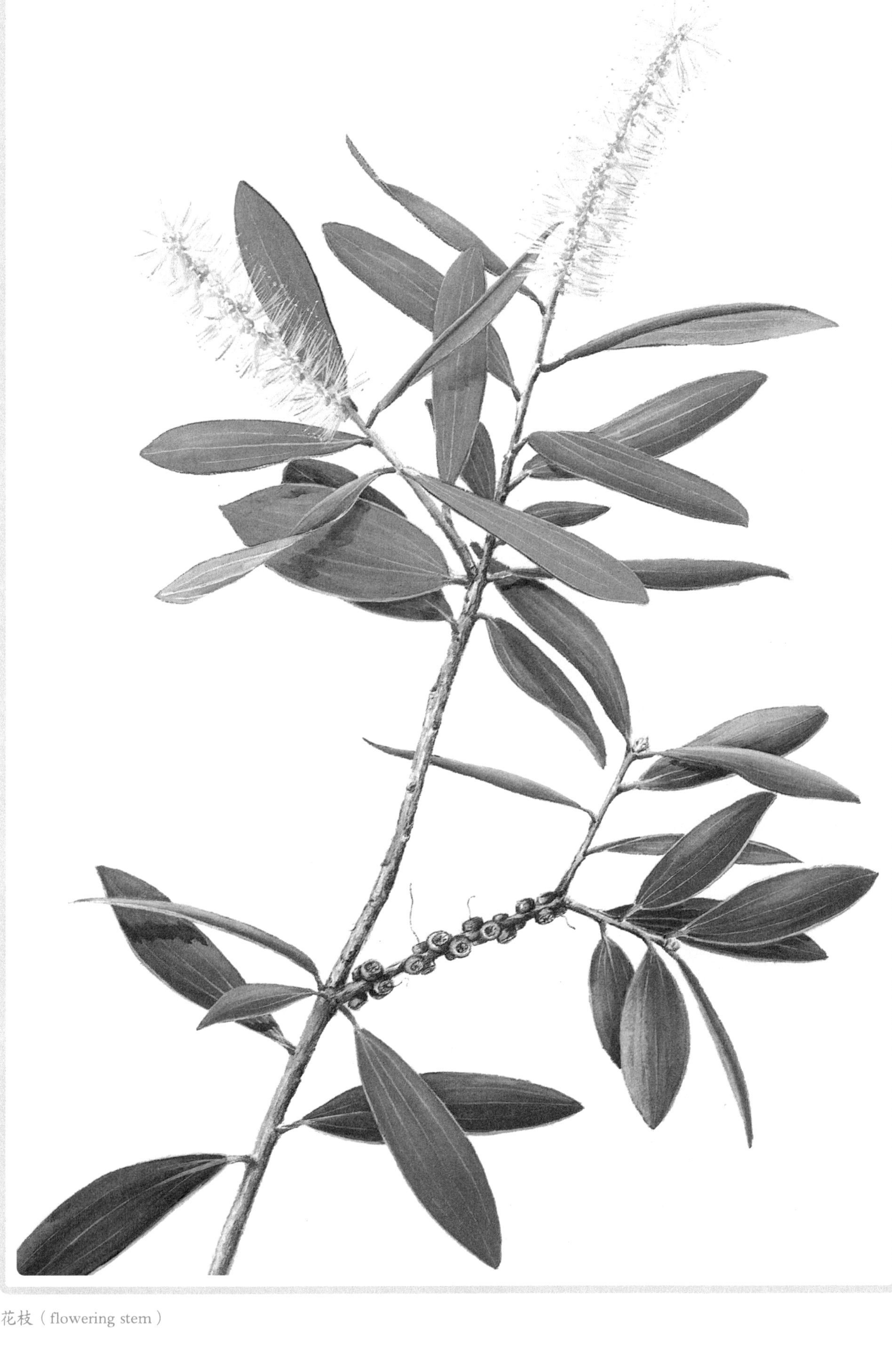

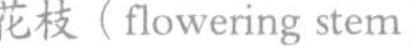

花枝（flowering stem）

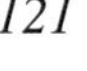

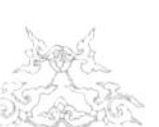

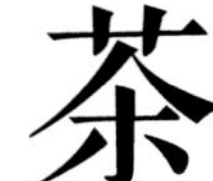

茶

Cha

Camellia sinensis

基　源　山茶科 Theaceae 山茶属 *Camellia* 植物茶 *Camellia sinensis* (L.) O. Ktze. 的干燥嫩叶或嫩芽。药材名为“茶叶”。

形态特征　常绿灌木。嫩枝、嫩叶具细柔毛。单叶互生；叶片薄革质，椭圆形或倒卵状椭圆形，先端短尖或钝尖，基部楔形，边缘有锯齿，下面无毛或微有毛。花两性，白色，芳香，通常单生或2朵生于叶腋；花梗向下弯曲；萼片5-6，圆形，宿存；花瓣5-8，宽倒卵形；雄蕊多数。蒴果近球形或扁形，果皮革质。

生境分布　原产我国南部，现长江流域及其以南各地广为栽培。

采收加工　4-6月采春茶及夏茶。加工方法因茶叶种类的不同而有差异，可分全发酵、半发酵、不发酵三大类。

性味功能　凉，苦、甘。清头目，除烦渴，消食，化痰，利尿，解毒。

主治用法　用于头痛，目昏，目赤，多睡善寐，感冒，心烦口渴，食积，口臭，痰喘，癫痫，小便不利，泻痢，喉肿，疮疡疖肠，水火烫伤。

化学成分　茶叶含有茶多酚（如儿茶素）、嘌呤类生物碱（如咖啡因、茶碱）、多糖、氨基酸（如茶氨酸）以及茶色素等。

备　注　依据制作工艺和品质不同，分为六大茶系，为绿茶、红茶、乌龙茶、黄茶、白茶和黑茶。

Source　It is the dried tender leaf or sprout of *Camellia sinensis* (L.) O. Ktze. (Theaceae). The medicinal material is called as “Chaye”.

Distribution　It is native to southern China. At present, it is widely cultivated in the Yangtze river basin and its southern regions.

Indications　It is used to treat headache, blurred vision, red eyes, profuse sleeping, common cold, vexation and thirst, food accumulation, fetid mouth odor, panting due to phlegm, epilepsy, dysuria, diarrhea, swollen throat, sore and ulcer, furuncles, and durn due to hot liquid or fire.

Chemical Constituents　It contains polyphenols (e.g., catechin), purine alkaloids (e.g., caffeine, theophylline), polysaccharides, amino acids (e.g., theanine), tea pigments, etc.

Note　Based on different production techniques and quality standards, Chinese tea can be divided into six major tea series, namely green tea, black tea, oolong tea, yellow tea, white tea and dark tea.

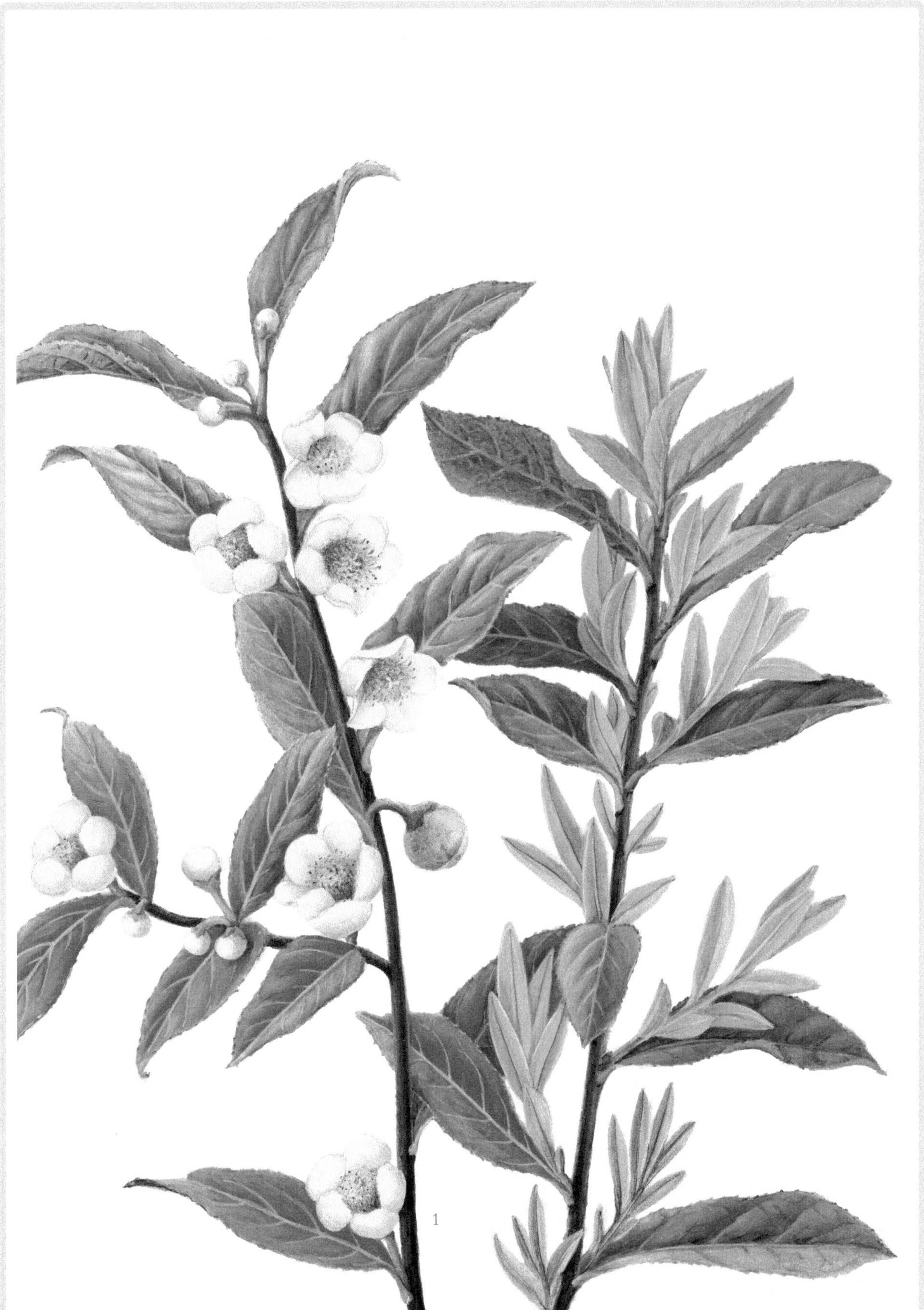

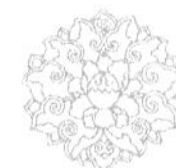

茶

1

2

1. 花枝（flowering stem）　2. 嫩枝（twig）

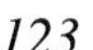

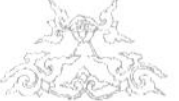

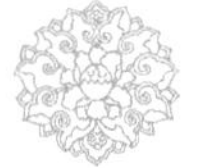

拟耧斗菜

Niloudoucai

Paraquilegia microphylla

基　　源　毛茛科 Ranunculaceae 拟耧斗菜属 *Paraquilegia* 植物拟耧斗菜 *Paraquilegia microphylla* (Royle) Drumm. et Hutch. 的干燥叶。药材名为“拟耧斗菜”。

形态特征　根状茎细圆柱形。二回三出复叶，轮廓三角状卵形，中央小叶宽菱形至肾状宽菱形，三深裂，每深裂片再 2-3 细裂。花葶直立；花萼淡紫色或淡紫红色，偶为白色，倒卵形至椭圆状倒卵形；花瓣倒卵形至倒卵状长椭圆形，顶端微凹，下部浅囊状；蓇葖直立。种子狭卵球形，褐色，一侧生狭翅，光滑。

生境分布　分布于我国西藏、云南、四川西部、甘肃西南部、青海、新疆。生于海拔 2700-4300 m 的高山山地石壁或岩石上。

采收加工　7-8 月采收，洗净泥沙，除去残叶、枯枝，晾干。

性味功能　寒，苦、涩。活血祛瘀，敛疮止血。

主治用法　主要用于跌打损伤，经闭，痛经，外伤出血，金疮，伤口久不愈合，崩漏下血。

化学成分　主要含有生物碱类、二萜类成分。

备　　注　拟耧斗菜为藏药。

Source　It is the dried leaf of *Paraquilegia microphylla* (Royle) Drumm. et Hutch. (Ranunculaceae). The medicinal material is called as “Niloudoucai”.

Distribution　*P. microphylla* is distributed in Tibet, Yunnan, western Sichuan, southerwestern Gansu, Qinghai and Xinjiang. It grows on cliffs or rocks on mountains of 2700–4300 m above sea level.

Indications　It is used to treat traumatic injury, amenorrhea, dysmenorrhea, bleeding due to external injury, incised wound, wounds that do not heal for a prolonged time, metrorrhagia and metrostaxis.

Chemical Constituents　It mainly contains alkaloids and diterpenoids.

Note　It is used in Tibetan medicine.

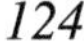

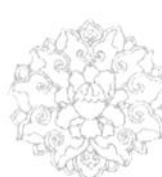

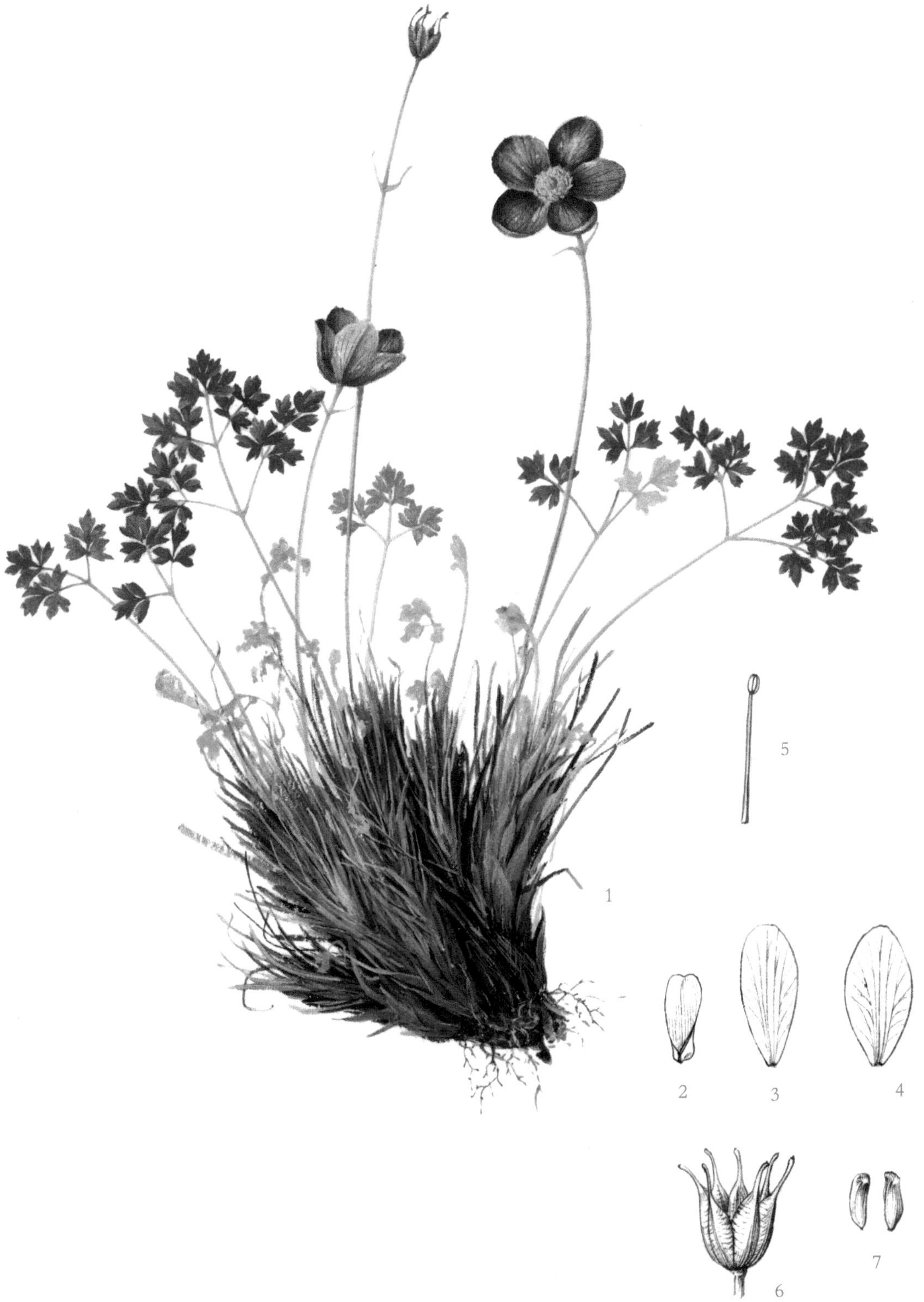

拟耧斗菜

1. 植株（plant） 2. 花萼（calyx） 3、4. 花瓣（petal） 5. 雄蕊（stamen） 6. 果实（fruit） 7. 种子（seed）

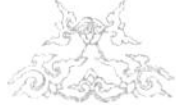

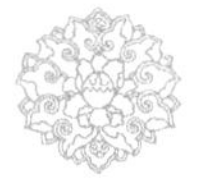

罗布麻

Luobuma

Apocynum venetum

基　　源　夹竹桃科 Apocynaceae 罗布麻属 *Apocynum* 植物罗布麻 *Apocynum venetum* L. 的干燥叶。药材名为“罗布麻叶”。

形态特征　直立半灌木，具乳汁。枝条圆筒形，淡红色。叶对生，叶片多为卵圆形，顶端具短尖头，叶缘具细牙齿。圆锥状聚伞花序，顶生或腋生；苞片膜质；花萼五深裂；花冠筒钟形，紫红色，两面密被颗粒状突起；雄蕊与副花冠裂片互生。蓇葖 2，平行或叉生，下垂，箸状圆筒形。种子顶端生有白色绢质的种毛。

生境分布　分布于我国秦岭 - 淮河、昆仑山以北各省区。生于盐碱荒地、冲积平原及荒漠戈壁上。

采收加工　夏季采收，除去杂质，干燥。

性味功能　凉，甘、苦。平肝安神，清热利水。

主治用法　用于肝阳眩晕，心悸失眠，浮肿尿少。

化学成分　主要含有槲皮素、金丝桃苷、羽扇豆醇棕榈酸酯、棕榈酸蜂花醇酯、延胡索酸、琥珀酸等。

备　　注　罗布麻的茎皮中富含纤维，可作为纺织原料。

Source　It is the dried leaf of *Apocynum venetum* L. (Apocynaceae). The medicinal material is called as “Luobumaye”.

Distribution　*A. venetum* is distributed in the provinces north of Qinling Mountains–Huaihe River and Kunlun Mountains. It grows on the salt alkaline wastelands, alluvial plain and desert.

Indications　It is used to treat vertigo due to ascendant hyperactivity of liver yang, palpitations and insomnia, edema and oliguria.

Chemical Constituents　It mainly contains quercetin, hyperoside, lupenyl palmitate, myricylpalmitate, fumaric acid, succinic acid, etc.

Note　The stem bark of *A. venetum* is rich in fibers and can be used as raw material for textiles.

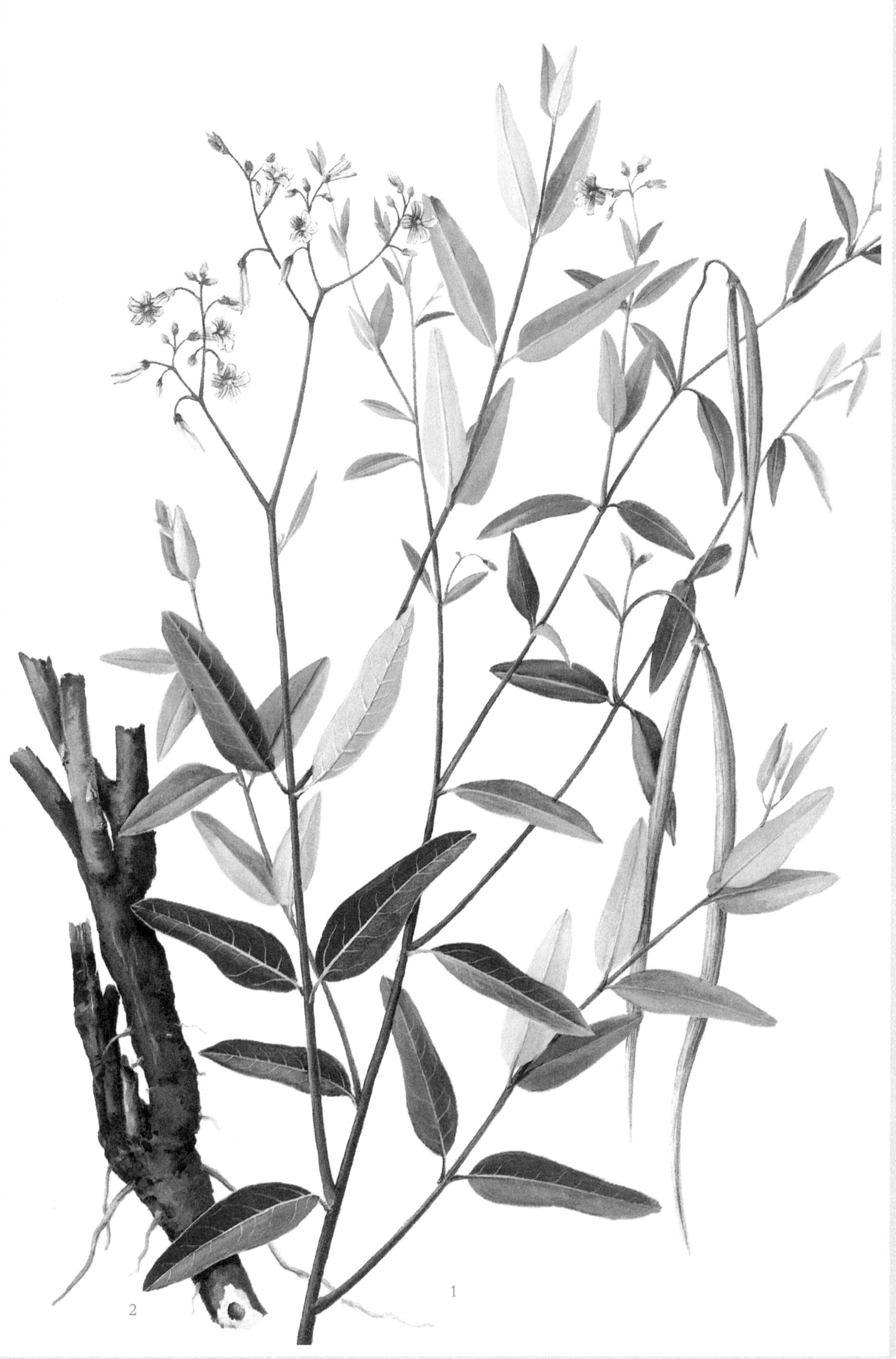

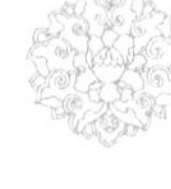

罗布麻

2

1

1. 花果枝（flowering and fruiting stem） 2. 根（root）

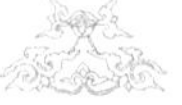

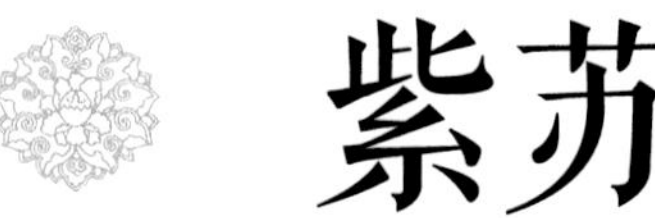

紫苏

Zisu
Perilla frutescens

基　　源　唇形科 Lamiaceae 紫苏属 *Perilla* 植物紫苏 *Perilla frutescens* (L.) Britt. 的干燥叶（或带嫩枝）。药材名为“紫苏叶”。

形态特征　一年生草本。茎绿色或紫色，钝四棱形，具四槽，密被长柔毛。叶阔卵形，边缘有粗锯齿，草质，绿色或紫色，或下面紫色；叶柄密被长柔毛。轮伞花序，由 2 花组成偏向一侧成假总状花序，顶生和腋生；花萼钟形；花冠白色至紫红色，冠檐近二唇形，上唇微缺，下唇三裂。小坚果近球形，灰褐色，具网纹。

生境分布　分布于我国华东、华南、西南、华北部分省区。生于山地、路旁、村边、荒地。栽培范围极广。

采收加工　夏季枝叶茂盛时采收，除去杂质，晒干。

性味功能　辛，温。解表散寒，行气和胃。

主治用法　用于风寒感冒，咳嗽呕恶，妊娠呕吐，鱼蟹中毒。不宜久煎。

化学成分　叶中主要含有挥发油类，如紫苏酮、异白苏烯酮。紫苏全草中含有紫苏醛、紫苏醇、薄荷醇、丁香油酚等挥发油类，以及黄芩素、野黑樱苷等成分。种子中含有氨基酸、棕榈酸、油酸、亚油酸等。

备　　注　紫苏原植物可见叶绿色，花白色的植株，习称“白苏”。紫苏叶亦可食用。紫苏的种子入药称“紫苏子”，可降气化痰，止咳平喘，润肠通便。紫苏的茎入药称“紫苏梗”，可理气宽中，止痛，安胎。

Source　It is the dried leaf or with twig of *Perilla frutescens* (L.) Britt. (Lamiaceae). The medicinal material is called as “Zisuye”.

Distribution　*P. frutescens* is distributed in some provinces of East, South, Southwest and North China. It grows in mountains, roadsides, villages or wastelands. It is cultivated widely.

Indications　It is used to treat wind–cold common cold, cough with nausea and retching, vomiting of pregnancy, and poisoning from fish and crabs. It is not to be decocted for prolonged period.

Chemical Constituents　The leaves mainly contain volatile oils, e.g., perillaketone and isoegomaketone. The whole herb contains volatile oil (e.g., perillaldehyde, perillyl alcohol, menthol, eugenol), baicalein, prunasin, etc. The seeds contain amino acids, palmitic acid, oleic acid, linoleic acid, etc.

Note　*P. frutescens* has green leaves with white flowers, which is known as “Baisu”. The leaves are also edible. The seed can be used as medicine, which is called Fructus Perillae, which has the function of descending qi and resolving phlegm, stopping cough and abating panting, and moistening intestines to relieve constipation. The stem can be used as medicine, which is called Caulis Perillae. It has the function of regulating qi to soothe the middle, relief of pain, and calm the fetus.

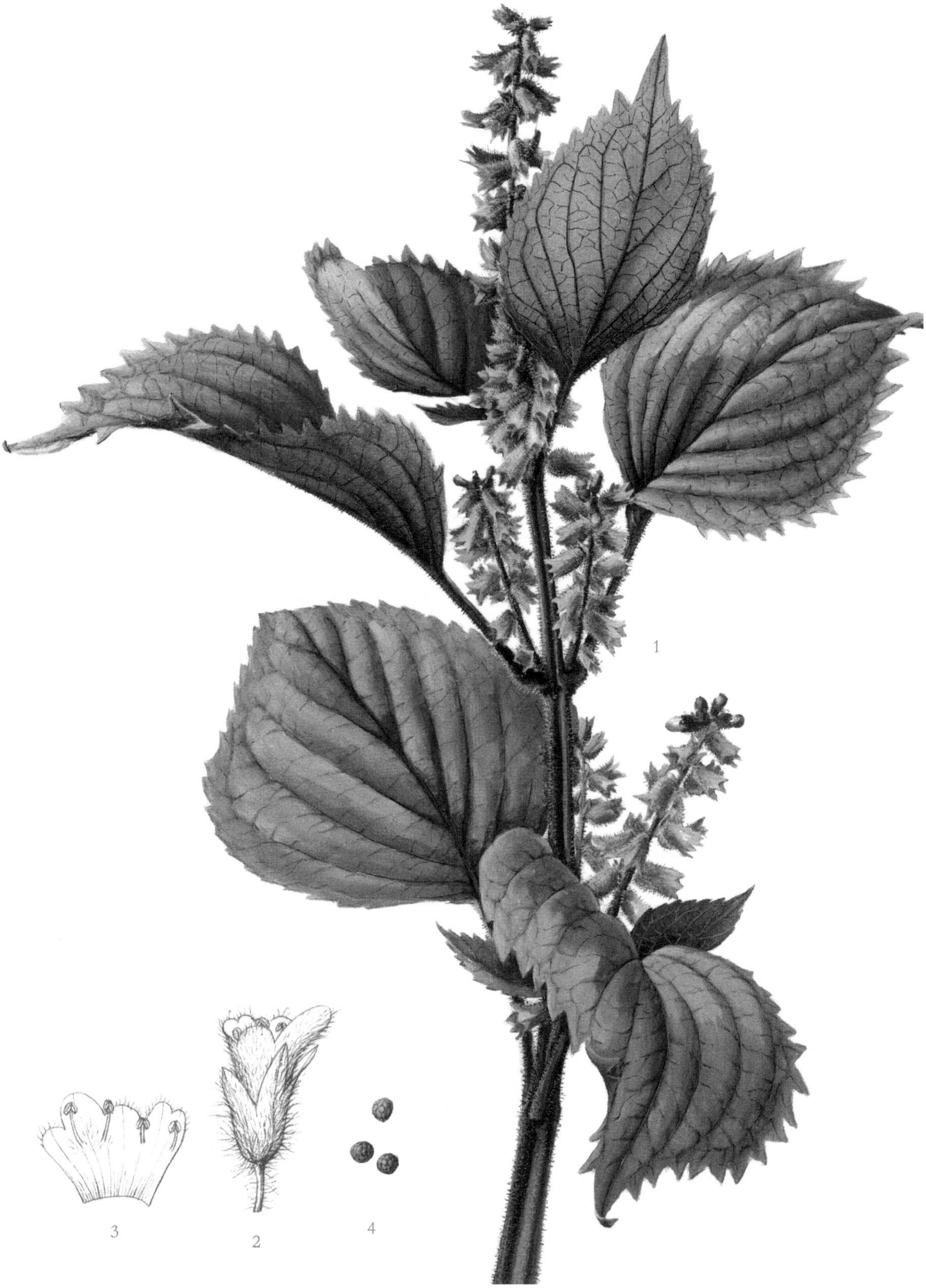

1

3 2 4

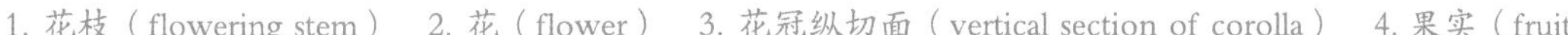

1. 花枝（flowering stem） 2. 花（flower） 3. 花冠纵切面（vertical section of corolla） 4. 果实（fruit）

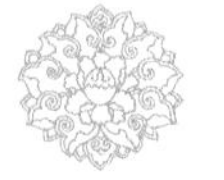

薄荷

Bohe

Mentha haplocalyx

基　源　唇形科 Lamiaceae 薄荷属 *Mentha* 植物薄荷 *Mentha haplocalyx* Briq. 的干燥地上部分。药材名为“薄荷”。

形态特征　多年生草本。茎下部具须根及匍匐茎，锐四棱形，具四槽，多分枝。叶片长圆状披针形，披针形，椭圆形或卵状披针形，边缘在基部以上疏生粗大的牙齿状锯齿。轮伞花序腋生，轮廓球形。花萼管状钟形，萼齿 5；花冠淡紫；雄蕊 4，二强。小坚果卵珠形，黄褐色。

生境分布　分布于我国南北各地。常生于低海拔的水边湿地。

采收加工　夏、秋二季茎叶茂盛或花开至三轮时，选晴天，分次采割，晒干或阴干。

性味功能　凉，辛。疏散风热，清利头目，利咽，透疹，疏肝行气。

主治用法　用于风热感冒，风温初起，头痛，目赤，喉痹，口疮，风疹，麻疹，胸胁胀闷。入汤剂宜后下。

化学成分　主要含有薄荷酮、薄荷脑、莰烯、柠檬烯、蒎烯、薄荷烯酮、乙酸薄荷酯等挥发油类成分；另还含有氨基酸、树脂、鞣质、迷迭香酸等。

备　注　全国各地薄荷栽培品种繁多；新鲜茎和叶经水蒸气蒸馏、冷冻等操作可制成薄荷素油和薄荷脑，可供医药原料及食品添加剂；幼嫩茎叶可作食用。现代植物分类研究已将薄荷的学名修订为 *Mentha canadensis* L.。

Source　It is the dried aerial part of *Mentha haplocalyx* Briq. (Lamiaceae). The medicinal material is called as “Bohe”.

Distribution　*M. haplocalyx* is distributed in all parts of northern and southern China. It commonly grows in the low-altitude waterside wetlands.

Indications　It is used to treat wind–heat cold, the onset of wind–warmth, headache, red eyes, pharyngitis, aphtha, rubella, measles, distention and oppression in chest and hypochondrium. It should be decocted later in decoction.

Chemical Constituents　It mainly contains menthone, menthol, camphene, limonene, pinene, piperitone, menthyl acetate and other volatile oils. It also contains amino acids, resins, tannins, rosmarinic acid, etc.

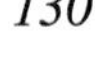

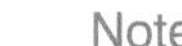

Note　There are many cultivated species all over China. The fresh stems and leaves can be made into peppermint oil and menthol by steam distillation and freezing, which can be used as medicinal raw materials and food additives. The young stems and leaves are edible. In modern plant taxonomic studies, the scientific name has been revised as *Mentha canadensis* L.

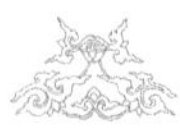

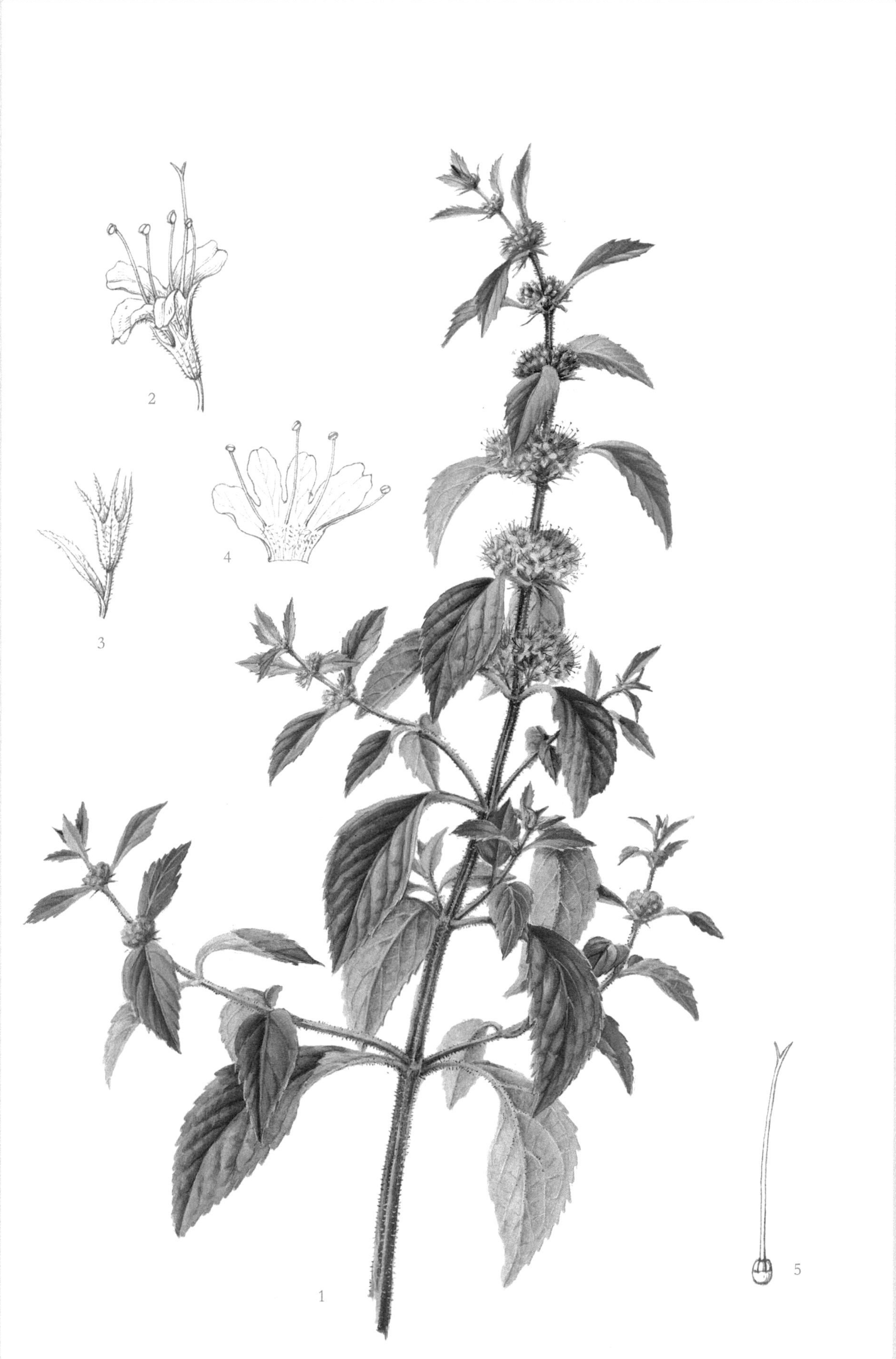

2

4

3

1

5

1. 花枝（flowering stem） 2. 花（flower） 3. 花萼（calyx） 4. 雄蕊（stamen） 5. 雌蕊（pistil）

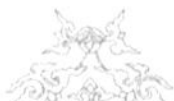

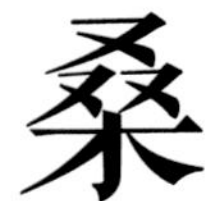

桑

Sang

Morus alba

基　　源　桑科 Moraceae 桑属 *Morus* 植物桑 *Morus alba* L. 的干燥叶。药材名为“桑叶”。

形态特征　多为乔木。冬芽红褐色，卵形，芽鳞覆瓦状排列。叶卵形或广卵形，边缘锯齿粗钝，有时叶各种分裂；表面鲜绿色，无毛，背面叶脉腋处有簇毛；托叶早落。花叶同放，单性，腋生或生于芽鳞腋内；花单性，雌雄异株；雌、雄花序均排列成穗状葇荑花序。瘦果，密集成长圆形聚合果，成熟时黑紫色或红色。

生境分布　分布于全国各地。生于山坡、田野、村庄等处。多为人工栽培。

采收加工　初霜后采收，除去杂质，晒干。

性味功能　寒，甘、苦。疏散风热，清肺润燥，清肝明目。

主治用法　用于风热感冒，肺热燥咳，头晕头痛，目赤昏花。

化学成分　叶中主要含有黄酮类、生物碱类、甾醇和多糖类等成分。

备　　注　桑除叶入药外，除去粗皮的根皮（桑白皮）、嫩枝（桑枝）、果实（桑椹）亦可入药。叶是重要的桑蚕饲料；桑树皮可用于制作桑皮纸，是高档的书画用纸，被用于故宫古书画修复；桑椹可供食用及酿酒。

Source　It is the dried leaf of *Morus alba* L. (Moraceae). The medicinal material is called as “Sangye”.

Distribution　*M. alba* is distributed all over China and grows in hillsides, fields, villages and other places. It is mostly cultivated nowadays.

Indications　It is used to treat wind–heat common cold, irritating dry cough due to lung heat, dizziness and headache, red eyes with blurred vision.

Chemical Constituents　The leaves mainly contain flavonoids, alkaloids, sterols and polysaccharides, etc.

Note　In addition to the leaves, the root bark (Cortex Mori), the tender branches (Ramulus Mori), and the fruit (Fructus Mori) can also be used as medicine. The leaves are important silkworm feed. Mulberry bark can be used to make mulberry paper, which is a high-grade painting and calligraphy paper, It is used for restoration of the ancient paintings of the Forbidden City. Fructus Mori is edible and can be used to brew alcohol.

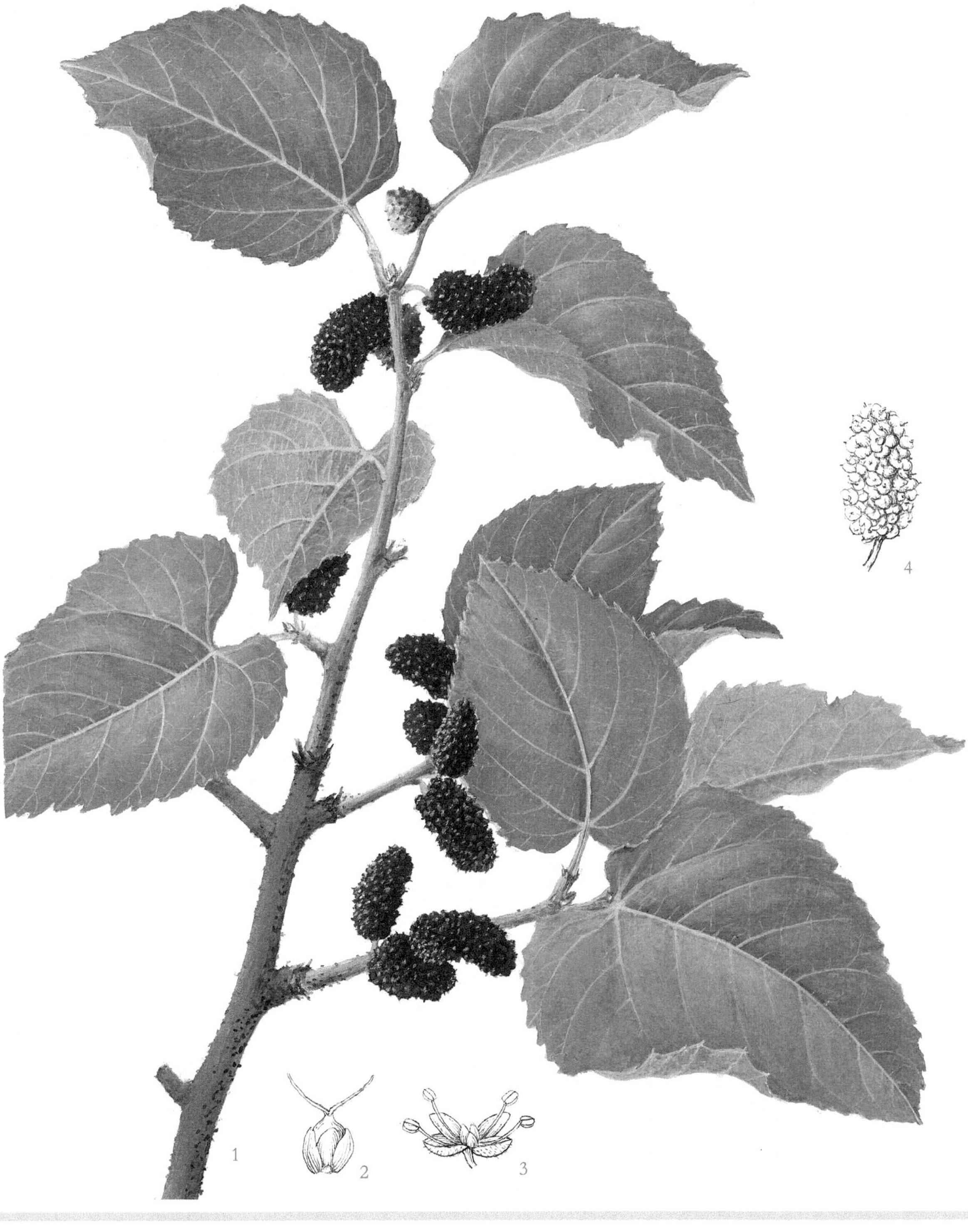

桑

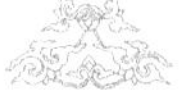

1. 果枝（fruiting stem） 2. 雌花（female flower） 3. 雄花（male flower） 4. 果实（fruit）

艾

Ai

Artemisia argyi

基　　源　菊科 Asteraceae 蒿属 *Artemisia* 植物艾 *Artemisia argyi* Lévl. et Van. 的干燥叶。药材名为“艾叶”。

形态特征　多年生草本，有浓烈香气。茎多为单生，有明显纵棱，上部有少数短的分枝，被灰色蛛丝状柔毛。叶厚纸质，上面被灰白色短柔毛，背面密被灰白色蛛丝状密绒毛；基生叶具长柄，花期萎谢；上部叶与苞片叶多分裂，常为椭圆形。头状花序多组合为穗状花序在茎上形成圆锥花序，下倾。瘦果长卵形。

生境分布　除极干旱与高寒地区外，分布遍及全国。常生于低海拔至中海拔地区的荒地、村落旁，也生于森林、草原，可形成群落优势种。

采收加工　夏季花未开时采摘，除去杂质，晒干。

性味功能　温，辛、苦；有小毒。温经止血，散寒止痛；外用祛湿止痒。

主治用法　用于吐血，衄血，崩漏，月经过多，胎漏下血，少腹冷痛，经寒不调，宫冷不孕；外治皮肤瘙痒。醋艾炭温经止血，用于虚寒性出血。

化学成分　主要含有挥发油类成分，如香叶烯、桉叶精、异龙脑、柠檬烯等；另还含有奎诺酸、异泽兰黄素等三萜类和黄酮类化合物。

备　　注　艾叶陈久者良，晒干舂绒为“艾绒”，用于制作艾条，供艾灸用；艾绒亦是制作传统印泥的原料。湖北蕲春为道地，所栽培的艾为栽培品种 *Artemisia argyi* “Qiai”。

Source　It is the dried leaf of *Artemisia argyi* Levl. et Van. (Asteraceae). The medicinal material is called as “Aiye”.

Distribution　*A. argyi* is distributed all over China, except for extremely arid and cold alpine areas. It mostly grows in wastelands, beside villages, in forests and on grasslands at low to middle elevation. It can become the dominant species in the ecosystem.

Indications　It is used to treat hematemesis, epistaxis, metrorrhagia and metrostaxis, hypermenorrhea, vaginal bleeding during pregnancy, cold and pain at lower abdomen, menstrual cold and disorder, uterine cold with infertility. It also can be used for the external treatment of pruritus. The scorch of Folium Artemisiae Argyi processed with vinegar has the function of warming meridians to stop hemorrhage, treating deficiency–cold-type bleeding.

Chemical Constituents　It mainly contains volatile oil, e.g., myrcene, eucalyptol, isoborneol, limonene; it also contains triterpenoids (e.g., quinovic acid, eupatilin) and flavonoids.

Note　Folium Artemisiae Argyi has an even better effect after long-term storage. It can be made into moxa wool after it is dried in the sun and pounded. Moxa wool is used to make moxa sticks for moxibustion and traditional ink paste. Qichun County of Hubei Province, China produces the authentic Folium Artemisiae Argyi, and the cultivated forma is *Artemisia argyi* “Qiai”.

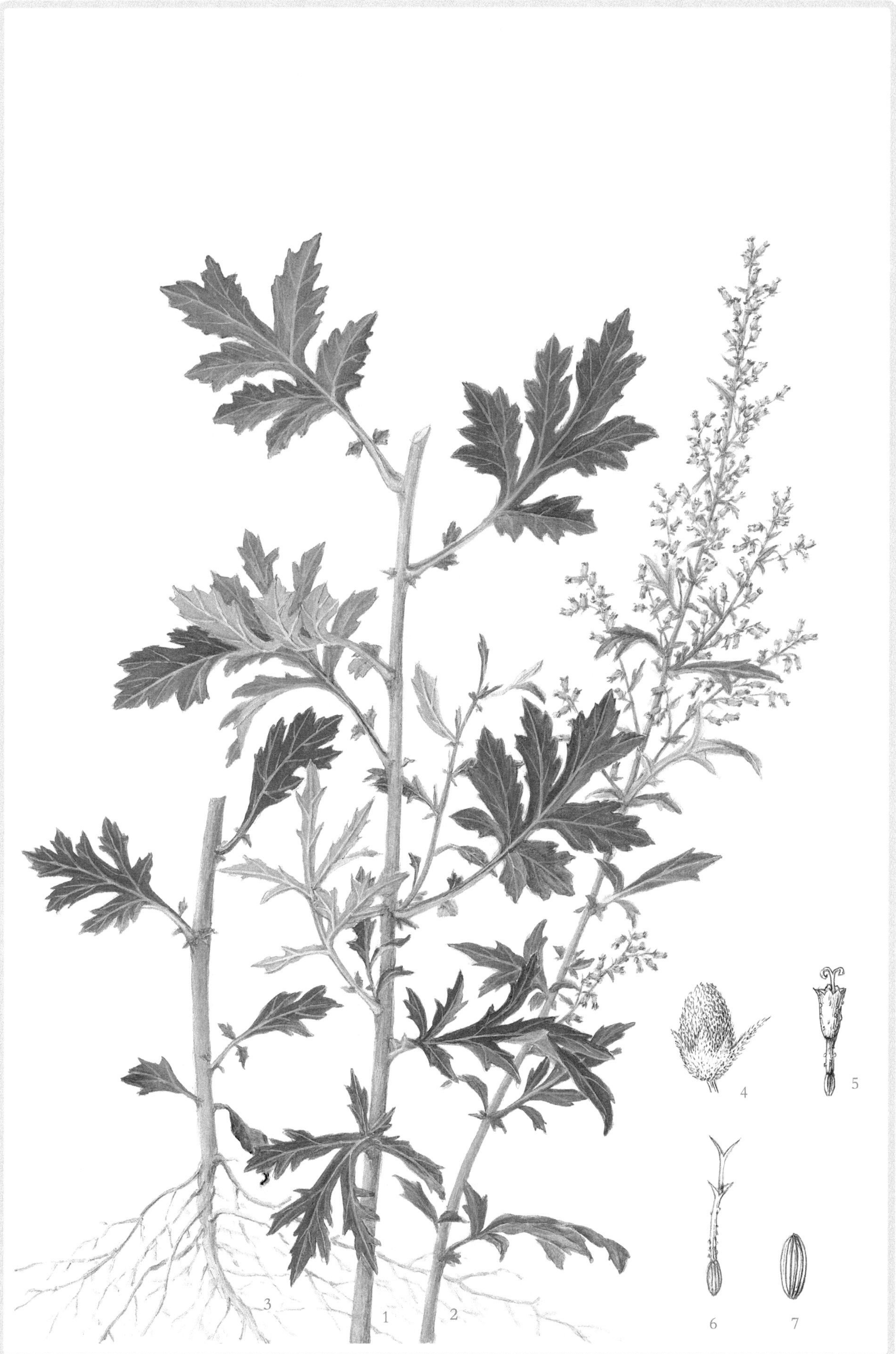

艾

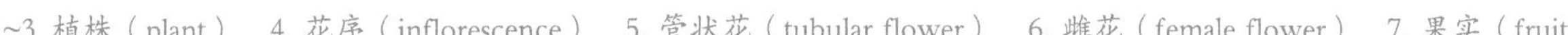

1~3. 植株（plant） 4. 花序（inflorescence） 5. 管状花（tubular flower） 6. 雌花（female flower） 7. 果实（fruit）

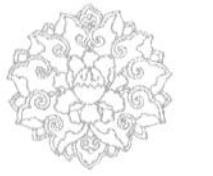

银杏

Yinxing

Ginkgo biloba

基　　源　银杏科 Ginkgoaceae 银杏属 *Ginkgo* 植物银杏 *Ginkgo biloba* L. 的干燥叶。药材名为“银杏叶”。

形态特征　乔木。叶扇形，有长柄，淡绿色，无毛，有多数叉状并列细脉，在短枝上常具波状缺刻，在长枝上常二裂；叶在长枝上螺旋状散生，短枝上簇生，落叶前变为黄色。雌雄异株，单性；雄球花柔荑花序状，下垂；雌球花具长梗，梗端常分两叉，每叉顶生一盘状珠座，胚珠着生其上，通常仅一个叉端的胚珠发育。种子具长梗，多近圆球形，外种皮肉质，熟时黄色，被白粉；中种皮白色，骨质，具 2-3 条纵脊；内种皮膜质，淡红褐色；胚乳肉质。

生境分布　我国特有的孑遗植物。现各地广泛栽培。

采收加工　秋季叶尚绿时采收，及时干燥。

性味功能　平，甘、苦、涩。活血化瘀，通络止痛，敛肺平喘，化浊降脂。

主治用法　用于瘀血阻络，胸痹心痛，中风偏瘫，肺虚咳喘，高脂血症。

化学成分　主要含有萜类内酯，如银杏内酯等；黄酮类，如山奈酚、槲皮素、异鼠李素、杨梅树皮素等。叶和种仁中含少量银杏酸、银杏酚、银杏醇等有毒物质。

备　　注　除去肉质外种皮的成熟种子习称“白果”，可供食用，亦可入药，具有敛肺定喘，止带缩尿的功效。银杏的外种皮汁液中含有致敏成分，成熟后具难闻气味。山东郯城县素有“天下银杏第一县”的美誉，定植银杏 700 万株以上，银杏植株也作为行道树树种，生长较慢，寿命极长。

Source　It is the dried leaf of *Ginkgo biloba* L. (Ginkgoaceae). The medicinal material is called as “Yinxingye”.

Distribution　*G. biloba* is a unique relict plant of China. It is widely cultivated nowadays.

Indications　It is used to treat static blood obstructing the collaterals, heart pain due to chest impediment, stroke marked by hemiplegia, dyspneic cough due to lung deficiency, and hyperlipemia.

Chemical Constituents　It mainly contains terpene lactones (e.g., ginkgolides), flavonoids (e.g., kaempferol, quercetin, isorhamnetin, myricetin). The leaves and kernels contain a small amount of ginkgolic acid, bilobol, ginnol and other toxic substances.

Note　The mature seeds without the fleshy testae are called Semen Ginkgo, which can be eaten and used as medicine. It has the effect of astringing lung, relieving dyspnea, controlling leukorrhea, and reducing urination. The episperm contains allergenic ingredients and has an unpleasant odor after maturation. Tancheng County of Shangdong Province is known as “The first county of *G. biloba* in the world”, where more than 7 million plants have been cultivated. *G. biloba* can be also used as street trees, which grow slowly and have a very long longevity.

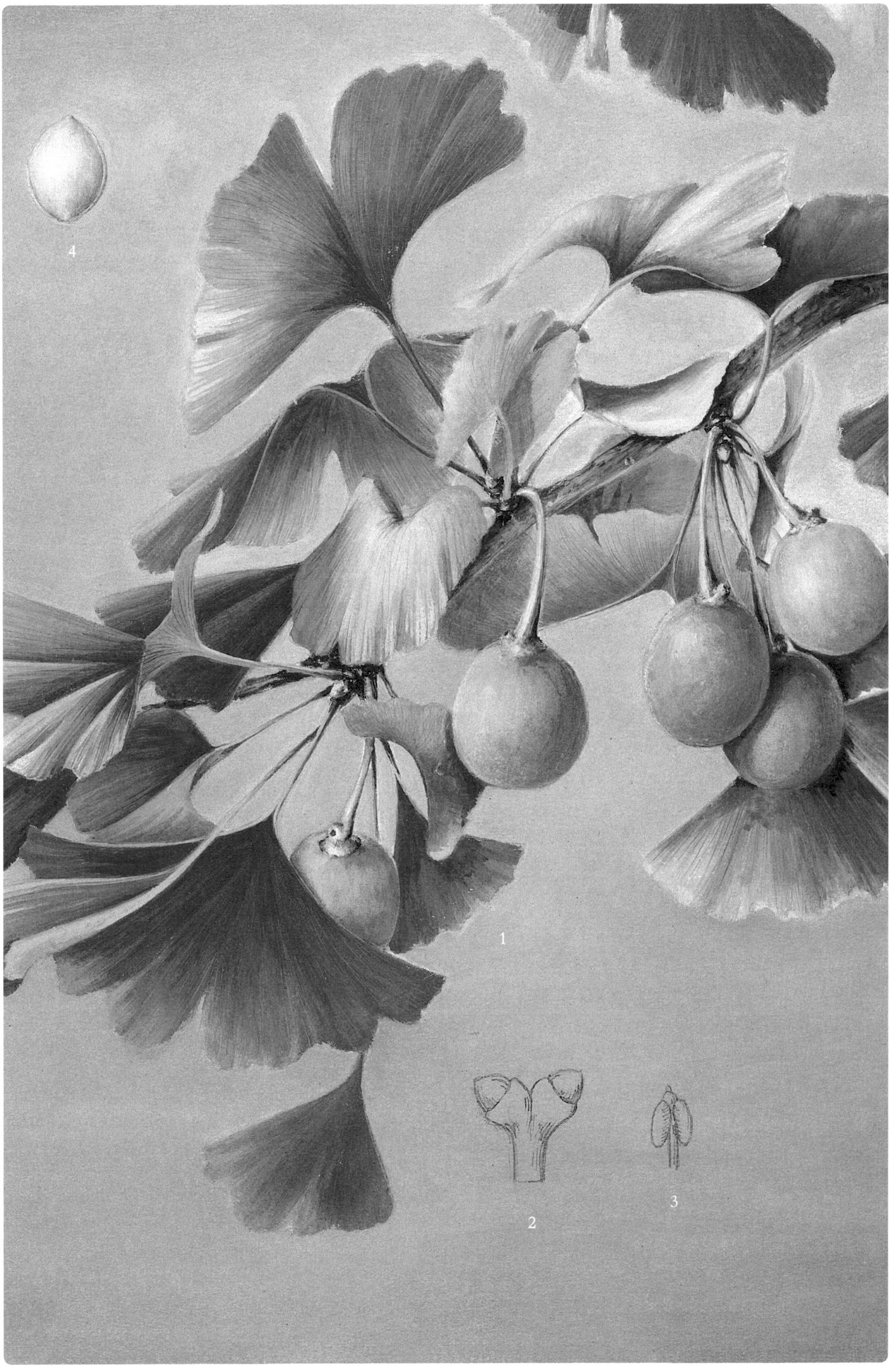

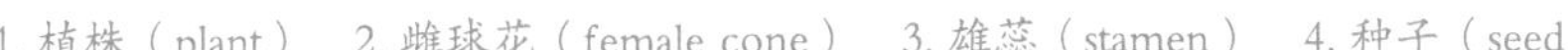

1. 植株（plant） 2. 雌球花（female cone） 3. 雄蕊（stamen） 4. 种子（seed）

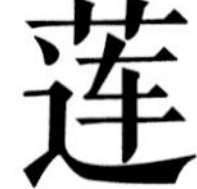

莲

Lian

Nelumbo nucifera

基　　源　睡莲科 Nymphaeaceae 莲属 *Nelumbo* 植物莲 *Nelumbo nucifera* Gaertn. 的干燥叶。药材名为“荷叶”。

形态特征　多年生水生草本。根状茎横生，节间膨大，内有孔道，节部缢缩。叶圆形，盾状，全缘稍呈波状，上面光滑，具白粉；叶柄中空，散生小刺。花大，芳香；花瓣红色至白色，多椭圆形，由外向内渐小。坚果卵形，果皮革质，坚硬，熟时黑褐色。种子（莲子）卵形或椭圆形，种皮红色或白色。

生境分布　分布于我国南北各省。常见栽培于池塘内。

采收加工　夏、秋二季采收，晒至七八成干时，除去叶柄，折成半圆形或折扇形，干燥。

性味功能　平，苦。清暑化湿，升发清阳，凉血止血。

主治用法　用于暑热烦渴，暑湿泄泻，脾虚泄泻，血热吐衄，便血崩漏。荷叶炭收涩化瘀止血，用于出血症和产后血晕。

化学成分　叶中主要含有荷叶碱、荷叶苷、琥珀酸、苹果酸等。种子中主要含有槲皮素、天门冬素、淀粉、糖类等。莲子心中主要含有莲心碱、莲心季铵碱、棕榈酸、叶绿素等。

备　　注　根状茎（藕）作蔬菜，也可制成藕粉；种子可供食用。莲不仅叶可入药，《中国药典》还收载有藕节、莲房、莲须、莲子和莲子心。莲花以其出淤泥而不染的高洁品格，被文人骚客赋予了“花中君子”的雅号，常出现在中国古代文学作品中。

Source　It is the dried leaf of *Nelumbo nucifera* Gaertn. (Nymphaeaceae). The medicinal material is called “Heye”.

Distribution　*N. nucifera* is distributed in north and south China. It is commonly cultivated in ponds.

Indications　It is used to treat extreme thirst with summer-heat, diarrhea due to summer heat and dampness, diarrhea due to spleen deficiency, hematemesis and epistaxis due to heat in blood, bloody stool with metrorrhagia and metrostaxis. The burnt Folium Nelumbinis has the function of astringing discharge, transforming stasis and hemostasis, which can be used to treat hemorrhage and postpartum fainting due to hemorrhage.

Chemical Constituents　The leaves mainly contain nuciferine, nelunboside, succinic acid, malic acid, etc. The seed mainly contains quercetin, asparagine, starch, saccharides, etc. Plumula Nelumbinis mainly contains liensinine, lotusine, palmitic acid, chlorophyll, etc.

Note　The rhizome (lotus root) is used as a vegetable and can also be made into lotus root powder. The seed is edible. Not only the leaves of *N. nucifera* can be used as medicine, but also Nodus Nelumbinis Rhizomatis, Receptaculum Nelumbinis, Stamen Nelumbinis, Semen Nelumbinis, and Plumula Nelumbinis are also listed in *Chinese Pharmacopoeia*. The lotus flower is viewed as “the gentleman of flowers” by men of literature and writing since it grows out of the mud unsoiled. Therefore, it often appears in ancient Chinese literature.

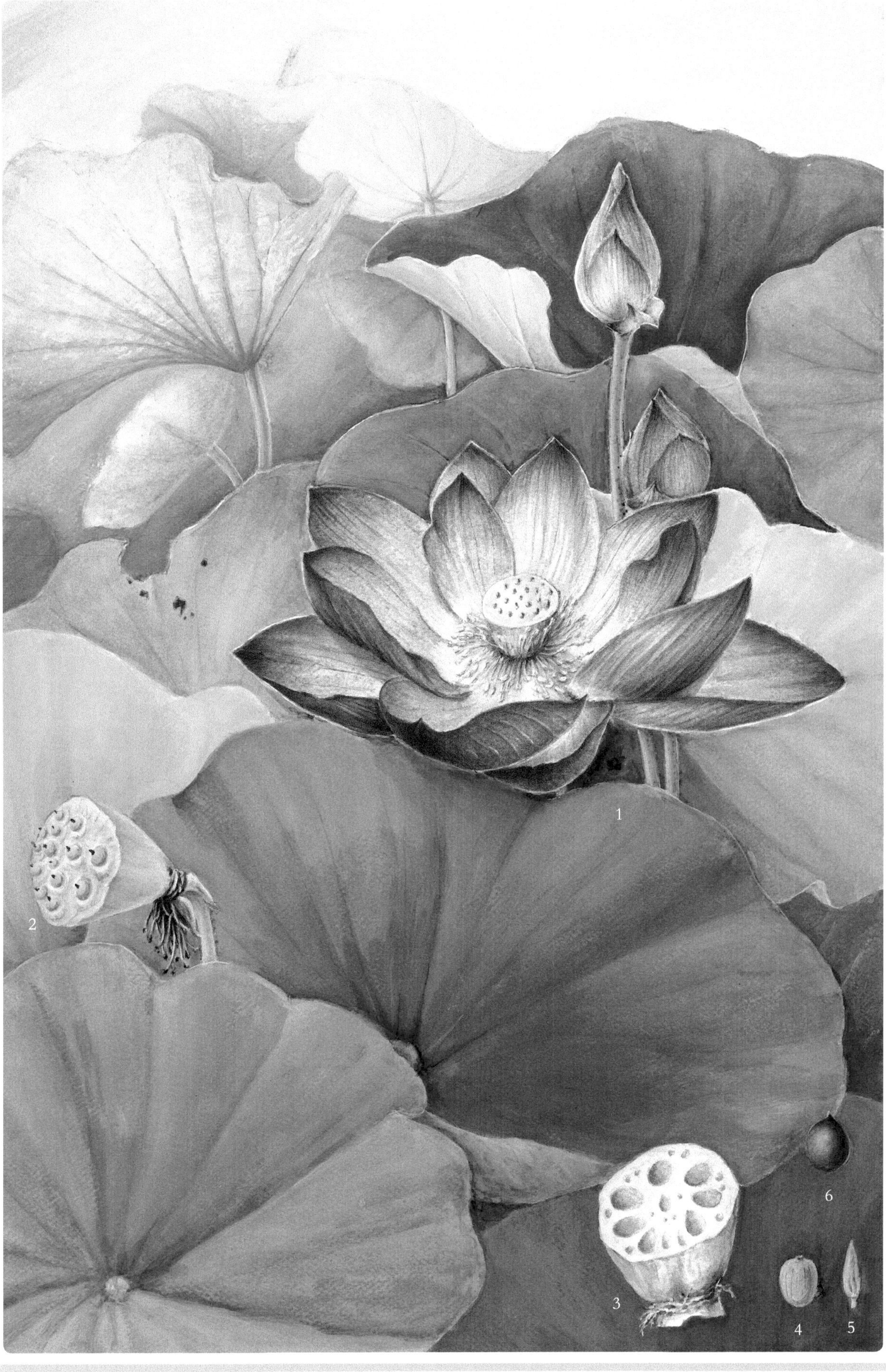

莲

1. 植株（plant） 2. 花托（receptacle） 3. 根状茎（rhizome） 4. 种子（seed） 5. 胚芽（plumule） 6. 成熟种子（ripe seed）

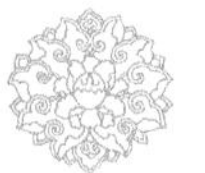

木芙蓉

Mufurong

Hibiscus mutabilis

基　　源　锦葵科 Malvaceae 木槿属 *Hibiscus* 植物木芙蓉 *Hibiscus mutabilis* L. 的干燥叶。药材名为“木芙蓉叶”。

形态特征　落叶灌木或小乔木。小枝、叶柄、花梗和花萼均密被星状毛与直毛相混的细绵毛。叶宽卵形至圆卵形，常 5-7 裂，裂片三角形；托叶早落。花单生于枝端叶腋间；花萼钟形；花初开时白色或淡红色，后变深红色，花瓣近圆形，外面被毛，基部具髯毛。蒴果扁球形，被淡黄色刚毛。种子肾形，背面被长柔毛。

生境分布　原产于我国湖南，现全国大部分省区均有栽培。

采收加工　夏、秋二季采收，干燥。

性味功能　平，辛。凉血，解毒，消肿，止痛。

主治用法　可用于治疗痈疽焮肿，缠身蛇丹，烫伤，目赤肿痛，跌打损伤。

化学成分　叶中含有黄酮苷类、酚类、氨基酸类、鞣质、还原糖等成分。

备　　注　木芙蓉花亦可入药，可用于清热解毒，凉血止血，消肿排脓。

Source　It is the dried leaf of *Hibiscus mutabilis* L. (Malvaceae). The medicinal material is called as “Mufurongye”.

Distribution　*H. mutabilis* is native to Hunan and cultivated in most provinces of China.

Indications　It is used to treat carbuncle, abscess, and swelling, herpes zoster, scalds, red eyes with swelling and pain, and traumatic injury.

Chemical Constituents　The leaves contain flavonoid glycosides, phenols, amino acids, tannins, reducing sugars, etc.

Note　The flower can also be used as medicine which has the function of clearing heat and removing toxin, cooling blood and stopping bleeding, and resolving swelling and expelling pus.

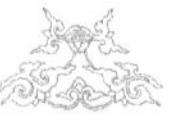

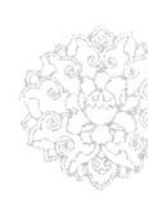

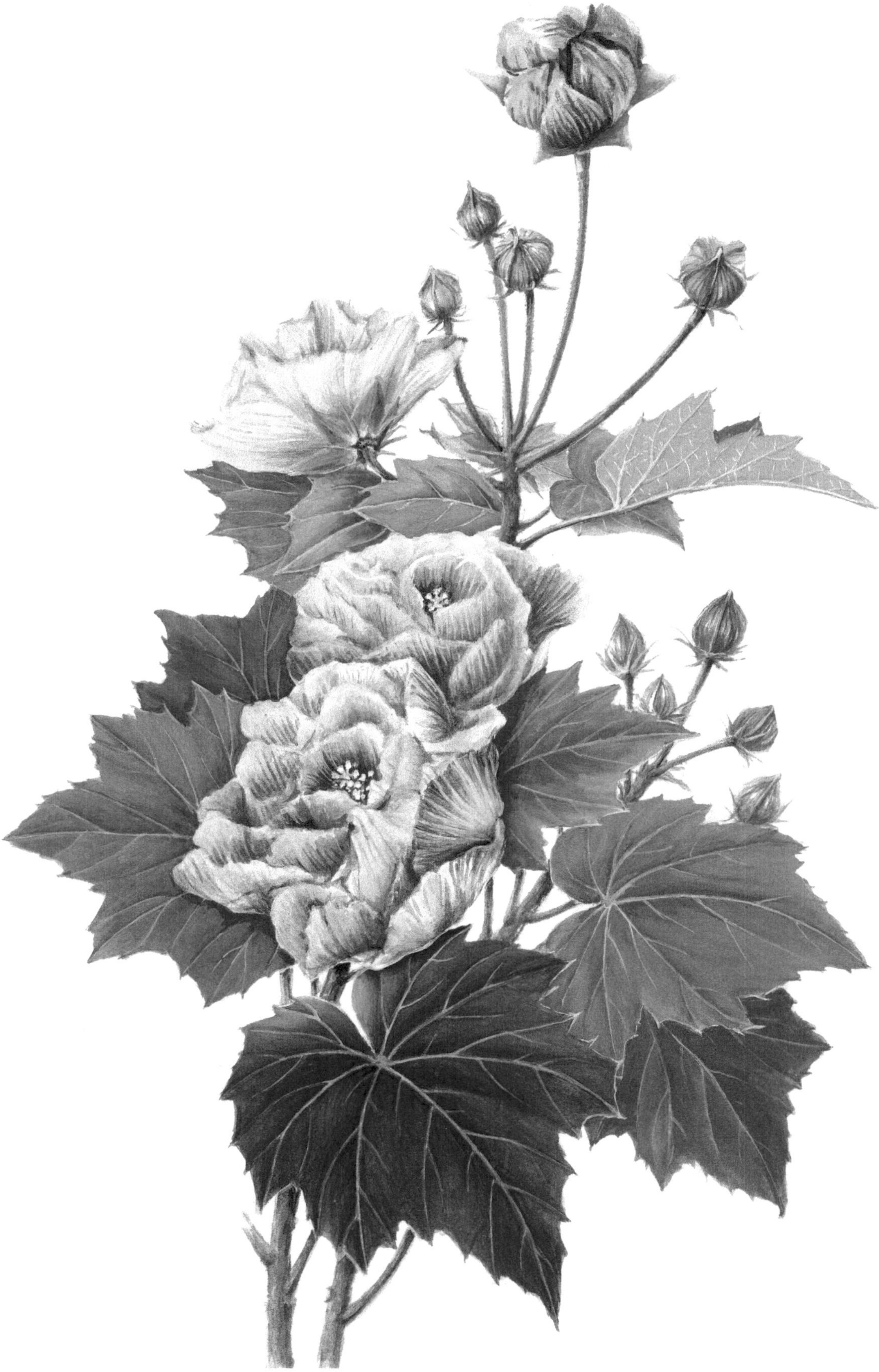

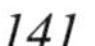

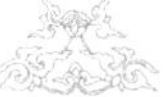

花枝（flowering stem）

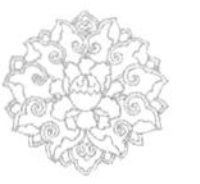

忍冬

Rendong

Lonicera japonica

基　　源　忍冬科 Caprifoliaceae 忍冬属 *Lonicera* 植物忍冬 *Lonicera japonica* Thunb. 的干燥花蕾或带初开的花。药材名为“金银花”。

形态特征　半常绿藤本。幼枝红褐色，密被柔毛。叶对生，纸质，卵形至矩圆状卵形，顶端渐尖，基部圆形，有糙缘毛。总花梗通常单生于小枝上部叶腋；花萼筒长约 2 mm；花冠白色，后变黄色，唇形，外被长腺毛。浆果球形，熟时蓝黑色，有光泽。种子卵圆形，褐色，中部有一凸起的脊，两侧有浅的横沟纹。

生境分布　分布于华东、中南、西南、华北部分省区。常生于山坡疏林、灌丛、村落旁，常见栽培。

采收加工　夏初花开放前采收，干燥。

性味功能　寒，甘。清热解毒，疏散风热。

主治用法　用于痈肿疔疮，喉痹，丹毒，热毒血痢，风热感冒，温病发热。

化学成分　主要含有绿原酸、异绿原酸、木犀草素、芳樟醇、蒎烯、异双花醇、香叶醇、丁香油酚等。

备　　注　茎枝入药称“忍冬藤”，可清热解毒，疏风通络。

Source　It is the dried alabastrum or blooming flowers of *Lonicera japonica* Thunb. (Caprifoliaceae). The medicinal material is called as “Jinyinhua”.

Distribution　*L. japonica* is distributed in East, South Central, Southwest and North China. It commonly grows in sparse forests on hillsides, shrubs, or beside villages. It is commonly cultivated at present.

Indications　It is used to treat swollen abscess, furuncle, sore, pharyngitis, erysipelas, hematodiarrhoea caused by heat toxin, wind–heat common cold, warm disease with fever.

Chemical Constituents　It mainly contains chlorogenic acid, isochlorogenic acid, luteolin, linalool, pinene, isoepoxylinalol, geraniol, eugenol, etc.

Note　The stem and branch can be used as medicine, which is called Caulis Lonicerae Japonicae. It has the function of clearing heat and removing toxin, and dispersing wind and unblocking collaterals.

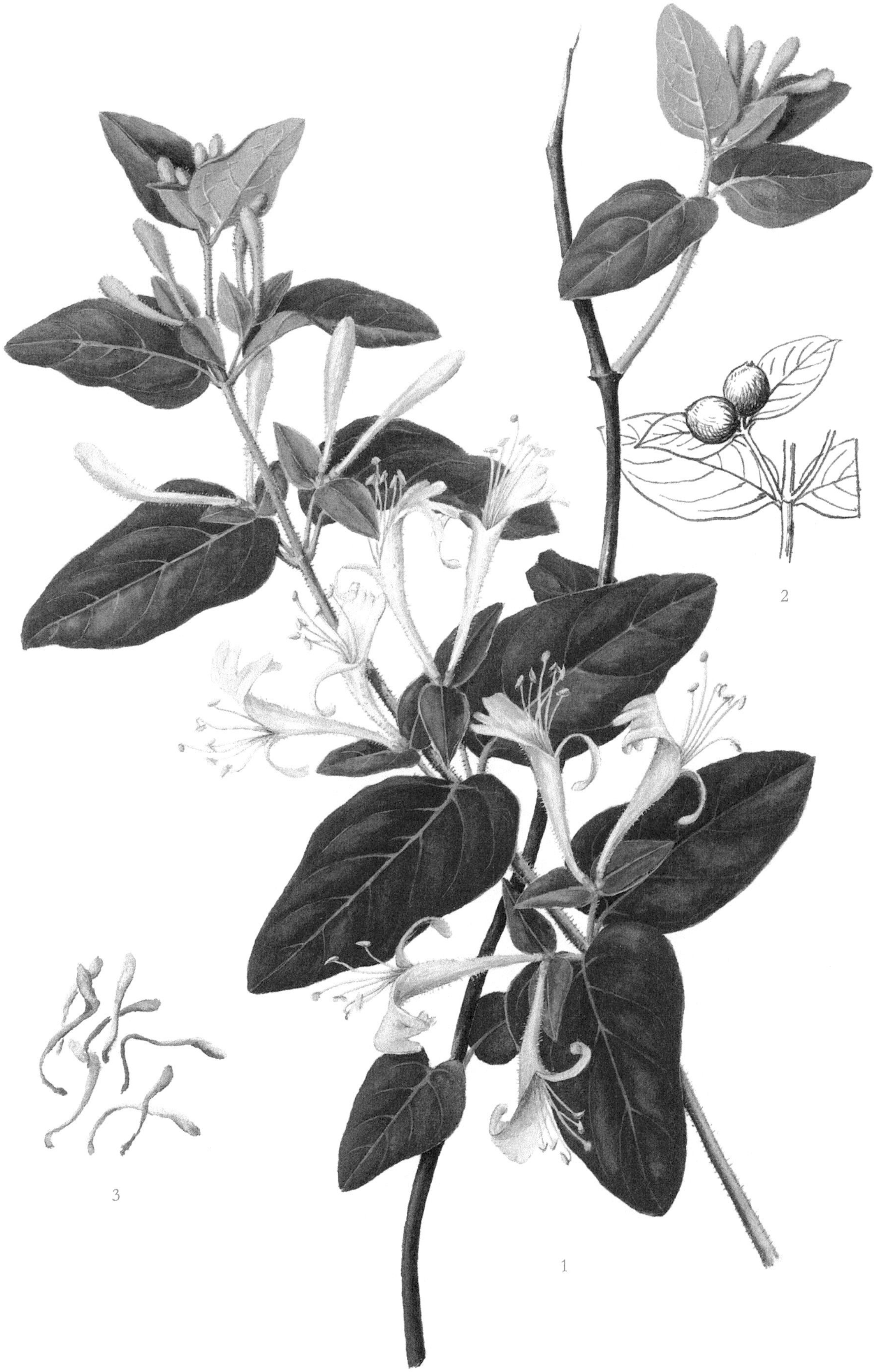

1

2

3

1. 花枝（flowering stem） 2. 果枝（fruiting stem） 3. 干花（dried flower）

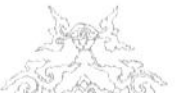

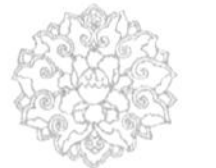

番红花

Fanhonghua

Crocus sativus

基　　源　鸢尾科 Iridaceae 番红花属 *Crocus* 植物番红花 *Crocus sativus* L. 的干燥柱头。药材名为"西红花"。

形态特征　多年生草本。球茎扁圆球形，外有黄褐色的膜质包被。叶基生，9-15 片，狭条形，绿色，边缘反卷；叶丛基部包有 4-5 片膜质的鞘状叶。花茎甚短；花 1-2 朵，多为粉红色；花被裂片 6，2 轮排列；雄蕊 3，直立；花柱橙红色，上部三分枝，分枝弯曲而下垂，柱头略扁。蒴果椭圆形，具三钝棱。

生境分布　原产欧洲南部至伊朗。药用西红花主产于伊朗和西班牙。现各地常见栽培，我国药用西红花来源主要栽培于上海。

采收加工　10-11 月下旬，晴天早晨日出时采花，再摘取柱头，随即晒干，或在 55-60℃下烘干。

性味功能　平，甘。活血化瘀，凉血解毒，解郁安神。

主治用法　用于经闭癥瘕，产后瘀阻，温毒发斑，忧郁痞闷，惊悸发狂。煎服或沸水泡服。孕妇慎用。

化学成分　主要含有西红花苷、番红花苦苷、番红花酸二甲酯、α - 番红花酸、番红花醛等成分。

备　　注　西红花又名藏红花，由伊朗进入西藏传入内地，并非西藏原产。

Source　It is the dried stigma of *Crocus sativus* L. (Iridaceae). The medicinal material is called as "Xihonghua".

Distribution　*C. sativus* is native to the regions of southern Europe to Islamic Republic of Iran. *C. sativus* for medicinal use is mainly cultivated in Islamic Republic of Iran and Kingdom of Spain. It is commonly cultivated nowaways and those for medicinal use is mainly from Shanghai.

Indications　It is used to treat amenorrhea with abdominal mass, postpartum stagnation of blood stasis, eruption caused by warm toxin, melancholy, and stuffiness sensation, palpitation due to fright, and mania. It should be decocted in water or brewed in boiling water. Pregnant women should use it with caution.

Chemical Constituents　It mainly contains crocin, picrocrocin, crocetin dimethyl ester, α-crocetin, safranal, etc.

Note　*C. sativus* was introduced from Islamic Republic of Iran to Tibet, and to inland. It is not native to Tibet.

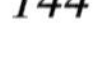

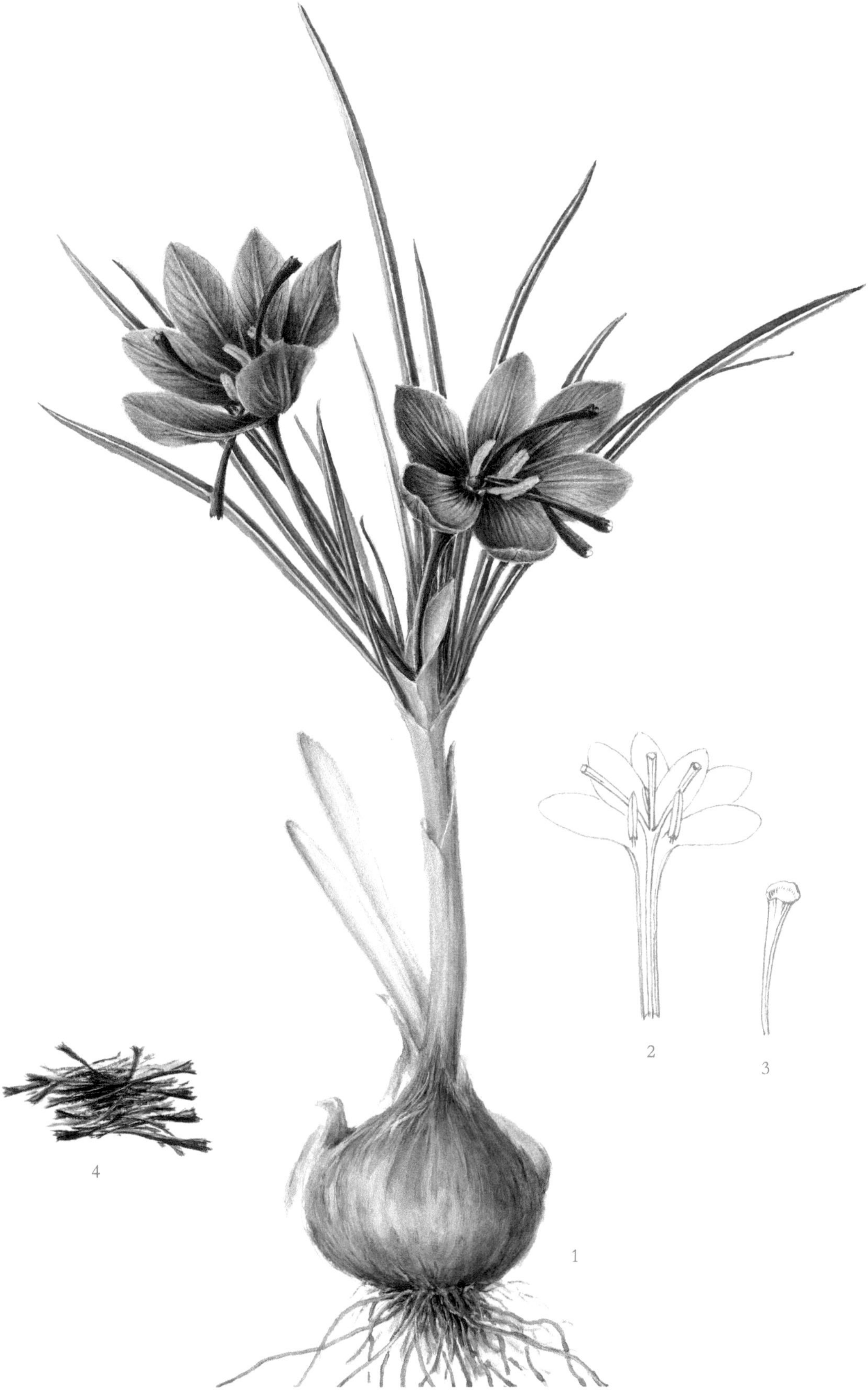

1

2

3

4

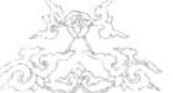

1. 植株（plant） 2. 花（flower） 3、4. 柱头（stigma）

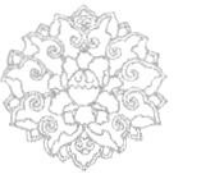

红花

Honghua

Carthamus tinctorius

基　　源　菊科 Asteraceae 红花属 *Carthamus* 植物红花 *Carthamus tinctorius* L. 的干燥花。药材名为“红花”。

形态特征　一年生草本。茎直立，上部分枝，全部茎枝淡白色，光滑，无毛。叶常披针形，边缘具锯齿，齿顶有针刺，质地坚硬，革质，两面无毛，基部无柄，半抱茎。头状花序多数，在茎顶排成伞房花序，为苞叶所围绕，苞片顶端和边缘具针刺。总苞片 4 层；小花橘红色，全部为两性。瘦果倒卵形，乳白色。

生境分布　原产中亚地区。现华北各地以及新疆广泛栽培。

采收加工　夏季花由黄变红时采摘，阴干或晒干。

性味功能　温，辛。活血通经，散瘀止痛。

主治用法　用于经闭，痛经，恶露不行，癥瘕痞块，胸痹心痛，瘀滞腹痛，胸胁刺痛，跌扑损伤，疮疡肿痛。孕妇慎用。

化学成分　主要含有羟基红花黄色素 A、红花苷、红花黄色素、红花醌苷、新红花苷、棕榈酸、肉豆蔻酸等。

备　　注　红花的花含色素，是我国古代印染红色织物的色素。红花种子油可供食用。

Source　It is the dried flower of *Carthamus tinctorius* L. (Asteraceae). The medicinal material is called as “Honghua”.

Distribution　*C. tinctorius* is native to central Asia. It is widely cultivated in North China and Xinjiang nowaways.

Indications　It is used to treat amenorrhea, dysmenorrhea, lochioschesis, abdominal mass, heart pain due to chest impediment, stasis with pain in the abdomen, stabbing pain in the chest and hypochondrium, traumatic injury, swelling and pain of sore and ulcer. Pregnant women should use it with caution.

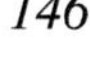

Chemical Constituents　It mainly contains hydroxyl safflow yellow A, carthamin, safflow yellow, carthamone, neocarthamin, palmitic acid, myristic acid, etc.

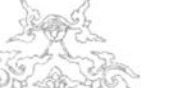

Note　The flower of *C. tinctorius* contains pigment which was used to dye red fabrics in ancient China. Its seed oil is edible.

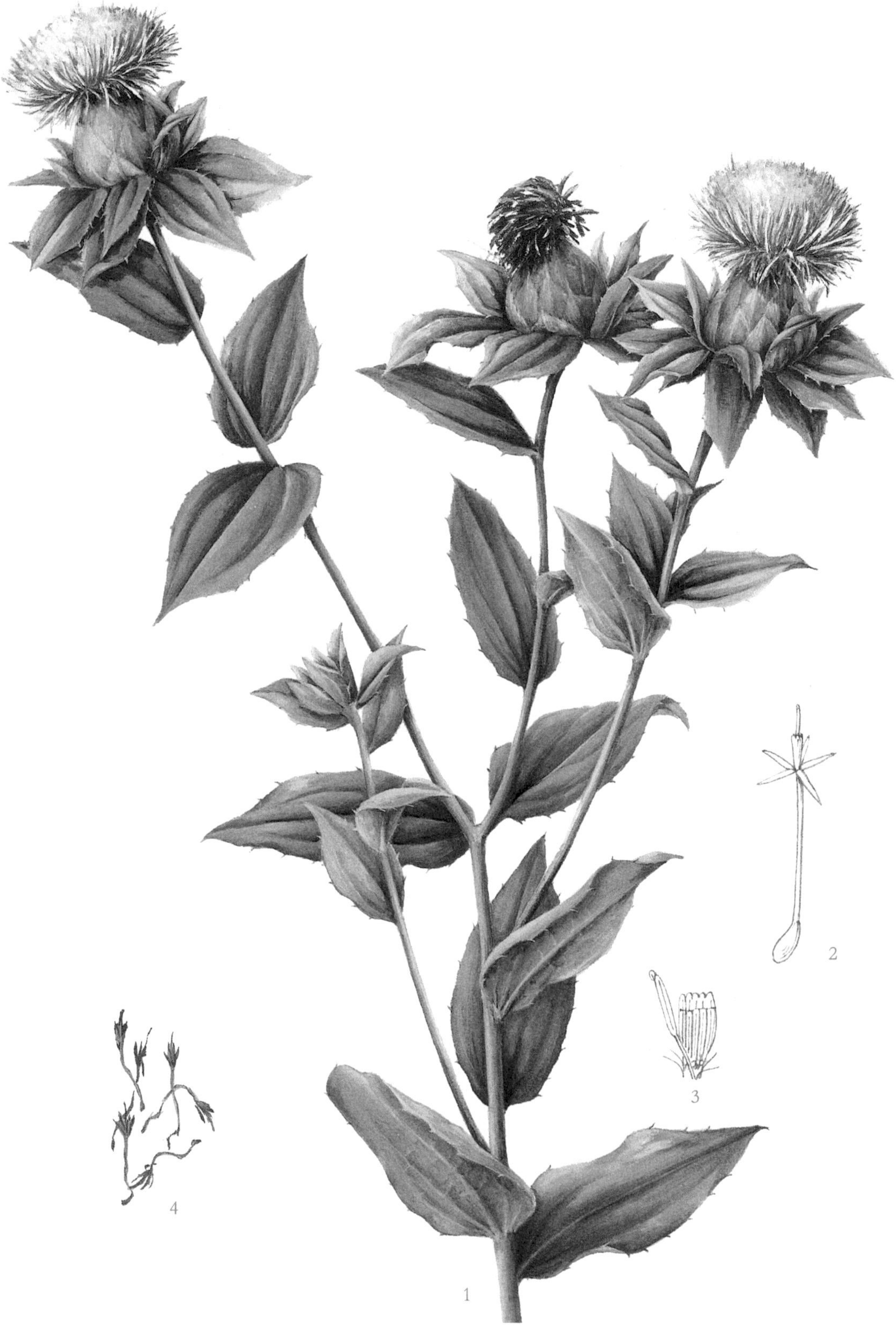

1. 花枝（flowering stem） 2. 花（flower） 3. 雌蕊及雄蕊（pistil and stamen） 4. 干花（dried flower）

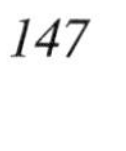

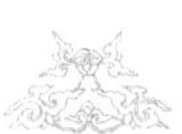

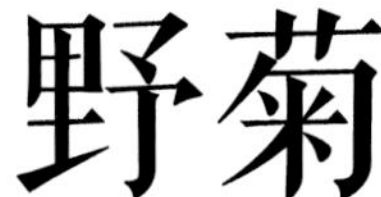

野菊

Yeju

Chrysanthemum indicum

基　　源　菊科 Asteraceae 菊属 *Chrysanthemum* 植物野菊 *Chrysanthemum indicum* L. 的干燥头状花序。药材名为“野菊花”。

形态特征　多年生草本。茎的分枝或仅在茎顶分枝；茎枝被稀疏的毛。基生叶和下部叶花期萎落；中部叶卵形或椭圆状卵形；羽状浅裂或分裂不明显而边缘有浅锯齿。头状花序，在茎枝顶端排成疏松的伞房圆锥花序或少数在茎顶排成伞房花序；苞片边缘白色或褐色宽膜质；舌状花黄色，顶端全缘或 2-3 齿。瘦果。

生境分布　广泛分布于东北、华北、华中、华南、西南各地。常生于山坡草地、灌丛、湿地、田野边及山路旁。

采收加工　秋、冬二季花初开放时采摘，晒干，或蒸后晒干。

性味功能　微寒，苦、辛。清热解毒，泻火平肝。

主治用法　主要用于疔疮痈肿，目赤肿痛，头痛眩晕。

化学成分　主要含有野菊花内酯、野菊花醇、野菊花酮、菊油环酮、密蒙花苷、熊果酸、亚油酸、刺槐苷、木犀草素、胡萝卜苷、豚草素等。

Source　It is the dried capitulum of *Chrysanthemum indicum* L. (Asteraceae). The medicinal material is called as “Yejuhua”.

Distribution　It is widely distributed in Northeast, North, Central, South, and Southwest China. It commonly grows on hillside grasslands, shrubs, wetlands, fields, and mountain roadsides.

Indications　It is used to treat boils, sore, swollen abscess, red eyes with swelling and pain, headache, and dizziness.

Chemical Constituents　It mainly contains handelin chrysanthelide, chrysanthemol, indicumenone, chrysanthenone, buddleoglucoside, ursolic acid, linoleic acid, acaciin, luteolin, daucosterol, curnambrin, etc.

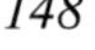

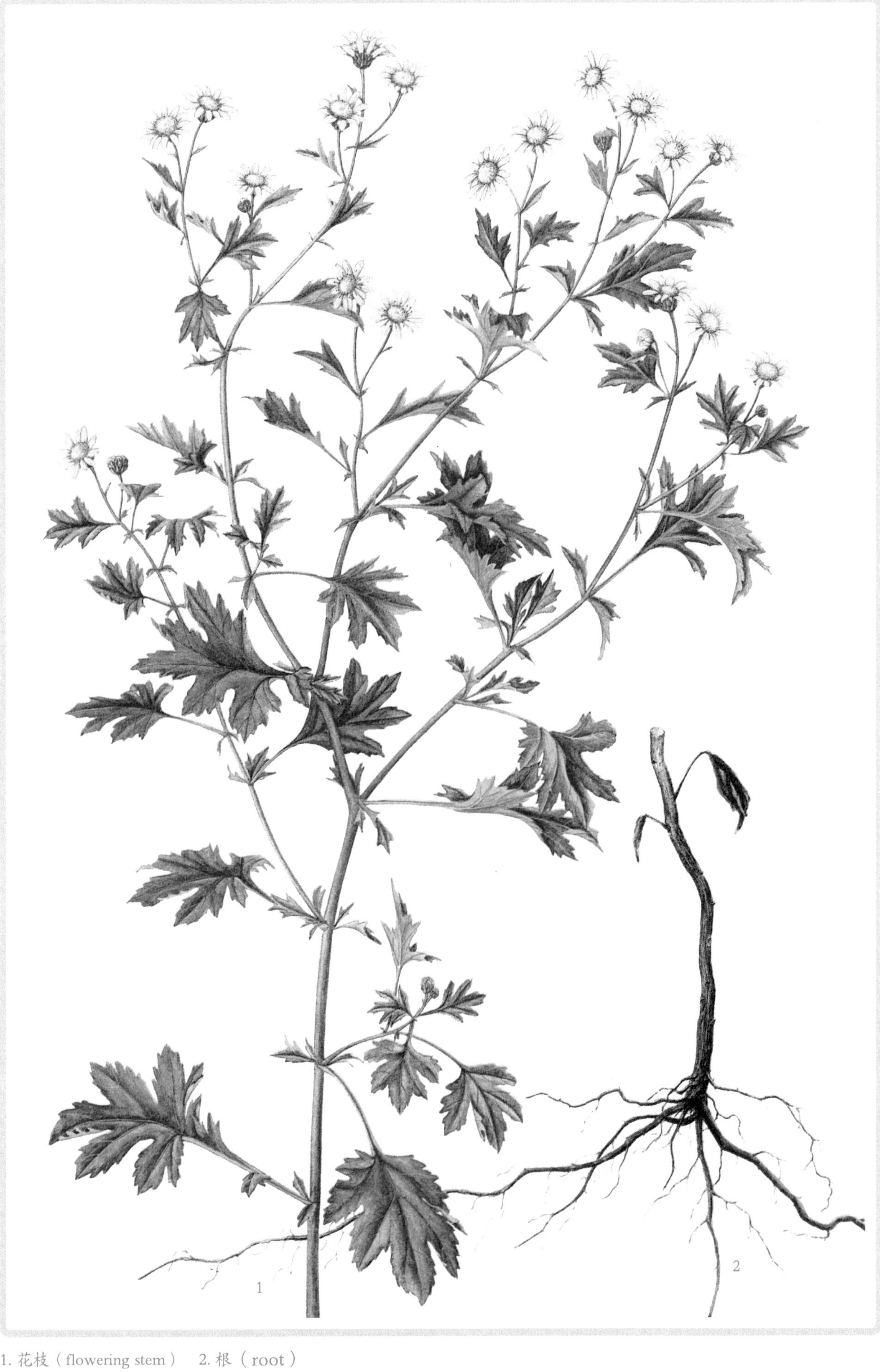

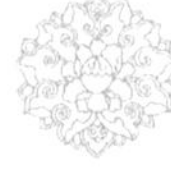

1

2

1. 花枝（flowering stem） 2. 根（root）

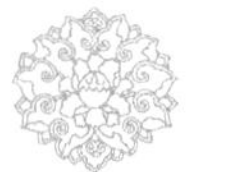

凌霄

Lingxiao

Campsis grandiflora

基　　源　紫葳科 Bignoniaceae 凌霄属 *Campsis* 植物凌霄 *Campsis grandiflora* (Thunb.) Schum. 的干燥花。药材名为“凌霄花”。

形态特征　木质攀援藤本。依靠气生根攀附。叶对生，奇数羽状复叶，小叶 7-9 枚，卵形至卵状披针形，顶端尾状渐尖，基部阔楔形，边缘有粗锯齿。枝条顶生疏散的短圆锥花序；花萼钟状，分裂至中部，裂片披针形；花冠内面鲜红色，外面橙黄色，长约 5cm，裂片半圆形。蒴果，顶端钝。

生境分布　分布于华东、中南及河北、四川、贵州等地。生于山谷及河边疏林内，攀援于树上或石壁上。常见庭院栽培。

采收加工　夏、秋二季花盛开时采摘，干燥。

性味功能　寒，甘、酸。活血通经，凉血祛风。

主治用法　主要用于月经不调，经闭癥瘕，产后乳肿，风疹发红，皮肤瘙痒，痤疮。孕妇慎用。

化学成分　主要含有 β-谷甾醇、辣红素、熊果酸、阿魏酸、水杨酸、芹菜素等。

Source　It is the dried flower of *Campsis grandiflora* (Thunb.) Schum. (Bignoniaceae). The medicinal material is called as “Lingxiaohua”.

Distribution　*C. grandiflora* is distributed in East China, Central China, and South China, Hebei, Sichuan, Guizhou, etc. It climbs on trees or stone walls, in valleys and sparse forests along riverside. It is commonly cultivated in courtyards.

Indications　It is used to treat menstrual irregularities, amenorrhea and abdominal mass, postpartum mammary swelling, red rubella, pruritus, and acne. Pregnant women should use it with caution.

Chemical Constituents　It mainly contains β-sitosterol, capsanthin, ursolic acid, ferulic acid, salicylic acid, apigenin, etc.

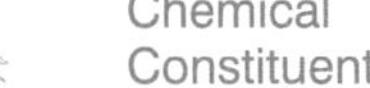

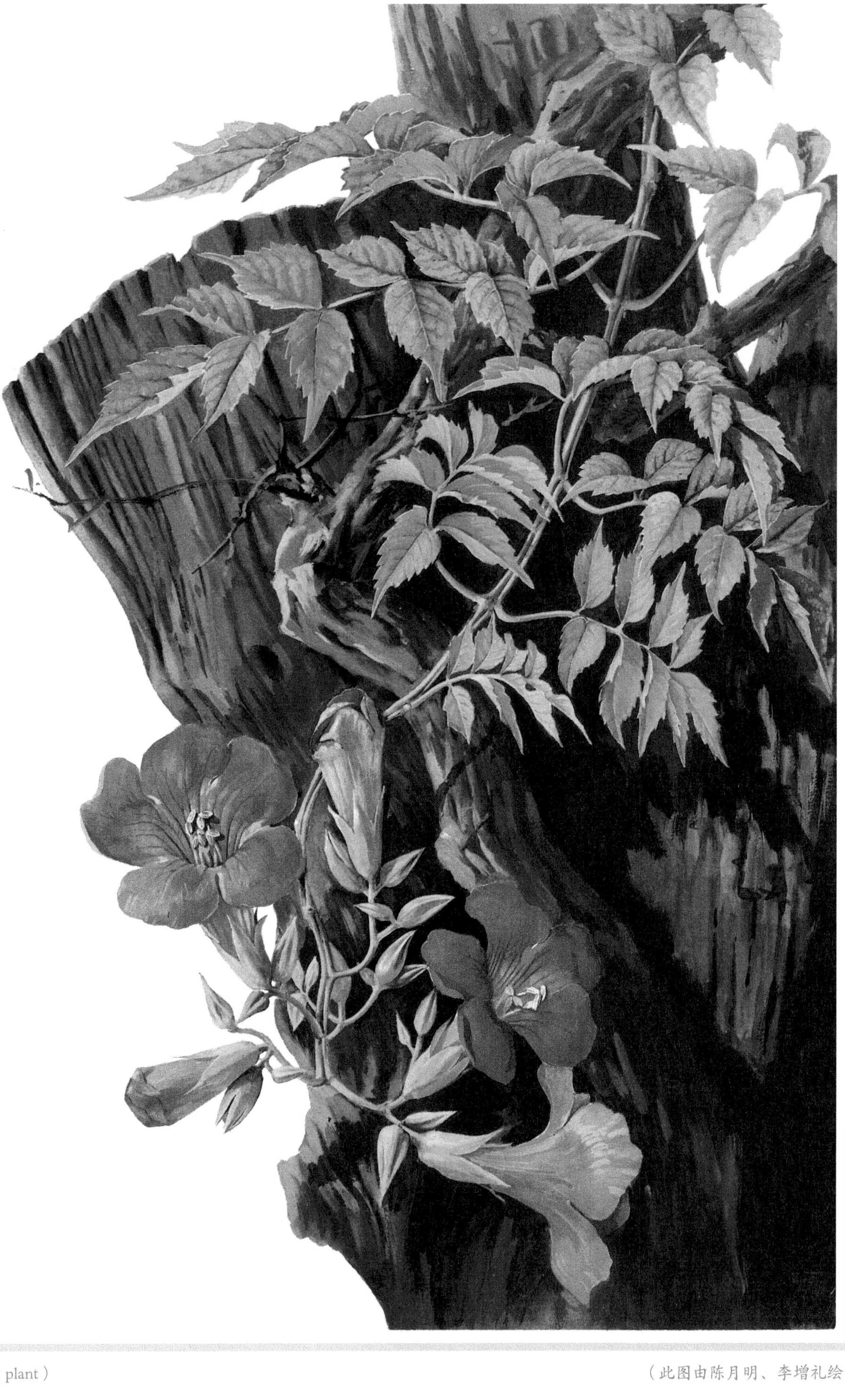

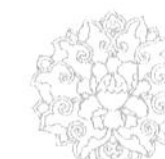

植株（plant）

（此图由陈月明、李增礼绘）

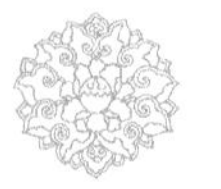

木槿

Mujin

Hibiscus syriacus

基　源　锦葵科Malvaceae木槿属*Hibiscus*植物木槿*Hibiscus syriacus* L.的干燥花。药材名为“木槿花”。

形态特征　落叶灌木。小枝密被黄色星状绒毛。叶菱形至三角状卵形，具深浅不同的三裂或不裂，先端钝，基部楔形，边缘具不整齐齿缺。花单生于枝端叶腋间，花梗被星状短绒毛；花萼钟形，密被星状短绒毛，裂片5，三角形；花钟形，淡紫色，直径3-6cm，花瓣倒卵形，外面疏被纤毛和星状长柔毛。蒴果卵圆形，密被黄色星状绒毛。种子肾形，背部被黄白色长柔毛。

生境分布　原产于我国中部各地。华东、中南、西南及河北、陕西、台湾等地均有栽培。

采收加工　夏、秋季选晴天早晨，花半开时采摘，晒干。

性味功能　凉，甘、苦。清热利湿，凉血解毒。

主治用法　主要用于肠风泻血，赤白下痢，痔疮出血，肺热咳嗽，咳血，烫伤等。

化学成分　含有皂草黄甙、肌醇和粘液质等。

Source　It is the dried flower of *Hibiscus syriacus* L. (Malvaceae). The medicinal material is called as “Mujinhua”.

Distribution　It is native to all parts of central China. It is cultivated in East China, Central South China, and Southwest China, as well as Hebei, Shanxi, Chinese Taiwan, etc.

Indications　It is used to treat bloody stool, dysentery with red and white secretions, bleeding from hemorrhoid, cough with lung heat, hemoptysis, scald, etc.

Chemical Constituents　It contains saponarin, inositol, mucilage, etc.

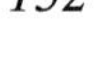

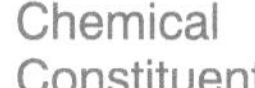

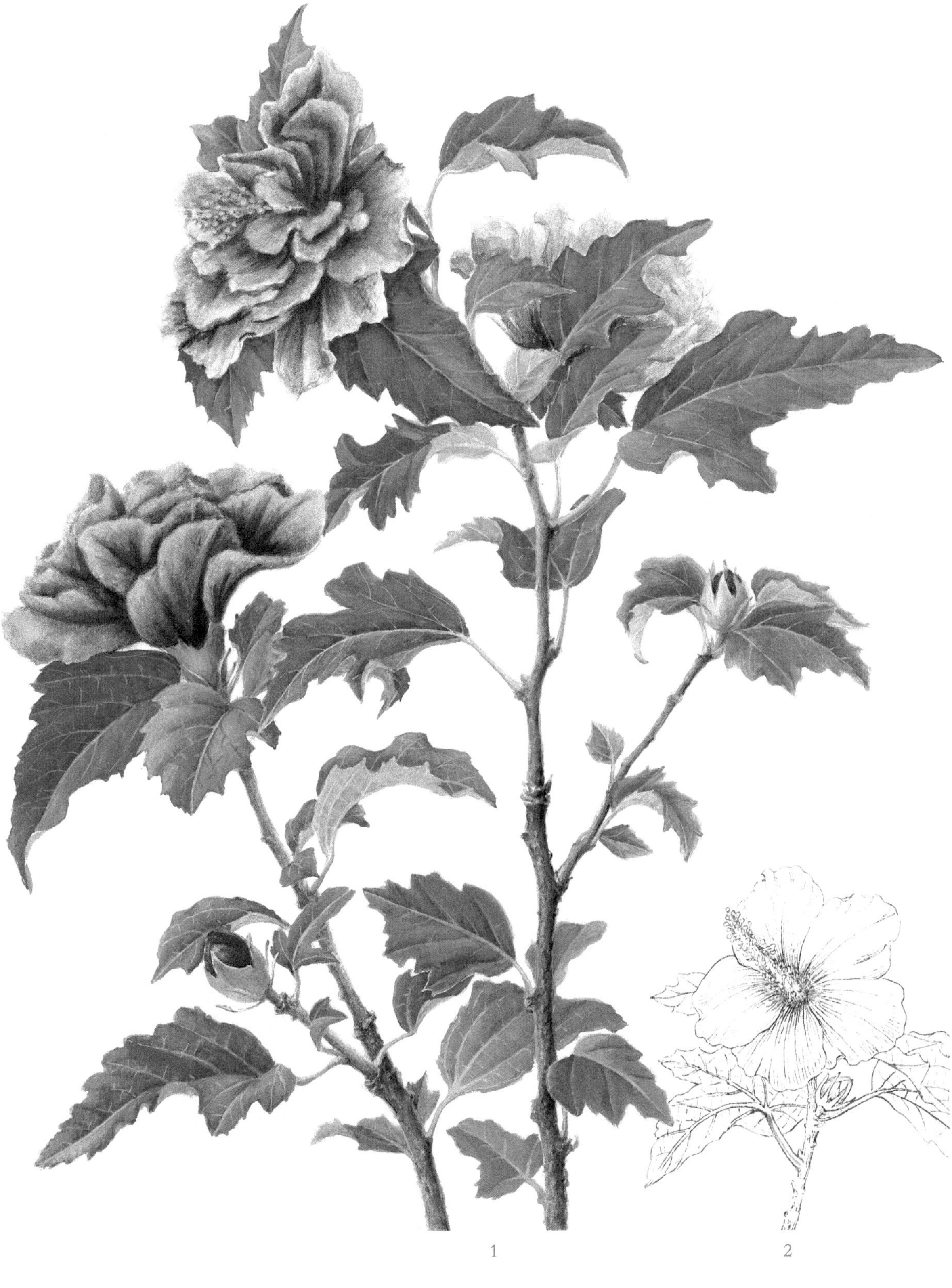

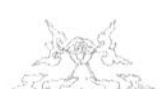

1、2. 花枝（flowering stem）

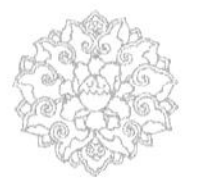

余甘子

Yuganzi

Phyllanthus emblica

基　　源　大戟科 Euphorbiaceae 叶下珠属 *Phyllanthus* 植物余甘子 *Phyllanthus emblica* L. 的干燥成熟果实。药材名为"余甘子"。

形态特征　乔木。叶片纸质至革质，排成二列，线状长圆形，顶端截平或钝圆，有锐尖头或微凹，基部浅心形而稍偏斜；托叶三角形，褐红色，边缘有睫毛。多朵雄花和 1 朵雌花组成聚伞花序；萼片 6；雄花萼片膜质，黄色，长倒卵形；雌花萼片长圆形。蒴果呈核果状，球形，外果皮肉质，淡黄白色，内果皮硬壳质。

生境分布　分布于中部、西南各省区，常生于河谷的山坡向阳处。现南方省区多栽培。

采收加工　冬季至次春果实成熟时采收，除去杂质，干燥。

性味功能　凉，甘、酸、涩。清热凉血，消食健胃，生津止咳。

主治用法　主要用于血热血瘀，消化不良，腹胀，咳嗽，喉痛，口干。

化学成分　果实主要含鞣质，如没食子酸、葡萄糖没食子鞣苷、鞣料云实素、原诃子酸、诃黎勒酸等。

备　　注　藏医常用药。

Source　It is the dried mature fruit of *Phyllanthus emblica* L. (Euphorbiaceae). The medicinal material is called as "Yuganzi".

Distribution　*P. emblica* is distributed in the central and southwest provinces. It commonly grows in the sunny hillside with sun expasure in river valleys. It is commonly cultivated in southern China nowaways.

Indications　It is used to treat heat in blood and blood stasis, indigestion, abdominal bloating, cough, sore throat, and dry mouth.

Chemical Constituents　The fruit mainly contains tannins, e.g., gallic acid, glucogallin, corilagin, terchebin, chebulagic acid, etc.

Note　It is commonly used in Tibetan medicine.

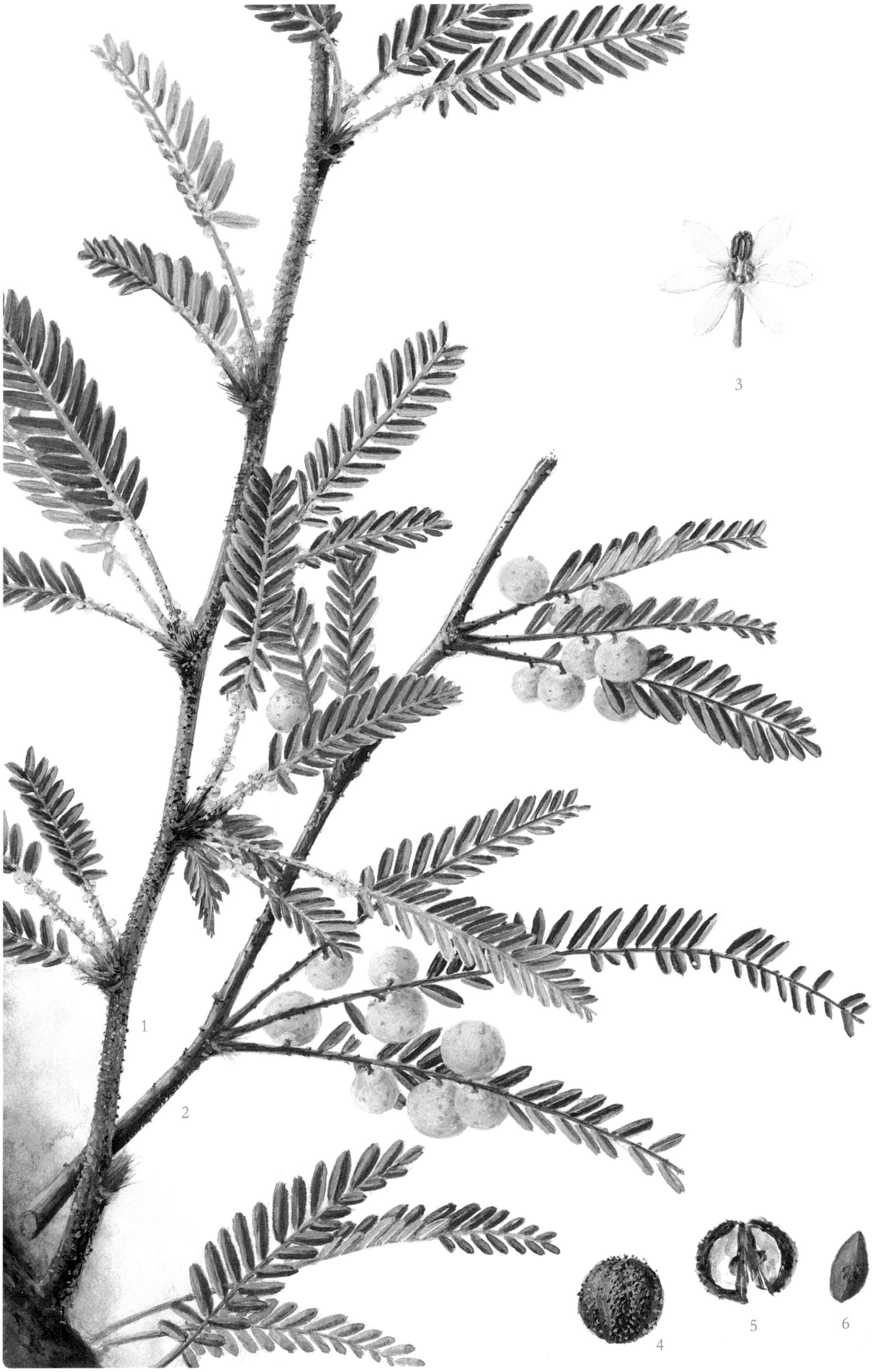

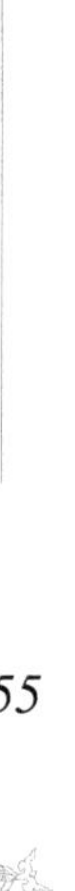

1. 花枝（flowering stem） 2. 果枝（fruiting stem） 3. 花（flower） 4. 果实（fruit） 5. 果实纵切面（vertical section of fruit）
6. 种子（seed）

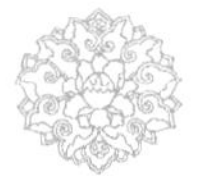

山茱萸

Shanzhuyu

Cornus officinalis

基　　源　山茱萸科 Cornaceae 山茱萸属 *Cornus* 植物山茱萸 *Cornus officinalis* Sieb. et Zucc. 的干燥成熟果肉。药材名为“山茱萸”。

形态特征　落叶乔木或灌木。叶对生，纸质，卵状椭圆形，全缘，上面绿色，下面浅绿色，脉腋密生淡褐色丛毛。伞形花序，生于枝侧，总苞片 4，卵形，革质，花后脱落；花小，先叶开放；花萼裂片 4；花瓣 4，舌状披针形，黄色，向外反卷。核果长椭圆形，紫红色。核骨质，狭椭圆形，有几条不整齐的肋纹。

生境分布　分布于我国华东、华中各省。生于山坡林中。常见栽培。道地药材产地为浙江。

采收加工　秋末冬初果皮变红时采收果实，用文火烘或置沸水中略烫后，及时除去果核，干燥。

性味功能　微温，酸、涩。补益肝肾，收涩固脱。

主治用法　用于眩晕耳鸣，腰膝酸痛，阳痿遗精，遗尿尿频，崩漏带下，大汗虚脱，内热消渴。

化学成分　主要含有环烯醚萜苷类，如马钱苷、山茱萸苷等；以及有机酸类，如没食子酸、苹果酸、酒石酸等；还含有氨基酸类、挥发油类、酚类、多糖类、鞣质等。

Source　It is the dried mature pulp of *Cornus officinalis* Sieb. et Zucc. (Cornaceae). The medicinal material is called as “Shanzhuyu”.

Distribution　*C. officinalis* is distributed in East and Central China. It grows in hillside forests and commonly cultivated. The source of authenic medicinal materials is Zhejiang.

Indications　It is used to treat dizziness with tinnitus, soreness and pain of the lower back and knee, impotence and seminal emission, enuresis and frequent urination, metrorrhagia and metrostaxis with leukorrhea, profuse sweating and prostration syndrome, internal heat and wasting thirst.

Chemical Constituents　It mainly contains iridoid glycosides (e.g., loganin, cornoside), organic acids (e.g., gallic acid, malic acid, tartaric acid), amino acids, volatile oils, phenols, polysaccharides, tannins, etc.

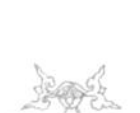

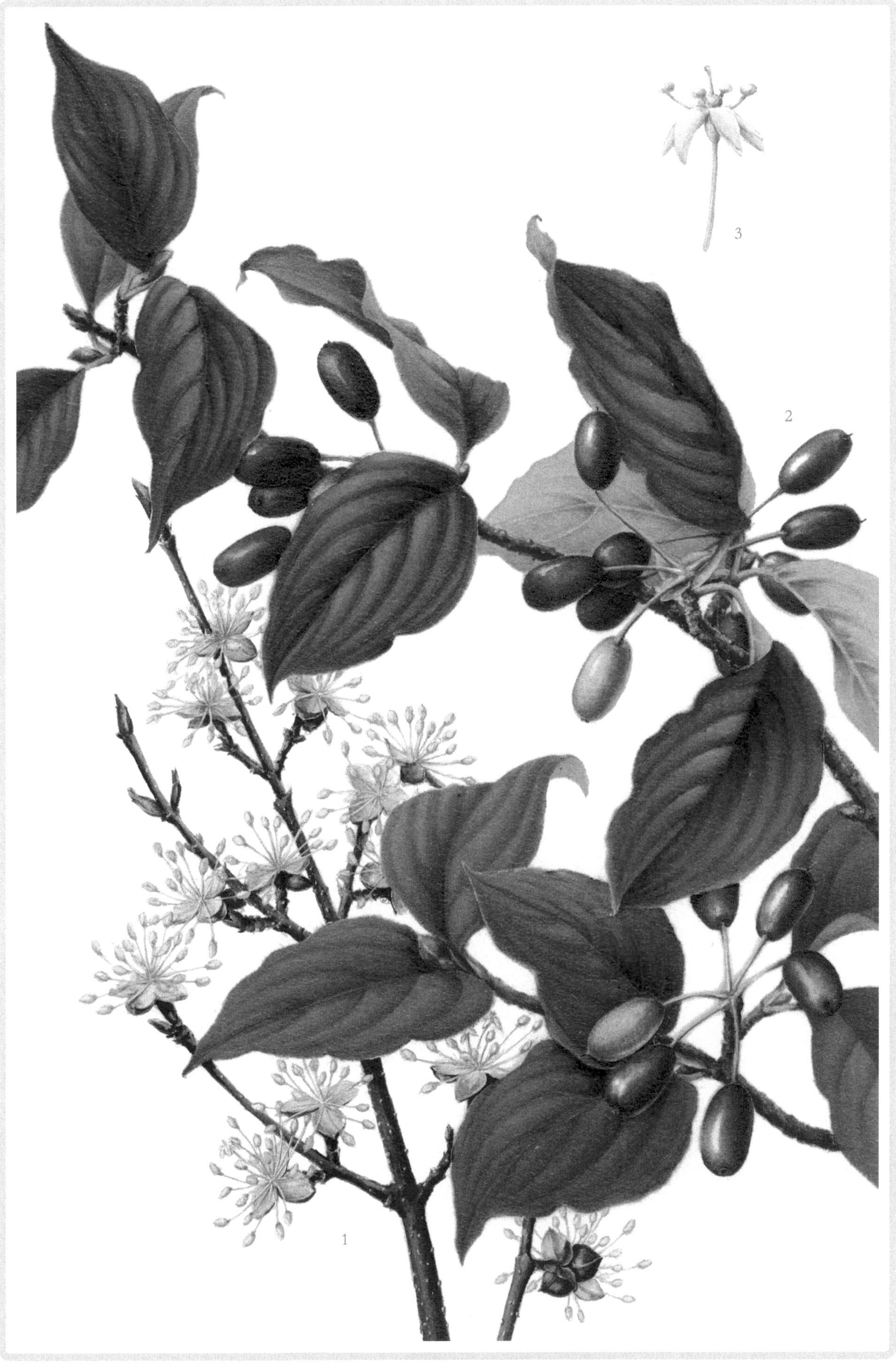

山茱萸

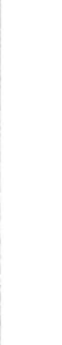

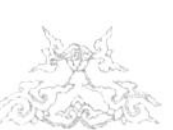

1. 花枝（flowering stem） 2. 果枝（fruiting stem） 3. 花（flower）

马兜铃

Madouling
Aristolochia debilis

基　源　马兜铃科 Aristolochiaceae 马兜铃属 *Aristolochia* 植物马兜铃 *Aristolochia debilis* Sieb. et Zucc. 的干燥成熟果实。药材名为“马兜铃”。

形态特征　草质藤本。根圆柱形。茎暗紫色或绿色。叶纸质，卵状三角形或戟形，顶端钝圆，基部心形。花单生或 2 朵聚生于叶腋；花被基部膨大呈球形，上部收狭成管状，管口扩大呈漏斗状，黄绿色，口部有紫斑；檐部一侧极短，另一侧延伸成舌片。蒴果近球形，具六棱。种子扁平，钝三角形，边缘具白色膜质宽翅。

生境分布　分布于长江流域以南各省区以及山东、河南等。生于海拔较低的山谷、路旁及山坡灌丛中。

采收加工　秋季果实由绿变黄时采收，干燥。

性味功能　微寒，苦。清肺降气，止咳平喘，清肠消痔。

主治用法　用于肺热咳喘，痰中带血，肠热痔血，痔疮肿痛。本品含马兜铃酸，可引起肾脏损害等不良反应；儿童及老年人慎用；孕妇、婴幼儿及肾功能不全者禁用。

化学成分　主要含有马兜铃酸、马兜铃内酰胺、木兰碱、马兜铃烯、青木香酮、树脂、鞣质等。

Source　It is the dried mature fruit of *Aristolochia debilis* Sieb. et Zucc. (Aristolochiaceae). The medicinal material is called as “Madouling”.

Distribution　*A. debilis* is distributed in regions on the south of Yangtze River Basin, Shandong, and Henan. It grows in valleys at a low altitude, roadsides and hillside thickets.

Indications　It is used to treat cough and panting due to heat in the lung, sputum containing blood, hemorrhoidal bleeding with intestine heat, and swelling and pain of hemorrhoids. It contains aristolochic acid, which can cause adverse effects such as kidney damage. Children and the elderly should use it with caution. Pregnant women, infants,, and those with renal impairment are prohibited to use it.

Chemical Constituents　It mainly contains aristolochic acid, aristolochialactam, magnoline, aristolene, debilone, resin, tannin, etc.

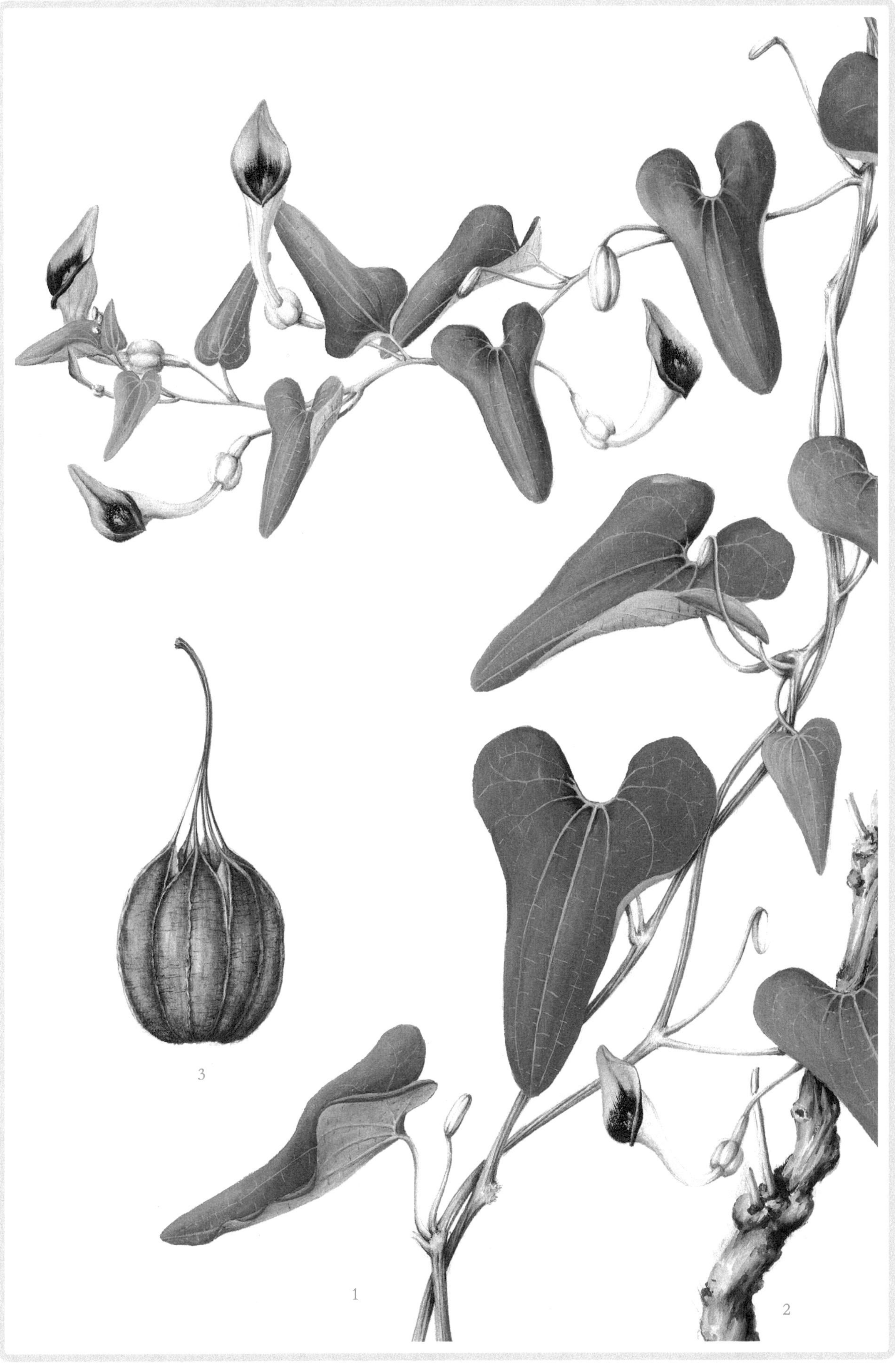

3

1

2

1. 花枝（flowering stem） 2. 根（root） 3. 果实（fruit）

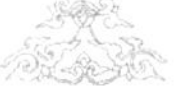

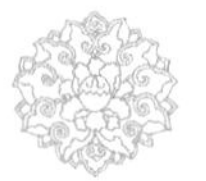

黄荆

Huangjing

Vitex negundo

基　　源　马鞭草科 Verbenaceae 牡荆属 *Vitex* 植物黄荆 *Vitex negundo* L. 的干燥果实。药材名为“黄荆子”。

形态特征　直立灌木。小枝四棱形。掌状复叶，小叶 5，小叶片长圆状披针形，常有少数粗锯齿，表面绿色，背面密被灰白色绒毛，中间小叶略大，两侧小叶渐小。聚伞花序排列呈圆锥状，顶生；花萼钟状，先端五齿裂，外面被灰白色绒毛；花冠淡紫色，外有微柔毛，先端五裂，二唇形。核果褐色，近球形，宿存花萼。

生境分布　分布于长江以南各地。常生于山坡、路旁或灌丛中。

采收加工　8-9 月采摘果实，干燥。

性味功能　温，辛、苦。祛风解表，止咳平喘，理气消食止痛。

主治用法　主要用于伤风感冒，咳嗽，哮喘，胃痛吞酸，消化不良，食积泻痢，胆囊炎，胆结石，疝气等。

化学成分　主要含有挥发油类成分，如含桉叶素、左旋香桧烯、α - 蒎烯、樟烯、β - 丁香烯、柠檬醛等；种子中含对羟基苯甲酸、蒿黄素、葡萄糖、脂肪酸等。

Source　It is the dried fruit of *Vitex negundo* L. (Verbenaceae). The medicinal material is called as “Huangjingzi”.

Distribution　*V. negundo* is distributed in the south of the Yangtze River. It commonly grows on hillsides, roadsides or in thickets.

Indications　It is used to treat common cold, cough, asthma, stomach pain with acid regurgitation, indigestion, food accumulation and diarrhea, cholecystitis, gallstone, hernia, etc.

Chemical Constituents　It mainly contains volatile oils, e.g., cineole, L-sabinene, α-pinene, camphene, β-caryophyllene, citral. The seed contains *p*-hydroxybenzoic acid, artemetin, glucose, fatty acids, etc.

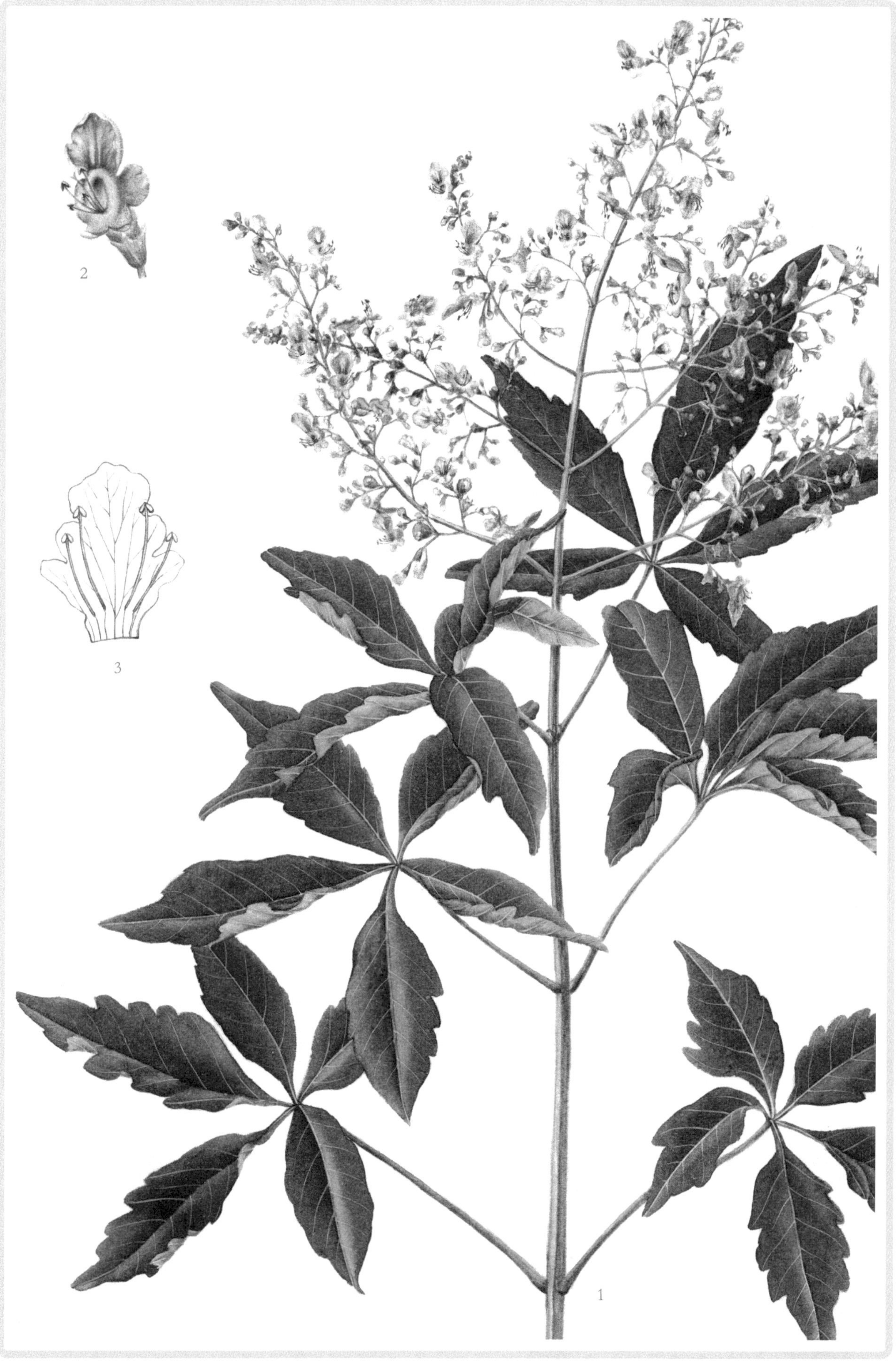

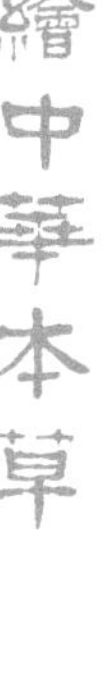

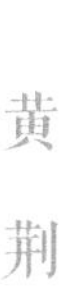

1. 花枝（flowering stem） 2. 花（flower） 3. 雄蕊（stamen）

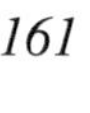

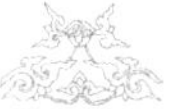

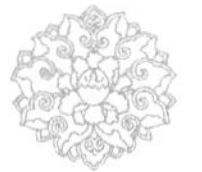

五味子

Wuweizi

Schisandra chinensis

基　　源　木兰科 Magnoliaceae 五味子属 *Schisandra* 植物五味子 *Schisandra chinensis* (Turcz.) Baill. 的干燥成熟果实。药材名为"五味子"，习称"北五味子"。

形态特征　落叶木质藤本。叶膜质，宽椭圆形、卵形、倒卵形或近圆形，先端急尖，基部楔形，上部边缘具疏浅锯齿，近基部全缘。雌雄异株；雄花花被片粉白色或粉红色，6-9 片，长圆形或椭圆状长圆形；雌花花被片和雄花相似。聚合果；小浆果红色，近球形或倒卵圆形，果皮具不明显腺点。种子 1-2 粒，肾形。

生境分布　分布于我国华北及东北各地，以及宁夏、甘肃。生于 1000 m 以上的山坡沟谷和路旁。

采收加工　秋季果实成熟时采摘，晒干或蒸后晒干，除去果梗和杂质。

性味功能　温，酸、甘。收敛固涩，益气生津，补肾宁心。

主治用法　主要用于久嗽虚喘，梦遗滑精，遗尿尿频，久泻不止，自汗盗汗，津伤口渴，内热消渴，心悸失眠。

化学成分　主要含有五味子甲素、五味子乙素、五味子丙素、五味子素、去氧五味子素、五味子醇甲、戈米辛、枸橼酸、苹果酸、酒石酸、琥珀酸、荜澄茄烯、防风根烯、芳樟醇、甾醇、柠檬醛等。

备　　注　五味子属现已独立成科，为五味子科 Schisandraceae。

Source　It is the dried mature fruit of *Schisandra chinensis* (Turcz.) Baill. (Magnoliaceae). The medicinal material is called as "Wuweizi".

Distribution　*S. chinensis* is distributed in North and Northeast China, Ningxia and Gansu. It commonly grows on hillsides, in valleys and roadsides at an altitude of over 1000 m.

Indications　It is used to treat deficiency-type dyspnea due to long-time cough, nocturnal emission, spermatorrhea, enuresis and frequent urination, chronic diarrhea, spontaneous sweating and night sweating, body fluid deficiency and thirst, internal heat and wasting thirst, and palpitation and insomnia.

Chemical Constituents　It mainly contains schisandrin A, schisandrin B, schisandrin C, deoxyschizandrin, schisandrol A, gomisin, citric acid, malic acid, tartaric acid, succinic acid, cadinene, bisabolane, linalool, sterol, citral, etc.

Note　The *Schisandra* genus now belongs to a family named Schisandraceae.

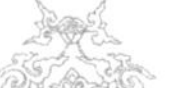

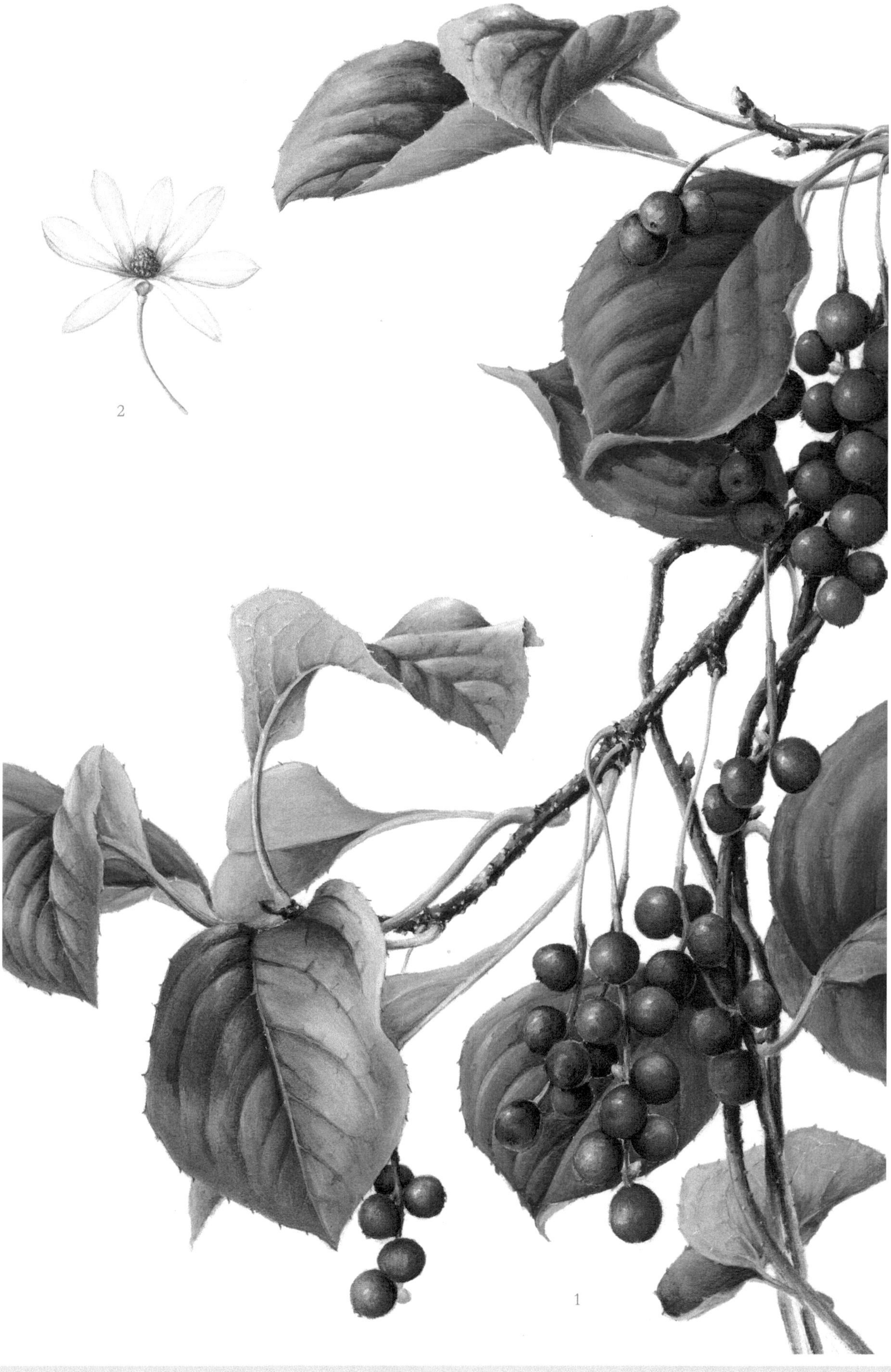

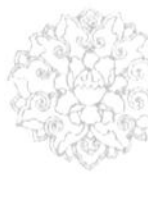

1. 果枝（fruiting stem） 2. 雌花（female flower）

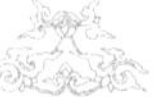

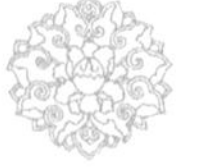

华中五味子

Huazhongwuweizi

Schisandra sphenanthera

基　　源　木兰科 Magnoliaceae 五味子属 *Schisandra* 植物华中五味子 *Schisandra sphenanthera* Rehd.et Wils. 的干燥成熟果实。药材名为“南五味子”。

形态特征　落叶木质藤本。小枝红褐色，具凸起的皮孔。叶纸质，倒卵形或倒卵状长椭圆形，干膜质边缘至叶柄成狭翅，上面深绿色，下面淡灰绿色，有白色点，边缘具疏齿；叶柄红色。花生于近基部叶腋，花梗纤细；花被片 5-9，橙黄色，椭圆形或长圆状倒卵形。雌雄异株。聚合果，成熟时红色。种子长圆形或肾形。

生境分布　分布于我国南方大部分省区。生于海拔 600-3000 m 的潮湿山坡或灌丛中。

采收加工　秋季果实成熟时采摘，晒干，除去果梗和杂质。

性味功能　温，酸、甘。收敛固涩，益气生津，补肾宁心。

主治用法　用于久嗽虚喘，梦遗滑精，遗尿尿频，久泻不止，自汗盗汗，津伤口渴，内热消渴，心悸失眠。

化学成分　主要含有木脂素类成分，如五味子酯甲、华中五味子酮、五味子醇甲、五味子醇乙等；另还含有挥发油类。

备　　注　五味子属现已独立成科，为五味子科 Schisandraceae。

Source　It is the dried mature fruit of *Schisandra sphenanthera* Rehd.et Wils. (Magnoliaceae). The medicinal material is called as “Nanwuweizi”.

Distribution　*S. sphenanthera* is distributed in most provinces of southern China. It commonly grows in damp hillsides or thickets at an altitude of 600–3000 m.

Indications　It is used to treat deficiency-type dyspnea due to long-time cough, nocturnal emission, spermatorrhea, enuresis and frequent urination, chronic diarrhea, spontaneous sweating and night sweating, body fluid deficiency and thirst, internal heat and wasting thirst, and palpitation and insomnia.

Chemical Constituents　It mainly contains lignans (e.g., schisantherin A, schisandron, schisandrol A, schisandrol B) and volatile oils.

Note　The *Schisandra* genus now belongs to a family named Schisandraceae.

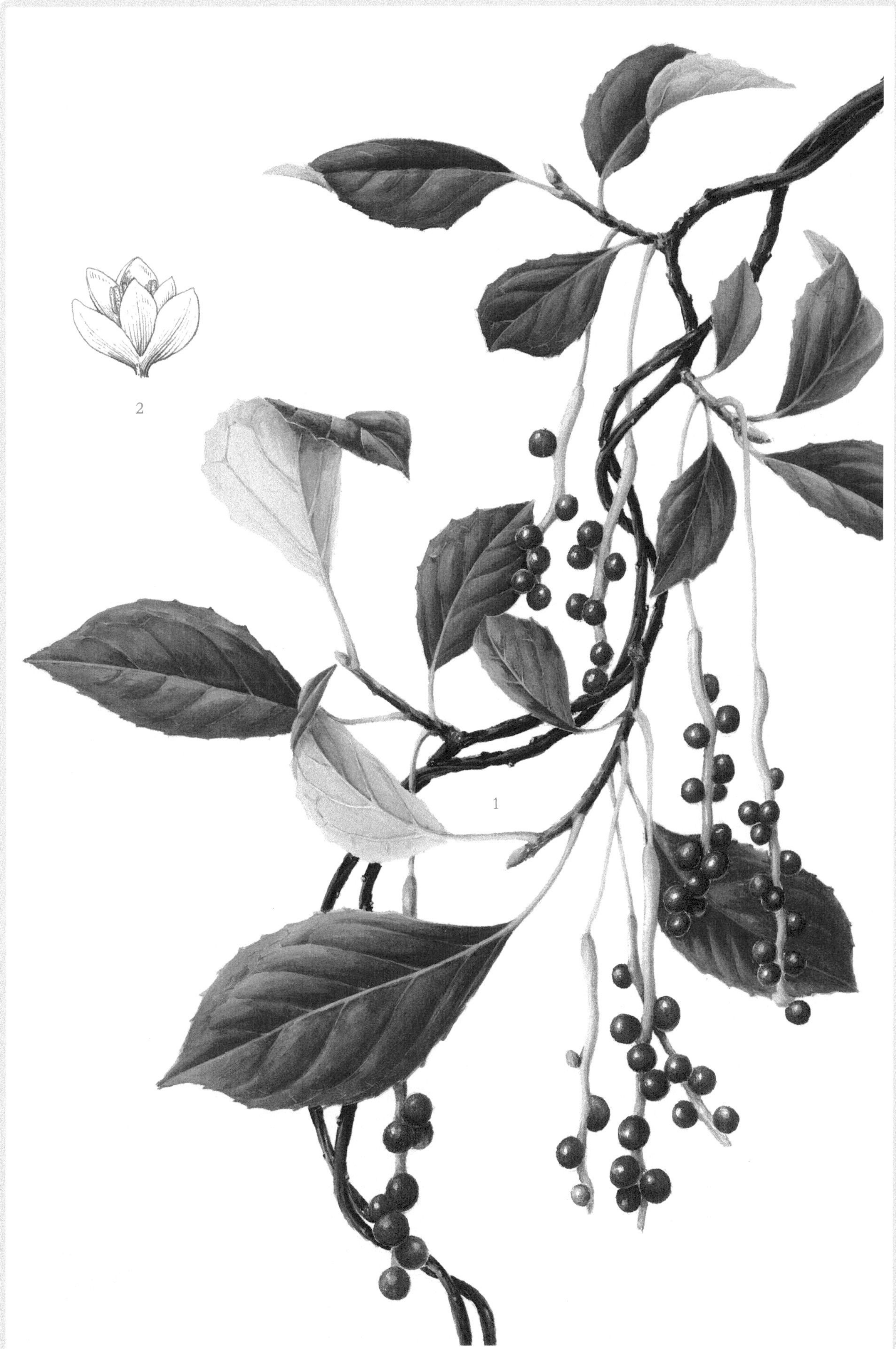

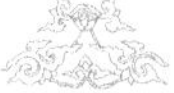

1. 果枝（fruiting stem）　2. 雄花（female flower）

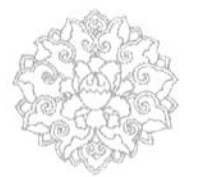

连翘

Lianqiao

Forsythia suspensa

基　源　木犀科 Oleaceae 连翘属 *Forsythia* 植物连翘 *Forsythia suspensa* (Thunb.) Vahl 的干燥果实。药材名为“连翘”。

形态特征　落叶灌木。枝条棕色或淡黄褐色，小枝灰褐色，略呈四棱形，疏生皮孔，节间中空，节部具实心髓。叶通常为单叶或三裂，叶片卵形或椭圆状卵形，叶缘除基部外具锐锯齿。花单生或2至数朵着生于叶腋，先于叶开放；花萼绿色；花冠黄色，裂片倒卵状长圆形。果实长椭圆形，先端喙状渐尖，表面疏生皮孔。

生境分布　分布于华北、华东、华中部分省区。生于海拔约数百米至 2000 m 的山坡灌丛、林下、山谷、山沟疏林中。我国除华南地区外，其他各地均有栽培。

采收加工　秋季果实初熟尚带绿色时采收，除去杂质，蒸熟，晒干，习称“青翘”；果实熟透时采收，晒干，除去杂质，习称“老翘”。

性味功能　微寒，苦。清热解毒，消肿散结，疏散风热。

主治用法　主要用于痈疽，瘰疬，乳痈，丹毒，风热感冒，温病初起，温热入营，高热烦渴，神昏发斑，热淋涩痛。

化学成分　主要含有连翘苷、连翘苷元、白桦脂酸、齐墩果酸、松脂素、熊果酸、挥发油、β-谷甾醇等。

Source　It is the dried fruit of *Forsythia suspensa* (Thunb.) Vahl. (Oleaceae). The medicinal material is called as “Lianqiao”.

Distribution　*F. suspensa* is distributed in some provinces of North China, East China, and Central China. It grows in hillside shrubs, forests, valleys, sparse forests at an altitude of several hundred meters to 2000 meters. It is cultivated in most parts of China, except for South China.

Indications　It is used to treat abscess and carbuncle, scrofula, acute mastitis, erysipelas, wind–heat common cold, initial stage of the warm disease, warm disease entering Ying untrients phase pattern, high fever with extreme thirst, unconsciousness with eruption, and unsmooth and painful urination seen in stranguria due to heat.

Chemical Constituents　It mainly contains phillyrin, phillygenin, betulinic acid, oleanolic acid, pinoresinol, ursolic acid, volatile oil, β-sitosterol, etc.

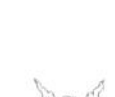

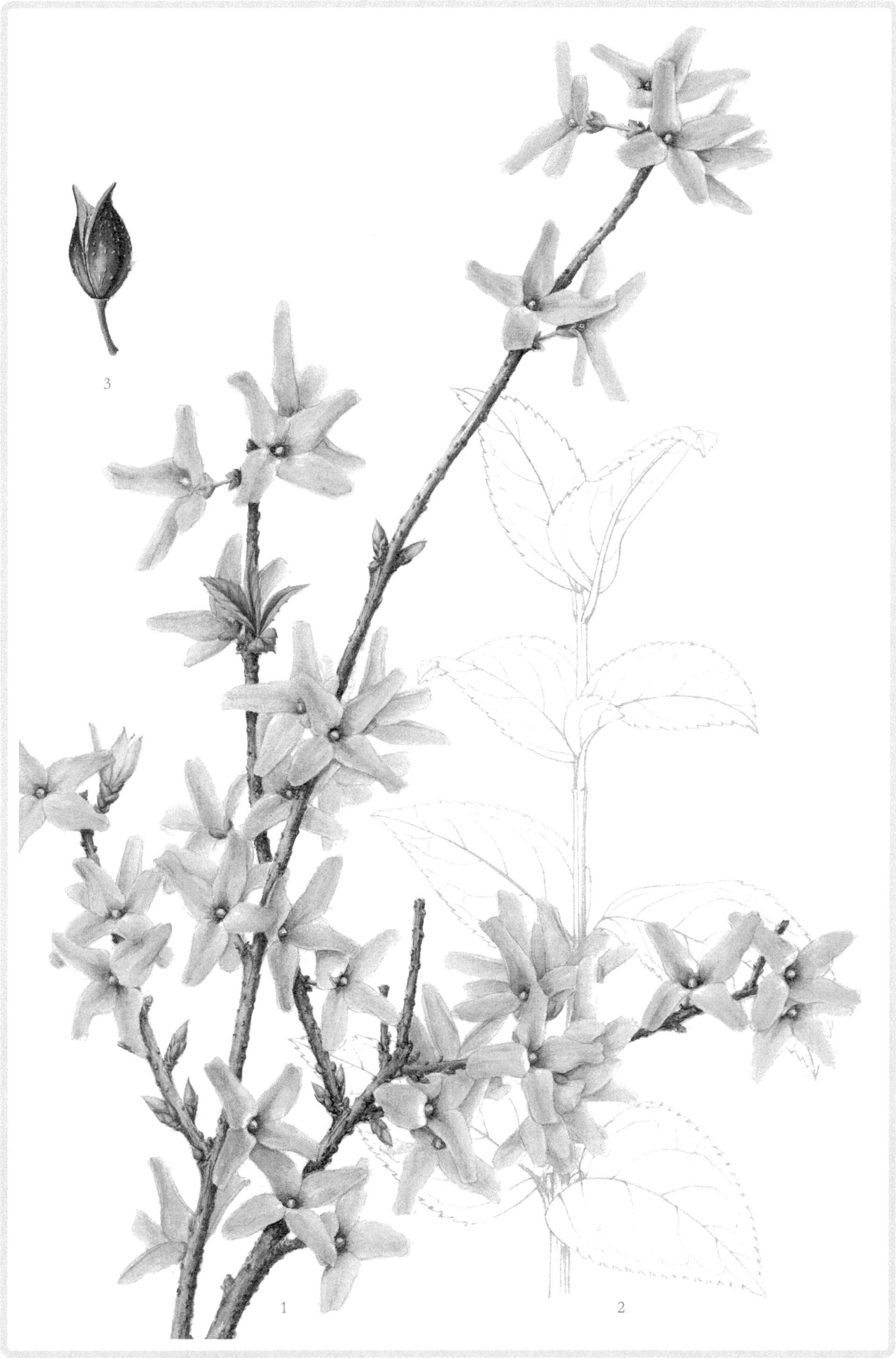

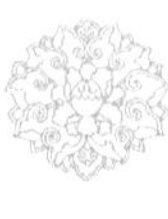

连翘

1. 花枝（flowering stem） 2. 枝条（vimen） 3. 果实（fruit）

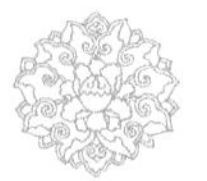

花椒

Huajiao

Zanthoxylum bungeanum

基　　源　芸香科 Rutaceae 花椒属 *Zanthoxylum* 植物花椒 *Zanthoxylum bungeanum* Maxim. 的干燥成熟果皮。药材名为“花椒”。

形态特征　落叶小乔木。茎干上的刺常早落，枝有短刺，当年生枝被短柔毛。叶有小叶 5-13 片，叶轴常有狭窄的叶翼；小叶对生，卵形，椭圆形；位于叶轴顶部的较大，叶缘有细裂齿，齿缝有油点。花序顶生或生于侧枝顶，花序轴常密被短柔毛；花被片 6-8 片，黄绿色。果紫红色，表面散生凸起的油点。种子黑色。

生境分布　分布于我国华北的部分省区，以及华东、华中和西南省区。生于山坡向阳干燥处，各地常见栽培。

采收加工　秋季采收成熟果实，晒干，除去种子和杂质。

性味功能　辛，温。温中止痛，杀虫止痒。

主治用法　用于脘腹冷痛，呕吐泄泻，虫积腹痛；外治湿疹，阴痒。

化学成分　主要含有挥发油类成分，如柠檬烯、1,8- 桉叶素等；另还含有白鲜碱、青椒碱等生物碱类成分，以及香柑内酯、甲氧基香豆素等香豆素类成分。

备　　注　为常用的香辛料。

Source　It is the dried mature pericarp of *Zanthoxylum bungeanum* Maxim. (Rutaceae). The medicinal material is called as “Huajiao”.

Distribution　*Z. bungeanum* is distributed in some provinces of North, East, Central Southwest China. It grows on sunny and dry hillsides. It is cultivated in various places.

Indications　It is used to treat cold pain in the stomach and abdomen, vomiting and diarrhea, and abdominal pain due to parasitic infestation. It is used externally to treat eczema and valual pruritus.

Chemical Constituents　It mainly contains volatile oils, e.g., limonene, 1,8-cineole. It also contains alkaloids (e.g., dictamnine, schinifoline) and coumarins (e.g., bergapten, herniarin).

Note　It is commonly used as spice.

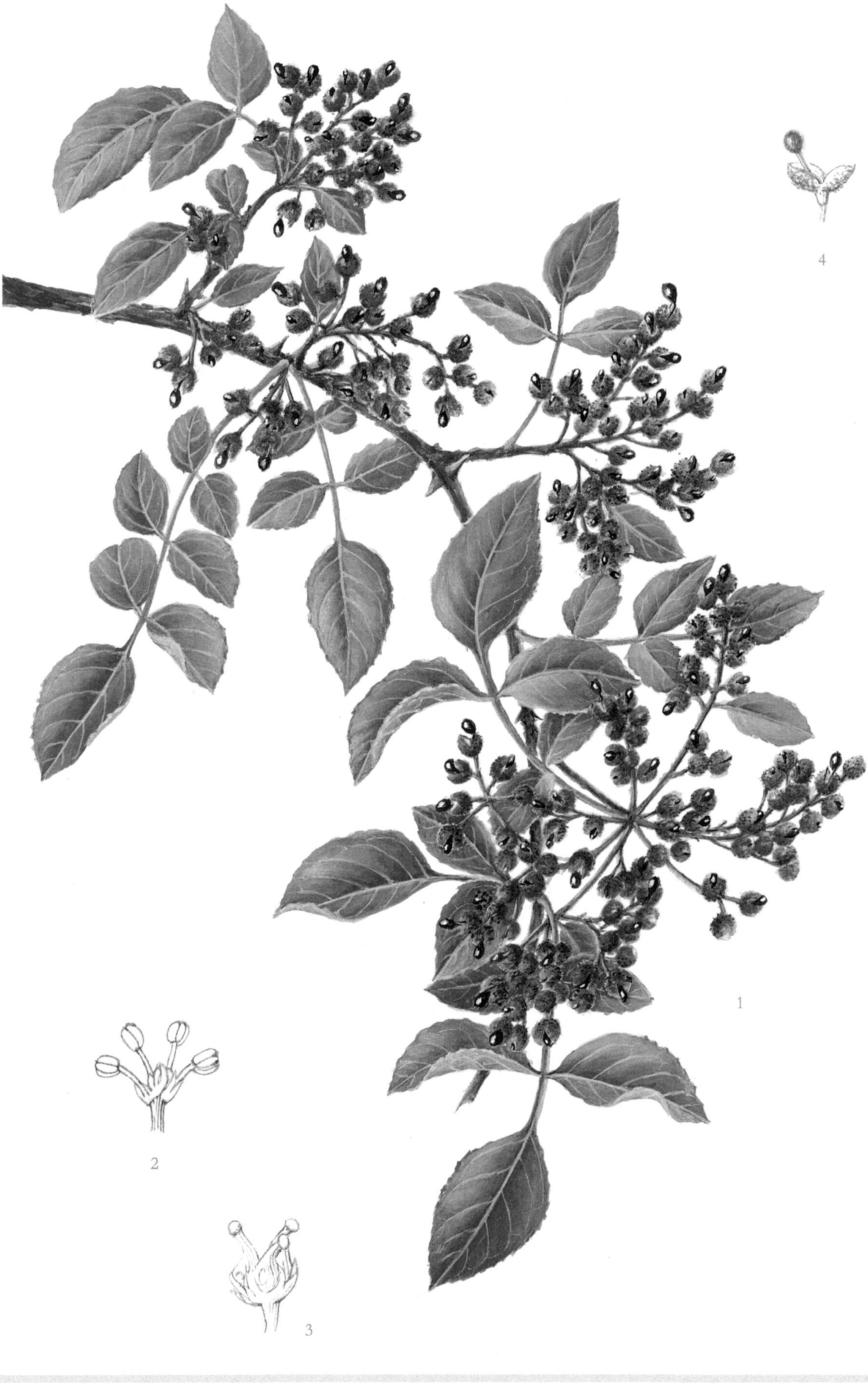

1. 果枝（fruiting stem）　2. 雄蕊（stamen）　3. 雌蕊（pistil）　4. 果实（fruit）

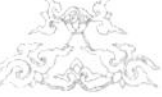

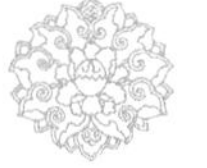

宁夏枸杞

Ningxiagouqi

Lycium barbarum

基　　源　茄科 Solanaceae 枸杞属 *Lycium* 植物宁夏枸杞 *Lycium barbarum* L. 的干燥成熟果实。药材名为“枸杞子”。

形态特征　灌木。分枝细密，有不生叶的短棘刺和生叶、花的长棘刺。叶互生或簇生，披针形或长椭圆状披针形，略带肉质。花在长枝上 1-2 朵生于叶腋，在短枝上 2-6 朵同叶簇生。花萼钟状，通常二中裂；花冠漏斗状，紫堇色，花开放时平展。浆果红色，果皮肉质，椭圆状至近球状。种子略成肾形，扁压，棕黄色。

生境分布　分布于我国华北地区。常生于土层深厚的沟岸、山坡和田埂旁。现宁夏、青海、新疆和天津栽培较广。

采收加工　夏、秋二季果实呈红色时采收，热风烘干，除去果梗，或晾至皮皱后，晒干，除去果梗。

性味功能　平，甘。滋补肝肾，益精明目。

主治用法　主要用于虚劳精亏，腰膝酸痛，眩晕耳鸣，阳萎遗精，内热消渴，血虚萎黄，目昏不明。

化学成分　主要含有多糖类，如枸杞多糖；维生素类，如胡萝卜素、核黄素等；氨基酸类，如天门冬氨酸、苏氨酸、谷氨酸等；另还含有生物碱类等。

备　　注　宁夏枸杞的根皮亦可入药，称“地骨皮”。

Source　It is the dried mature fruit of *Lycium barbarum* L. (Solanaceae). The medicinal material is called as “Gouqizi”.

Distribution　*L. barbarum* is distributed in North China. It commonly grows on the banks, hillsides and ridges of field deep soil layers. It is widely cultivated in Ningxia, Qinghai, Xinjiang, and Tianjin nowaways.

Indications　It is used to treat consumptive disease with damage of essence, soreness and pain of the lower back and knee, vertigo with tinnitus, impotence and seminal emission, internal heat and wasting thirst, shallow yellow due to blood deficiency, and blurred vision.

Chemical Constituents　It mainly contains polysaccharides (e.g., *L. barbarum* polysaccharide), vitamins (e.g., carotene, riboflavin), and amino acids (e.g., aspartic acid, threonine, glumatic acid). It also contains alkaloids, etc.

Note　The root bark can also be used as medicine, known as Cortex Lycii.

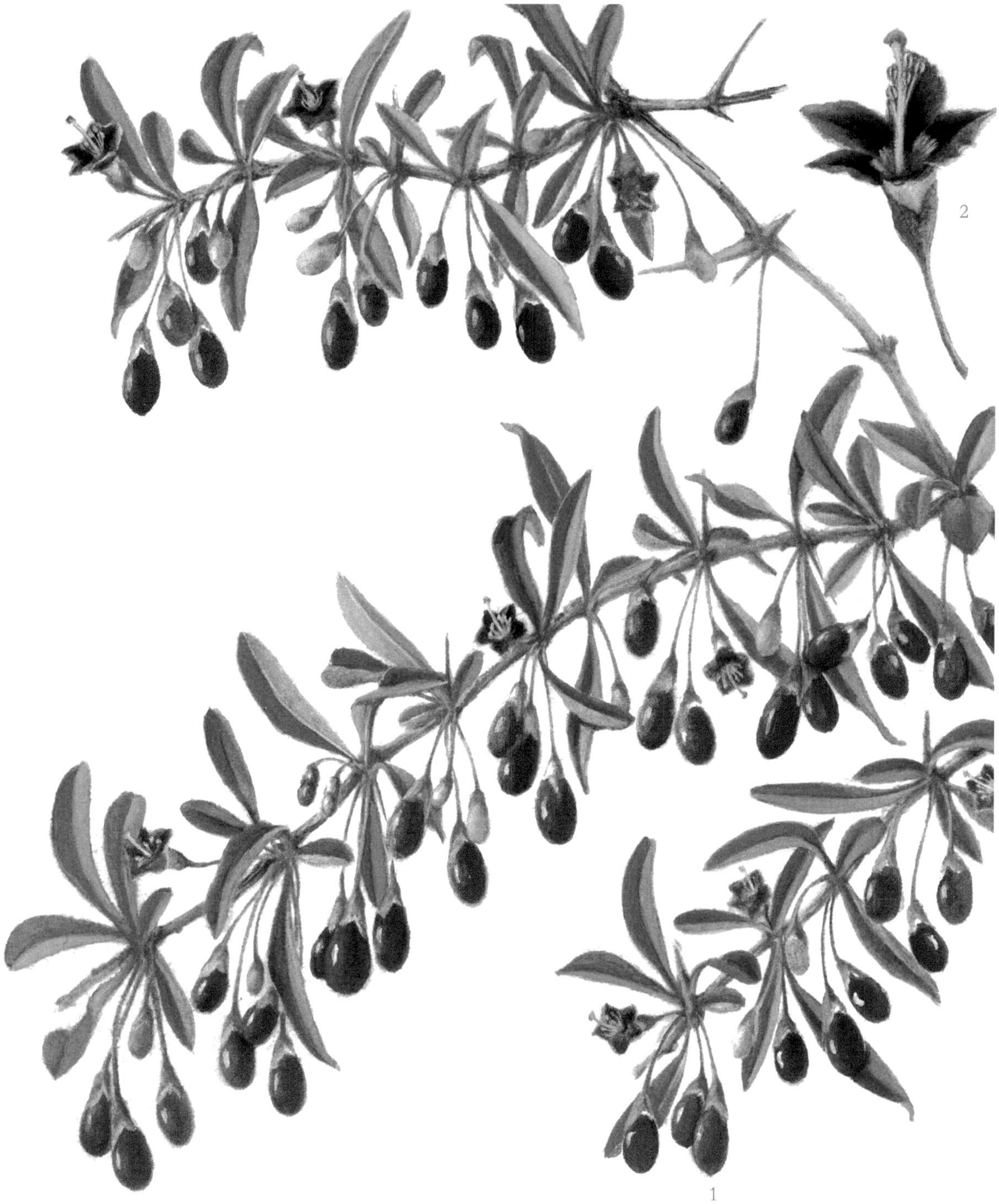

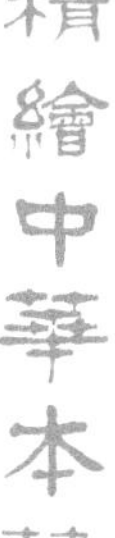

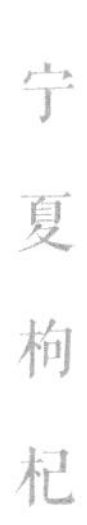

1. 果枝（fruiting stem） 2. 花（flower）

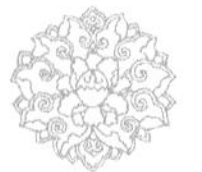

栀子

Zhizi

Gardenia jasminoides

基　源　茜草科 Rubiaceae 栀子属 *Gardenia* 植物栀子 *Gardenia jasminoides* Ellis 的干燥成熟果实。药材名为“栀子”。

形态特征　灌木。叶对生，革质，少为 3 枚轮生，叶形多样，通常为长圆状披针形或椭圆形，上面亮绿，下面色较暗；托叶膜质。花芳香，通常单朵生于枝顶，萼檐结果时增长，宿存；花冠白色或乳黄色，高脚碟状。果实长卵形或长圆形，黄色或橙红色，有翅状纵棱 5-9 条；种子多数，扁，近圆形而稍有棱角。

生境分布　分布于我国中南、西南以及东南部分省区。常生于丘陵山地和山坡灌丛中。

采收加工　9-11 月果实成熟呈红黄色时采收，除去果梗和杂质，蒸至上气或置沸水中略烫，取出，干燥。

性味功能　寒，苦。泻火除烦，清热利湿，凉血解毒；外用消肿止痛。

主治用法　主要用于热病心烦，湿热黄疸，淋证涩痛，血热吐衄，目赤肿痛，火毒疮疡；外治扭挫伤痛。

化学成分　主要含有环烯醚萜类，如栀子苷、异羟栀子苷、山栀子苷、栀子酮苷等；有机酸类，如奎宁酸、绿原酸等；挥发油类，如棕榈酸、丹皮酚等；黄酮类，如栀子素等；三萜类，如栀子花酸等；另还含有多糖、胆碱、熊果酸、D- 甘露醇等。

Source　It is the dried mature fruit of *Gardenia jasminoides* Ellis (Rubiaceae). The medicinal material is called as “Zhizi”.

Distribution　*G. jasminoides* is distributed in some provinces of south central, southwest and southeast China. It commonly grows in shrubs on hilly mountains and hillside.

Indications　It is used to treat vexation due to febrile disease, jaundice due to dampness–heat, strangury, hematemesis and epistaxis due to heat in blood, difficult and painful urination, hematemesis and epistaxis due to heat in blood, red eyes with swelling and pain, sore and ulcer due to fire-toxin. It can be applied externally for twist and contusion.

Chemical Constituents　It mainly contains iridoids (e.g., gardenoside, geniposide, shanzhiside, gardoside), organic acid (e.g., quinic acid, chlorogenic acid), volatile oils (e.g., palmitic acid, paeonol), flavonoids (e.g., gardenin), and triterpenoids (e.g., gradenolic acid). It also contains polysaccharides, choline, ursolic acid, D-manitol, etc.

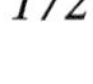

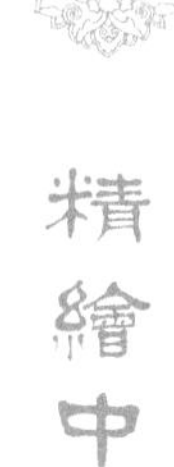

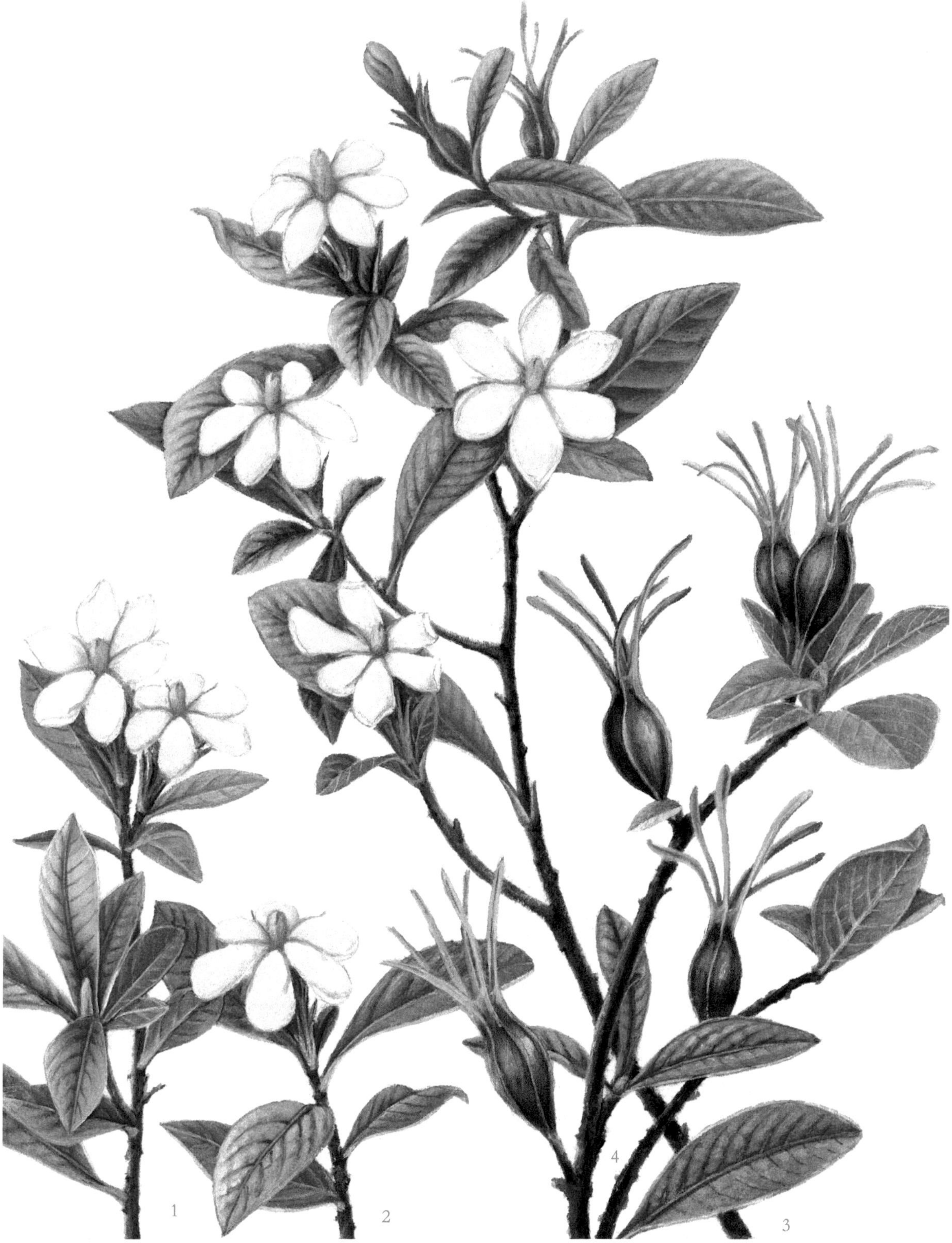

1～3. 花枝（flowering stem） 4. 果枝（fruiting stem）

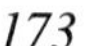

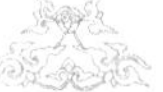

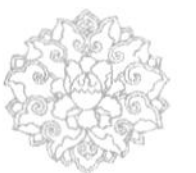

沙棘

Shaji

Hippophae rhamnoides

基　　源　胡颓子科 Elaeagnaceae 沙棘属 *Hippophae* 植物沙棘 *Hippophae rhamnoides* L. 的干燥成熟果实。药材名为“沙棘”。

形态特征　落叶灌木或乔木，棘刺较多。嫩枝密被银白色而带褐色鳞片。单叶通常近对生，纸质，狭披针形或矩圆状披针形，上面绿色，初被白色盾形毛或星状柔毛，下面银白色或淡白色，被鳞片。果实圆球形，橙黄色或橘红色。种子小，阔椭圆形至卵形，有时稍扁，黑色，有光泽。

生境分布　分布于华北、西北部分省区，黄土高原常见。常生于海拔 800-3600 m 的多砾石的向阳山坡或干涸的河床上。

采收加工　秋、冬二季果实成熟或冻硬时采收，除去杂质，干燥或蒸后干燥。

性味功能　温，酸、涩。健脾消食，止咳祛痰，活血散瘀。

主治用法　用于脾虚食少，食积腹痛，咳嗽痰多，胸痹心痛，瘀血经闭，跌扑瘀肿。

化学成分　主要含有黄酮、甾醇、类胡萝卜素、脂肪酸、维生素等成分。

备　　注　蒙古族、藏族习用药材。

Source　It is the dried mature fruit of *Hippophae rhamnoides* L. (Elaeagnaceae). The medicinal material is called as “Shaji”.

Distribution　*H. rhamnoides* is distributed in some provinces of North China and Northwest China, commonly found in Loess Plateau. It commonly grows on the hillside with gravel and sun exposure or dry riverbed at an altitude of 800–3600 m.

Indications　It is used to treat spleen deficiency with decreased food intake, food accumulation and abdominal pain, cough with profuse sputum, heart pain due to chest impediment, static blood and amenorrhea, and stasis with swelling caused by traumatic injury.

Chemical Constituents　It mainly contains flavonoids, sterols, carotenoids, fatty acids, vitamins, etc.

Note　It is commonly used by the Mongols and Tibetans.

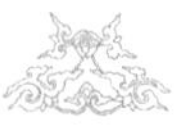

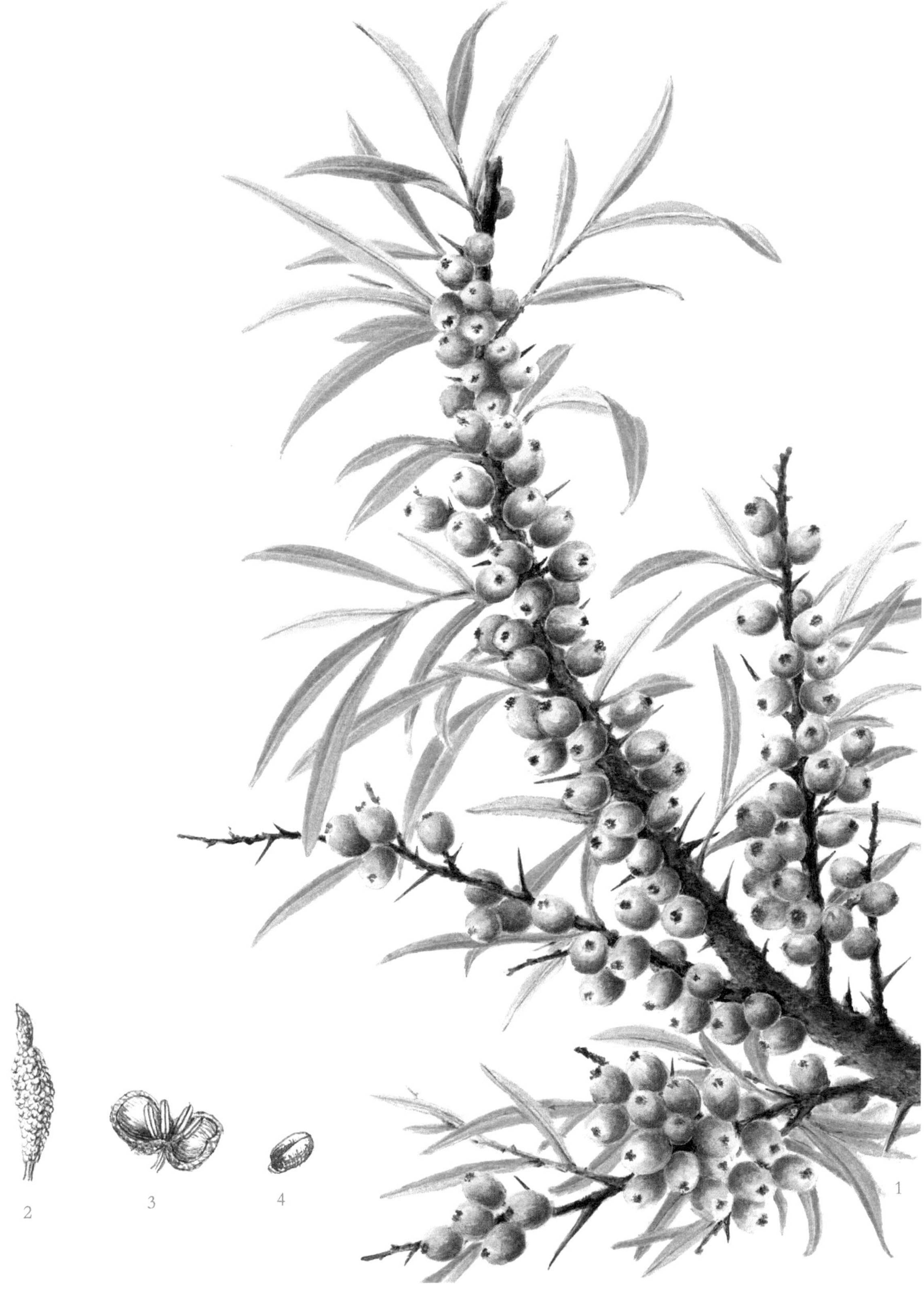

1. 果枝（fruiting stem） 2. 雌花（female flower） 3. 雄花（male flower） 4. 种子（seed）

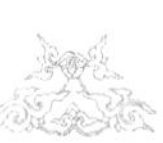

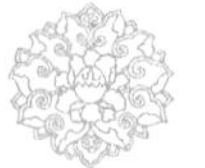

大高良姜

Dagaoliangjiang
Alpinia galanga

基　　源　姜科 Zingiberaceae 山姜属 *Alpinia* 植物大高良姜 *Alpinia galanga* (L.) Willd. 的干燥成熟果实。药材名为“红豆蔻”。

形态特征　多年生草本。根状茎有香气。叶片长圆形或披针形，顶端渐尖，基部渐狭，两面均无毛或叶背被长柔毛；叶柄短；叶舌近圆形。圆锥花序，花序轴被毛，分枝多，每一分枝上有花 3-6 朵；花绿白色，有异味；侧生退化雄蕊细齿状至线形，紫色；唇瓣倒卵状匙形，白色而有红线条，深二裂。果长圆形，熟时棕色。种子 3-6 粒。

生境分布　分布于我国广东、广西、云南、台湾等地。常见生于海拔 100-1300 m 的山谷溪边。

采收加工　秋季果实变红时采收，除去杂质，阴干。

性味功能　温，辛。散寒燥湿，醒脾消食。

主治用法　主要用于脘腹冷痛，食积胀满，呕吐泄泻，饮酒过多。

化学成分　主要含有挥发油类成分，如桂皮酸甲酯、樟脑等。

备　　注　大高良姜的根状茎亦可入药，可温胃止呕，散寒止痛。

Source　It is the dried mature fruit of *Alpinia galanga* (L.) Willd. (Zingiberaceae). The medicinal material is called as “Hongdoukou”.

Distribution　*A. galanga* is distributed in Guangdong, Guangxi, Yunnan and Chinese Taiwan, etc. It commonly grows beside streams in the valley at an altitude of 100–1300 m.

Indications　It is used to treat cold pain in the stomach and abdomen, food accumulation with abdominal distention and fullness, vomiting and diarrhea, excessive liquor consumption.

Chemical Constituents　It mainly contains volatile oils, e.g., methyl cinnamate, camphor.

Note　The rhizome can also be used as medicine, which has the function of warming the stomach and alleviating vomiting, and dissipating cold to kill pain.

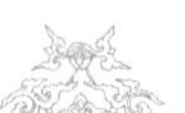

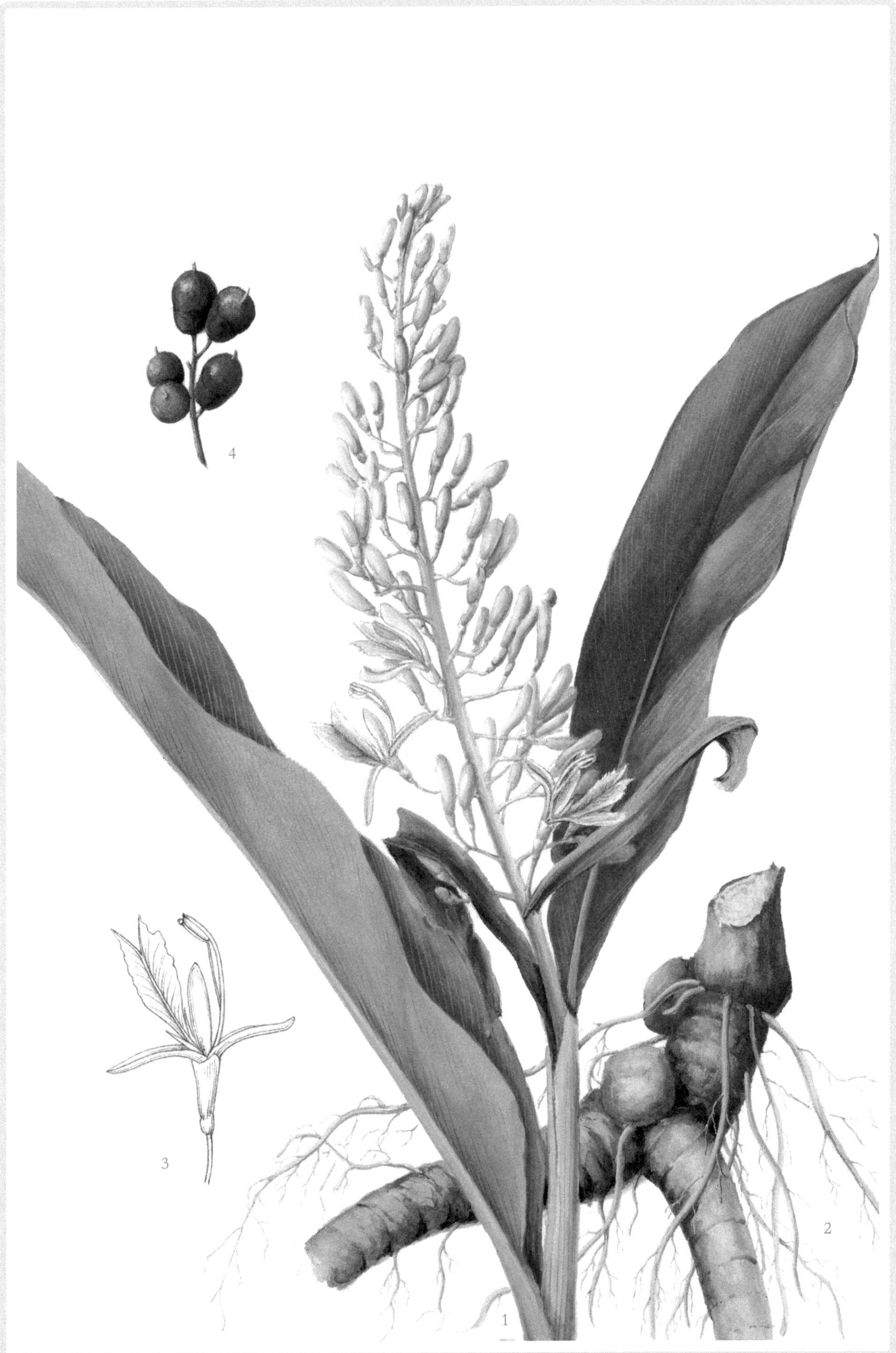

1. 花枝（flowering stem） 2. 根状茎（rhizome） 3. 花（flower） 4. 果实（fruit）

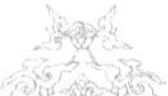

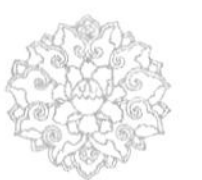

草豆蔻

Caodoukou

Alpinia katsumadai

基　　源　姜科 Zingiberaceae 山姜属 *Alpinia* 植物草豆蔻 *Alpinia katsumadai* Hayata 的干燥近成熟种子。药材名为“草豆蔻”。

形态特征　多年生草本。叶片狭椭圆形，有缘毛，两面近无毛。总状花序顶生，直立，花序轴密被粗毛；小苞片乳白色，阔椭圆形；花萼钟状，白色；花冠白色，裂片 3，长圆形，上方裂片较大，先端二浅裂，边缘具缺刻，前部具红黑色条纹，后部具淡紫红色斑点。蒴果近圆形，外被粗毛，熟时黄色。

生境分布　分布于广东、广西和海南。生于山地密林中。

采收加工　夏、秋二季采收，晒至九成干，或用水略烫，晒至半干，除去果皮，取出种子团，晒干。

性味功能　温，辛。燥湿行气，温中止呕。

主治用法　用于寒湿内阻，脘腹胀满冷痛，嗳气呕逆，不思饮食。

化学成分　主要含有挥发油类成分，如反 - 桂皮醛、桉叶素、芳樟醇等；另还含有山奈酚、熊竹素、山姜素、乔松素、小豆蔻明、桤木酮等。

备　　注　为常用的香辛料。

Source　It is the dried nearly mature seed of *Alpinia katsumadai* Hayata (Zingiberaceae). The medicinal material is called as “Caodoukou”.

Distribution　*A. katsumadai* is distributed in Guangdong, Guangxi and Hainan. It grows in dense mountainous forests.

Indications　It is used to treat internal obstruction by cold–dampness, abdominal fullness and distention with cold pain, belching and vomiting, and loss of appetite.

Chemical Constituents　It mainly contains volatile oils, e.g., *trans*-cinnamaldehyde, cineole, linalool. It also contains kaempferol, kumatakenin, alpinetin, pinocembrin, cardamonin, alnustone, etc.

Note　It is a commonly-used spice.

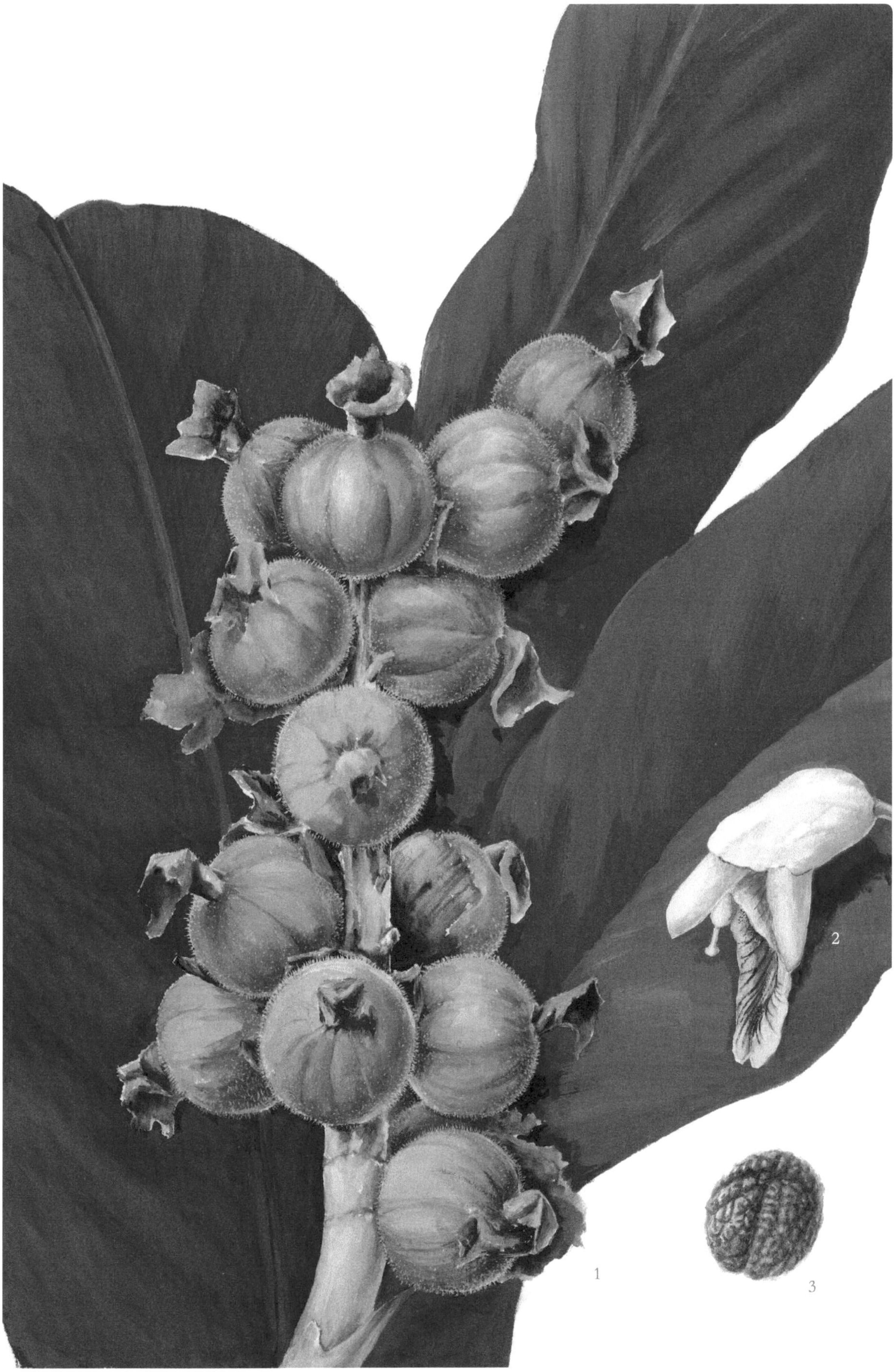

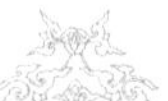

1. 果枝（fruiting stem）　2. 花（flower）　3. 种子（seed）

益智

Yizhi

Alpinia oxyphylla

基　源　姜科 Zingiberaceae 山姜属 *Alpinia* 植物益智 *Alpinia oxyphylla* Miq. 的干燥成熟果实。药材名为“益智”。

形态特征　多年生草本。茎丛生。根茎短。叶片披针形，顶端渐狭，具尾尖；叶柄短；叶舌膜质，二裂。总状花序包于一帽状总苞中，总苞花时脱落；花萼筒状，一侧开裂，先端具三齿裂；花冠裂片长圆形，后方 1 枚稍大，白色；唇瓣倒卵形，粉白色具红纹，先端皱波状。蒴果球形，有条纹。种子扁圆形，被淡黄色假种皮。

生境分布　分布于广东、广西、海南，常生于山林阴湿处。现多栽培。

采收加工　夏、秋间果实由绿变红时采收，晒干或低温干燥。

性味功能　辛，温。暖肾固精缩尿，温脾止泻摄唾。

主治用法　主要用于肾虚遗尿，小便频数，遗精白浊，脾寒泄泻，腹中冷痛，口多唾涎。

化学成分　主要含有桉油精、4- 萜品烯醇、α - 桉叶醇等挥发油类；以及氨基酸类、脂肪酸类、黄酮类，另含有益智酮甲、益智酮乙、益智醇等成分。

Source　It is the dried mature fruit of *Alpinia oxyphylla* Miq. (Zingiberaceae). The medicinal material is called as “Yizhi”.

Distribution　*A. oxyphylla* is distributed in Guangdong, Guangxi and Hainan. It commonly grows in shady and damp mountain forests. It is commonly cultivated nowdays.

Indications　It is used to treat enuresis due to deficiency in the kidney, frequent urination, seminal emission with gonorrhea, spleen cold and diarrhea, cold pain in the abdomen and excessive saliva.

Chemical Constituents　It mainly contains volatile oils (e.g., eucalyptol, 4-terpineol, α-eudesmol), amino acids, fatty acids, flavonoids, yakuchinone A, yakuchinone B, oxyphyllacinol, etc.

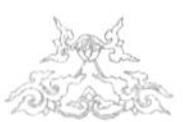

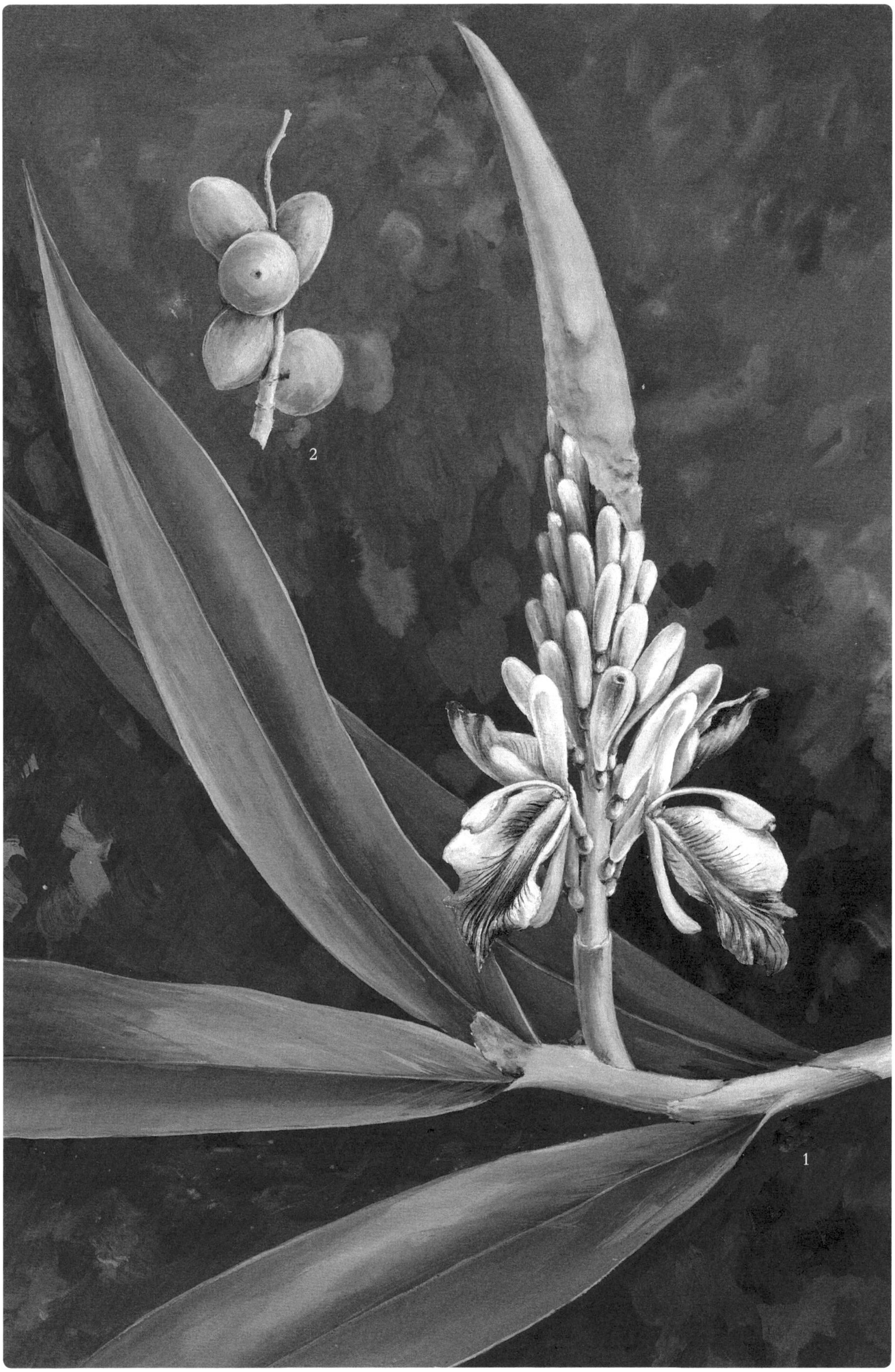

益智

1. 花枝（flowering stem） 2. 果序（infructescence）

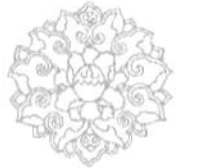

爪哇白豆蔻

Zhaowabaidoukou

Amomum compactum

基　　源　姜科 Zingiberaceae 豆蔻属 *Amomum* 植物爪哇白豆蔻 *Amomum compactum* Soland ex Maton 的干燥成熟果实。药材名为“白豆蔻”，习称“印尼白蔻”。

形态特征　多年生草本。根茎延长。茎基叶鞘红色。叶片披针形，顶端尾尖，具缘毛；叶舌二裂，圆形。穗状花序；苞片长圆形，具纵条纹及缘毛，宿存；花萼管与花冠管等长，被毛；花冠近白色，裂片长圆形；唇瓣椭圆形，淡黄色，中脉有带紫边的橘红色带，被毛。果扁球形，干时具 9 条棱槽，被疏长毛。种子为不规则多面体。

生境分布　原产印度尼西亚，我国海南、云南有栽培。生长于肥沃、潮湿的热带林下。

采收加工　果实成熟时，剪下果穗，晒干或烤干。

性味功能　温，辛。化湿行气，温中止呕，开胃消食。

主治用法　主要用于湿浊中阻，不思饮食，湿温初起，胸闷不饥，寒湿呕逆，胸腹胀痛，食积不消。后下。

化学成分　种子含有挥发油类成分，如 1,8- 桉叶油素、葛缕酮、α - 蒎烯、芳樟醇、香桧烯、月桂烯、月桂烯醇、柠檬烯、樟脑、龙脑等。

Source　It is the dried mature fruit of *Amomum compactum* Soland ex Maton (Zingiberaceae). The medicinal material is called as “Baidoukou”.

Distribution　*A. compactum* is native to Indonesia. It is also cultivated in Hainan and Yunnan, China. It grows in fertile and humid tropical forests.

Indications　It is used to treat dampness retained in the middle-jiao, loss of appetite, onset of dampness–warm, stuffiness in the chest and no hunger, vomiting due to cold–dampness, distention and pain in the chest and abdomen, food accumulation with indigestion. It should be decocted later.

Chemical Constituents　The seed contains volatile oils, e.g., 1,8-eucalyptol, carvone, α-pinene, linalool, sabinene, myrcene, myrcenol, limonene, camphor, borneol, etc.

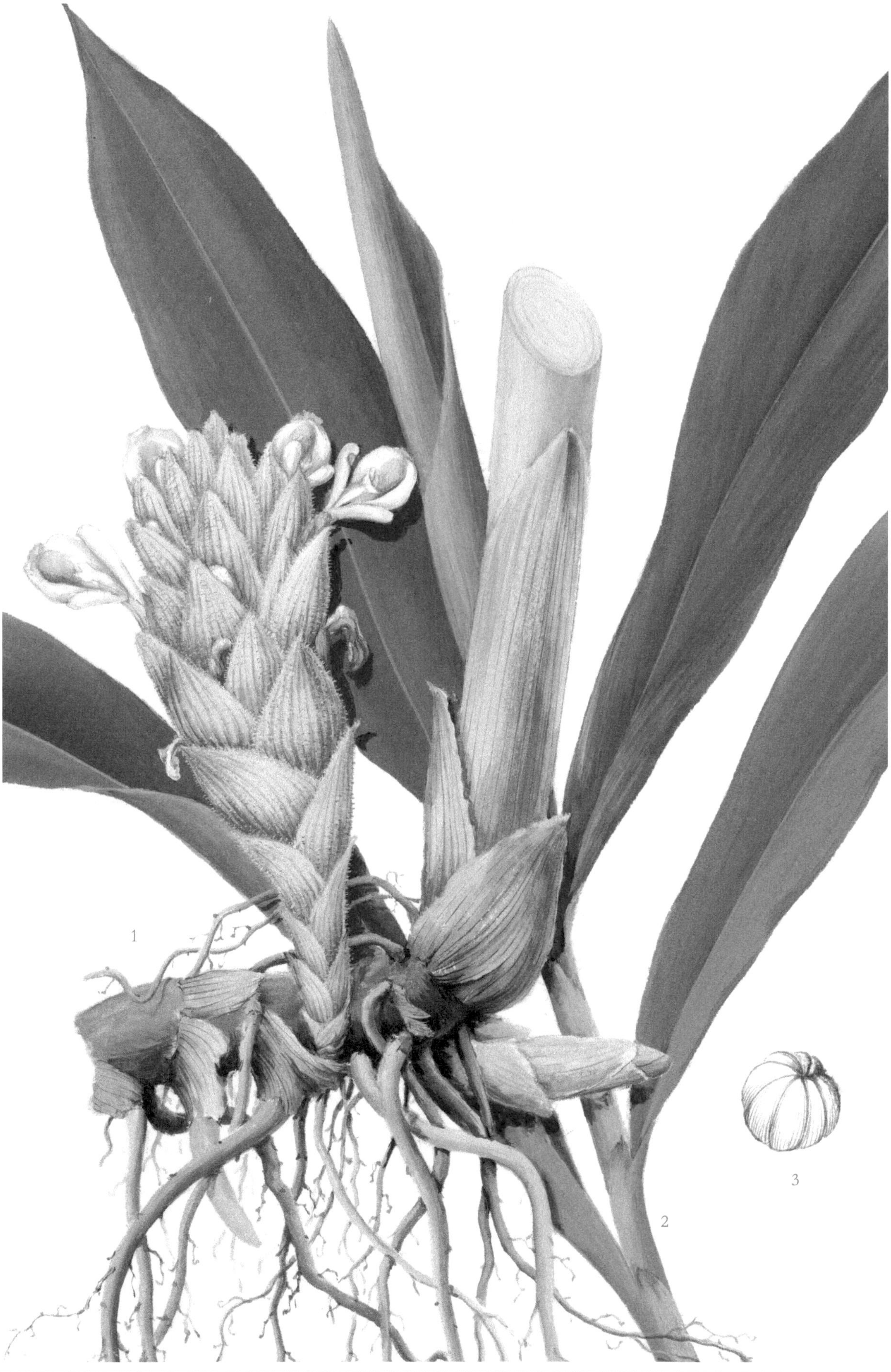

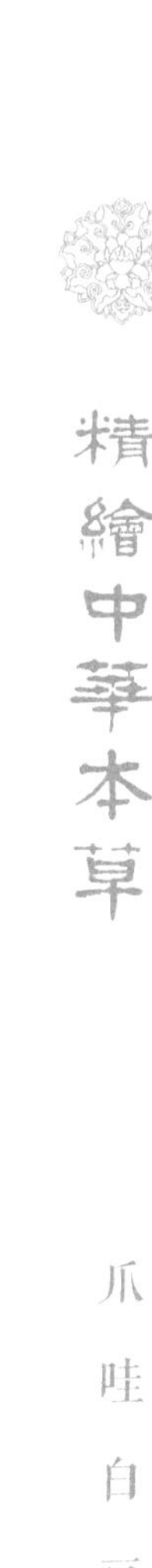

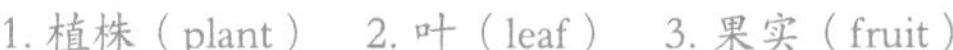
1. 植株（plant） 2. 叶（leaf） 3. 果实（fruit）

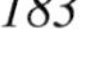

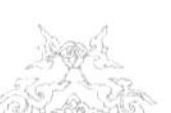

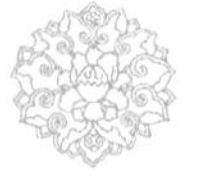

阳春砂

Yangchunsha

Amomum villosum

基　　源　姜科 Zingiberaceae 豆蔻属 *Amomum* 植物阳春砂 *Amomum villosum* Lour. 的干燥成熟果实。药材名为“砂仁”。

形态特征　多年生草本。根茎匍匐地面。叶片长披针形至线形，顶端尾尖；叶舌半圆形；叶鞘上有方格状网纹。穗状花序椭圆形，被褐色短绒毛；花萼管顶端具三浅齿，白色；花冠管裂片倒卵形，白色；唇瓣圆匙形，白色，顶端具黄色的小尖头，中脉凸起，基部具 2 个紫色斑点。蒴果椭圆形，紫红色，被柔刺。种子多角形。

生境分布　分布于福建、广东、广西、云南。生于山林阴湿处。现多栽培。道地药材产自广东阳春。

采收加工　夏、秋二季果实成熟时采收，晒干或低温干燥。

性味功能　温，辛。化湿开胃，温脾止泻，理气安胎。

主治用法　主要用于湿浊中阻、脘痞不饥、脾胃虚寒、呕吐泄泻、妊娠恶阻、胎动不安。后下。

化学成分　种仁含有挥发油类，如乙酰龙脑酯、樟脑、柠檬烯、樟烯、α - 蒎烯、β - 蒎烯、龙脑、月桂烯、α - 水芹烯、芳樟醇、金合欢烯、棕榈酸等。

备　　注　为常用的香辛料。

Source　It is the dried mature fruit of *Amomum villosum* Lour. (Zingiberaceae). The medicinal material is called as “Sharen”.

Distribution　*A. villosum* is distributed in Fujian, Guangdong, Guangxi and Yunnan. It grows in shady and damp mountain forests. It is commonly cultivated nowday. Authentic medicinal materials are produced in Yangchun, Guangdong.

Indications　It is used to treat dampness retained in the middlejiao, stomach stuffiness with loss of appetite, deficiency-cold of spleen and stomach, vomiting and diarrhea, morning sickness, and threatened abortion. It should be decocted later.

Chemical Constituents　The kernel contains volatile oils, e.g., bornyl acetate, camphor, limonene, camphene, α-pinene, β-pinene, borneol, myrcene, α-phellandrene, linalool, farnesene, palmitic acid, etc.

Note　It is a commonly-used spice.

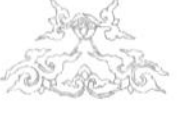

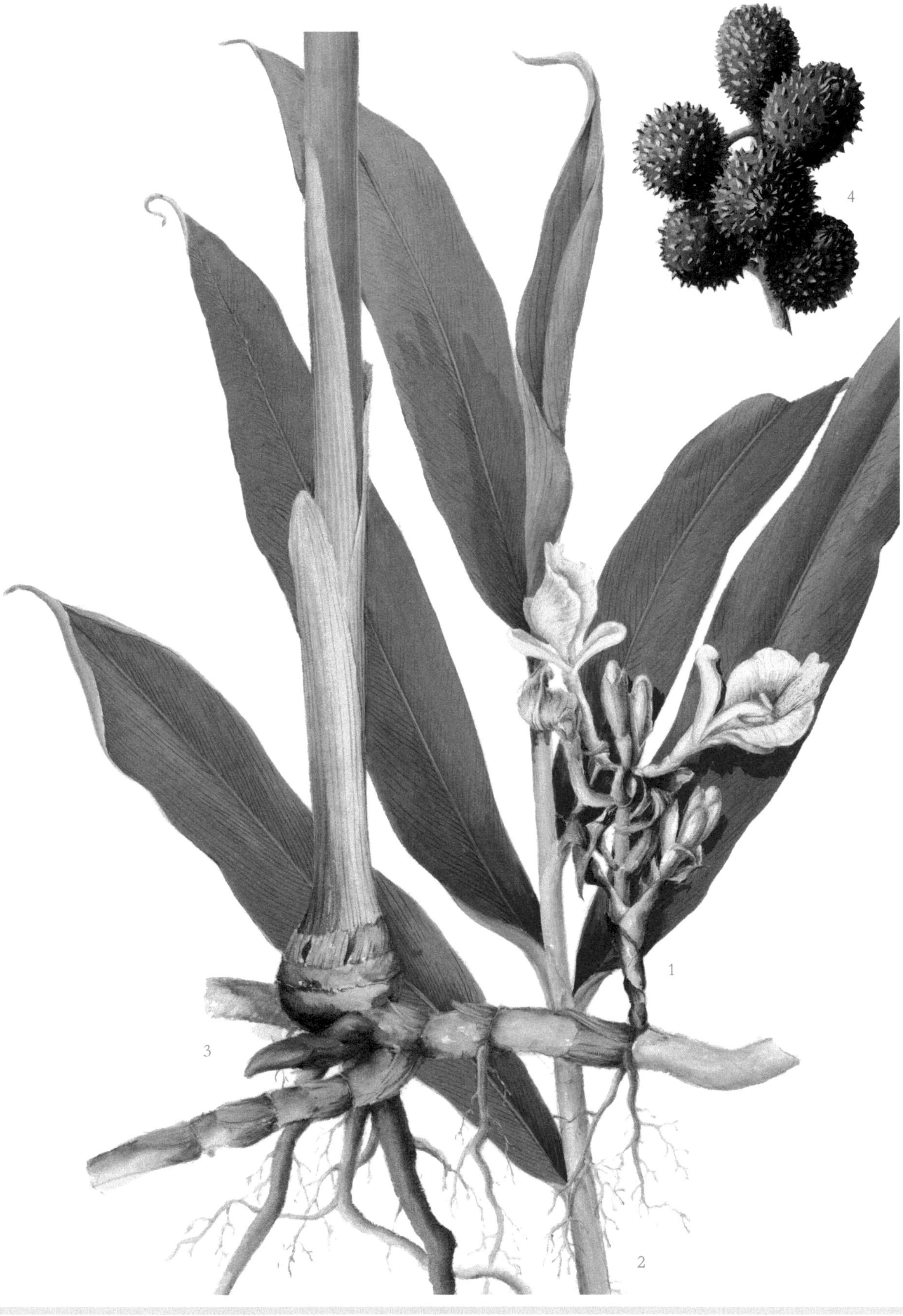

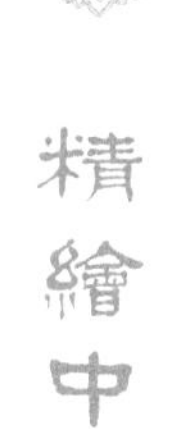

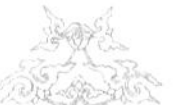

1. 花序（inflorescence） 2. 叶（leaf） 3. 根及根状茎（root and rhizome） 4. 果序（infructescence）

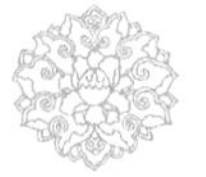

红草果

Hongcaoguo

Amomum hongtsaoko

基　源　姜科 Zingiberaceae 豆蔻属 *Amomum* 植物红草果 *Amomum hongtsaoko* C. F. Liang et D. Fang, 的干燥成熟果实。药材名为“红草果”。

形态特征　多年生草本。植株高大。叶片长圆状披针形至卵形；叶舌带紫色，叶舌及叶鞘边缘近革质。穗状花序柱状长卵形；苞片淡红色，长圆形；花浅橙色；花萼三齿裂，一侧浅裂；花冠管裂片长圆形，后方的一枚较大，兜状；唇瓣长圆状倒卵形，边缘多皱褶，中脉两侧各有一条红色条纹。蒴果成熟时暗紫色，近球形。种子多数。

生境分布　分布于广西南部，生于山沟边林下。

采收加工　秋季果实成熟时采收，除去杂质，晒干或低温干燥。

性味功能　温，辛。燥湿温中，截疟除痰。

主治用法　主要用于寒湿内阻，脘腹胀痛，痞满呕吐，疟疾寒热，瘟疫发热。

化学成分　主要含有挥发油类成分，如 α - 蒎烯、β - 蒎烯、芳樟醇、橙花叔醇、橙花醛、香叶醇等。

Source　It is the dried mature fruit of *Amomum hongtsaoko* C. F. Liang et D. Fang. (Zingiberaceae). The medicinal material is called as “Hongcaoguo”.

Distribution　*A. hongtsaoko* is distributed in the south of Guangxi. It grows under the beside ravines in the forests.

Indications　It is used to treat internal obstruction by cold–dampness, distention and pain in stomach forests and abdomen, stuffiness and fullness with vomiting, alternating chills and fever due to malaria, and fever due to pestilence.

Chemical Constituents　It mainly contains volatile oils, e.g., α-pinene, β-pinene, linalool, nerolidol, citral, geraniol, etc.

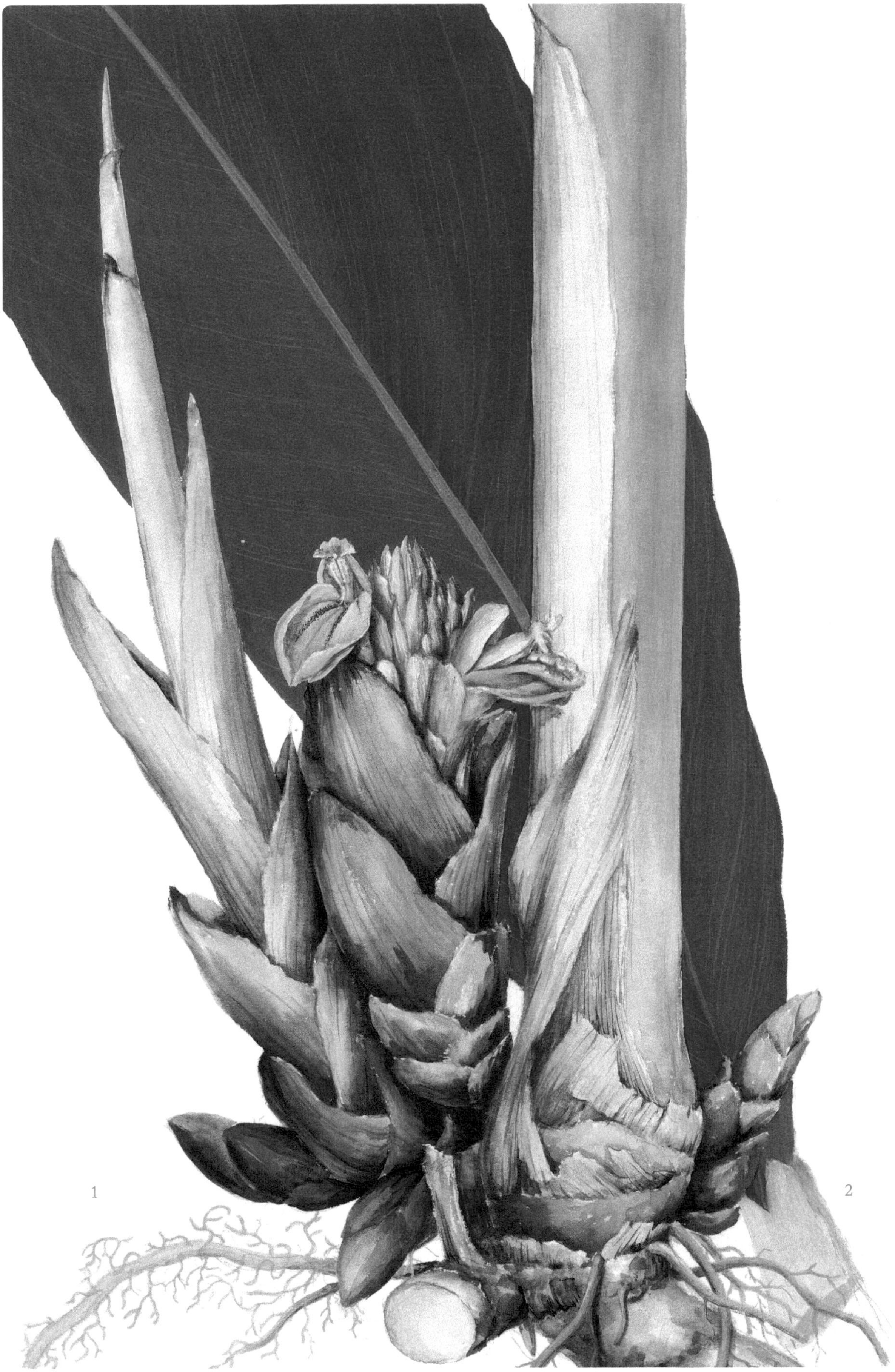

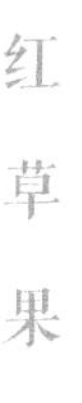

1

2

1. 植株（plant） 2. 叶（leaf）

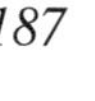

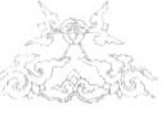

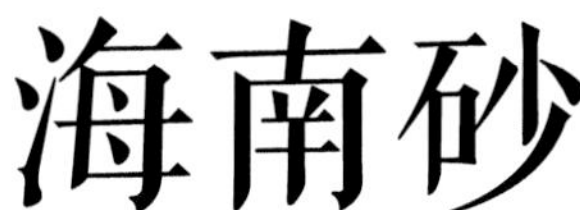

海南砂

Hainansha

Amomum longiligulare

基　　源　姜科 Zingiberaceae 豆蔻属 *Amomum* 植物海南砂 *Amomum longiligulare* T. L. Wu 的干燥成熟果实。药材名为“砂仁”。

形态特征　多年生草本。叶片线状披针形，顶端具尾尖，基部渐狭，两面无毛；叶舌披针形，长 2-4.5cm，薄膜质。总花梗被宿存鳞片；萼管白色，顶端三齿裂；花冠管较萼管略长，裂片长圆形；唇瓣圆匙形，白色，顶端具突出、二裂的黄色尖头，中脉隆起，紫色。蒴果卵圆形，具钝三棱，被短柔刺。种子紫褐色，被膜质假种皮。

生境分布　分布于海南，现广东、海南大量栽培。生于山谷密林下。

采收加工　夏、秋二季果实成熟时采收，晒干或低温干燥。

性味功能　温，辛。化湿开胃，温脾止泻，理气安胎。

主治用法　主要用于湿浊中阻，脘痞不饥，脾胃虚寒，呕吐泄泻，妊娠恶阻，胎动不安。后下。

化学成分　主要含有樟脑、龙脑、乙酸龙脑酯、柠檬烯等挥发油类成分；另还含有黄酮类成分。

备　　注　为常用的香辛料。

Source　It is the dried mature fruit of *Amomum longiligulare* T. L. Wu (Zingiberaceae). The medicinal material is called as “Sharen”.

Distribution　*A. longiligulare* is distributed in Hainan. It is cultivated in large amounts in Guangdong and Hainan nowdays. It grows on the floor of dense forest in the valley.

Indications　It is used to treat dampness retained in the middlejiao, stomach stuffiness with loss of appetite, deficiency-cold of spleen and stomach, vomiting and diarrhea, morning sickness, and threatened abortion. It should be decocted later.

Chemical Constituents　It mainly contains camphor, borneol, bornyl acetate, limonene and other volatile oils. It also contains flavonoids.

Note　It is a commonly-used spice.

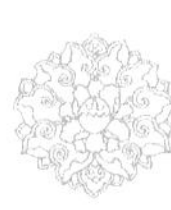

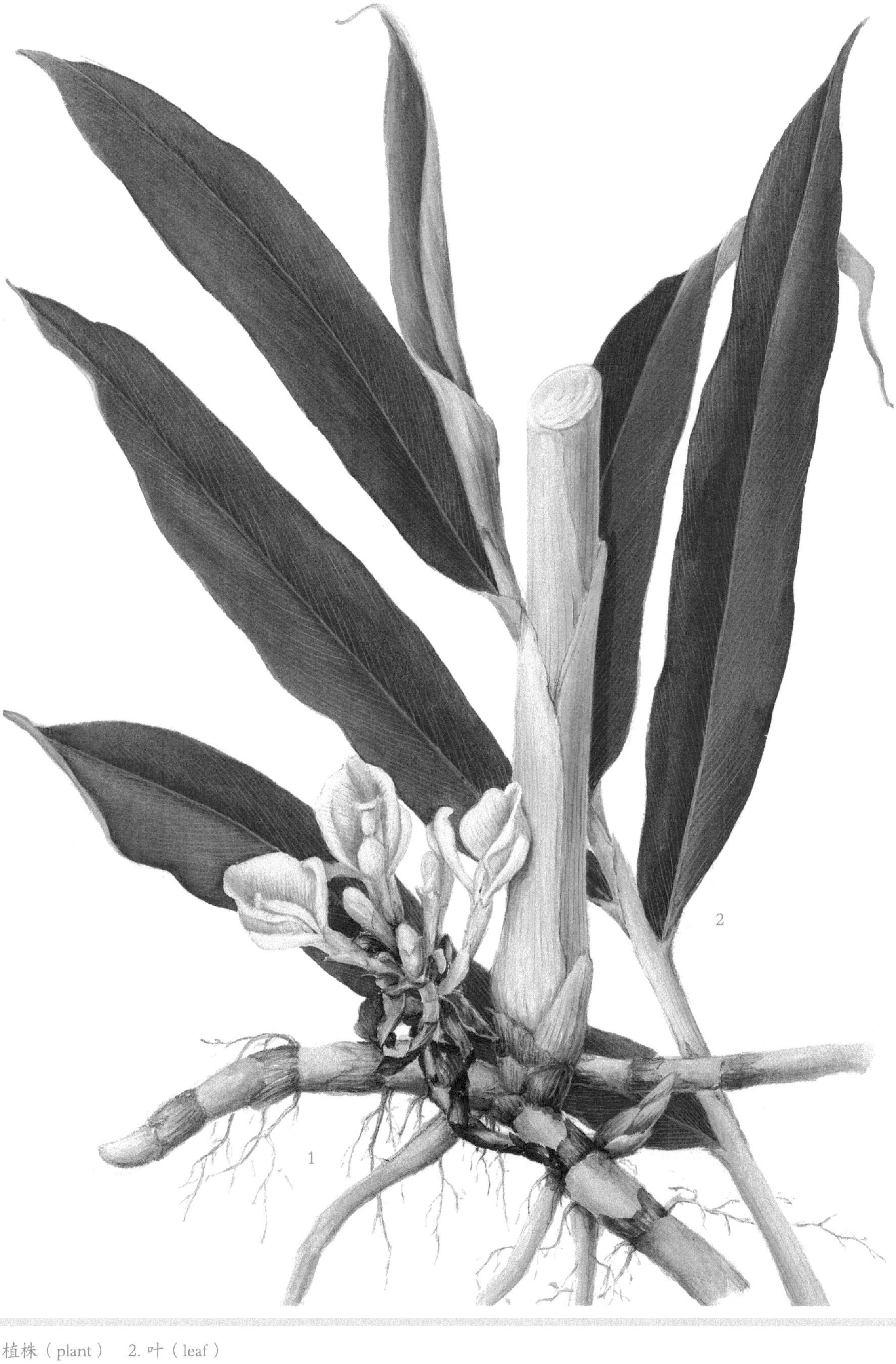

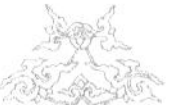

1. 植株（plant） 2. 叶（leaf）

水飞蓟

Shuifeiji

Silybum marianum

基　源　菊科 Asteraceae 水飞蓟属 *Silybum* 植物水飞蓟 *Silybum marianum* (L.) Gaertn. 的干燥成熟果实。药材名为“水飞蓟”。

形态特征　一年生或二年生草本。茎直立，覆白粉，被稀疏的蛛丝毛。莲座状基生叶与下部茎叶有叶柄，中部与上部茎叶渐小，羽状浅裂或羽状深裂，半抱茎，最上部叶披针形，心形抱茎。叶绿色，具大型白色花斑，边缘及顶端有坚硬的黄色针刺。头状花序多个，生枝端；小花红紫色，少有白色。瘦果压扁，长椭圆形，褐色。冠毛多层，刚毛状，白色。

生境分布　原产于南欧至北非，现华北和西北地区有栽培。生于通风、干燥和向阳的荒地或盐碱地。

采收加工　秋季果实成熟时采收果序，晒干，打下果实，除去杂质，晒干。

性味功能　凉，苦。清热解毒，疏肝利胆。

主治用法　主要用于肝胆湿热，胁痛，黄疸。供配制成药用。

化学成分　主要含有黄酮类，如槲皮素、二氢山奈酚等；甾醇类，如豆甾醇、菜油甾醇、胆甾醇等；有机酸类，如油酸、亚油酸、亚麻酸等；另还含有水飞蓟宾、次水飞蓟宾、氨基酸等。

Source　It is the dried mature fruit of *Silybum marianum* (L.) Gaertn. (Asteraceae). The medicinal material is called as “Shuifeiji”.

Distribution　*S. marianum* is native from Southern Europe to North Africa. It is cultivated in North and Northwest China nowdays. It grows in ventilated, dry wasteland or alkalized land with sun esposure.

Indications　It is used to treat dampness-heat in liver and gallbladder, hypochondriac pain, and jaundice. Dosage form formulation is usually seen.

Chemical Constituents　It mainly contains flavonoids (e.g., quercetin, dihydrokaempferol) sterols (e.g., stigmasterol, campesterol, cholesterol), and organic acids (e.g., oleic acid, linoleic acid, linolenic acid). It also contains isosilybin, silybin, amino acids, etc.

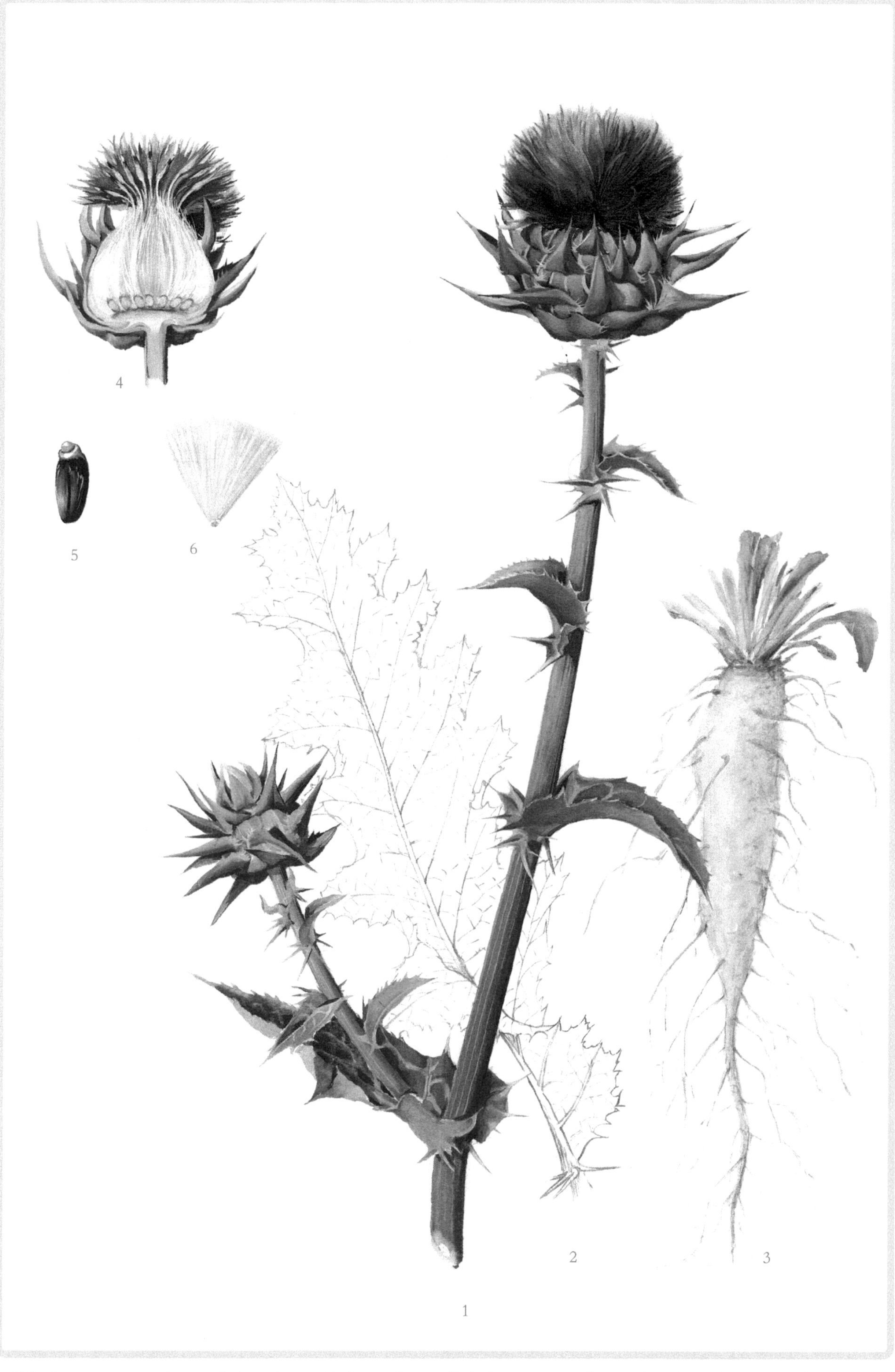

1. 花枝（flowering stem） 2. 叶（leaf） 3. 根（root） 4. 花序（inflorescence） 5. 种子（seed） 6. 冠毛（aigret）

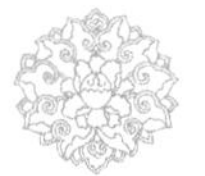

木鳖子

Mubiezi

Momordica cochinchinensis

基　　源　葫芦科 Cucurbitaceae 苦瓜属 *Momordica* 植物木鳖子 *Momordica cochinchinensis* (Lour.) Spreng. 的干燥成熟种子。药材名为“木鳖子”。

形态特征　藤本。根块状。叶柄粗壮；叶片卵状心形，3-5 中裂至深裂，基部心形。卷须粗壮，不分歧。雌雄异株；雄花顶端生一苞片；花萼筒漏斗状；花冠黄色，裂片卵状长圆形；雌花近中部生一苞片，形同雄花。果实卵球形，成熟时红色，密生具刺尖的突起。种子多数，卵形，边缘有齿，两面稍拱起，具雕纹。

生境分布　分布于我国华东、华南、西南诸省。常生于海拔 500-1000 m 的潮湿山沟及林缘。

采收加工　冬季采收成熟果实，剖开，晒至半干，除去果肉，取出种子，干燥。

性味功能　凉，苦、微甘；有毒。散结消肿，攻毒疗疮。

主治用法　主要用于疮疡肿毒，乳痈，瘰疬，痔瘘，干癣，秃疮。

化学成分　主要含有木鳖子皂苷、木鳖子定等皂苷类，以及木鳖糖蛋白、α - 菠菜甾醇、木鳖子酸、木鳖子素等。

Source　It is the dried mature seed of *Momordica cochinchinensis* (Lour.) Spreng. (Cucurbitaceae). The medicinal material is called as “Mubiezi”.

Distribution　*M. cochinchinensis* is distributed in East China, South China, and Southwest China. It commonly grows in the damp ravines and forest edges at an altitude of about 500–1000 m.

Indications　It is used to treat sore and ulcer and pyogenic toxin, acute mastitis, scrofula, hemorrhoid and fistula, tinea, and sore on baid scalp.

Chemical Constituents　It mainly contains saponins (e.g., momordica saponin, momordin), momorcochin, α-chondrillasterol, momordic acid, cochinchinin, etc.

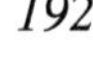

木鳖子

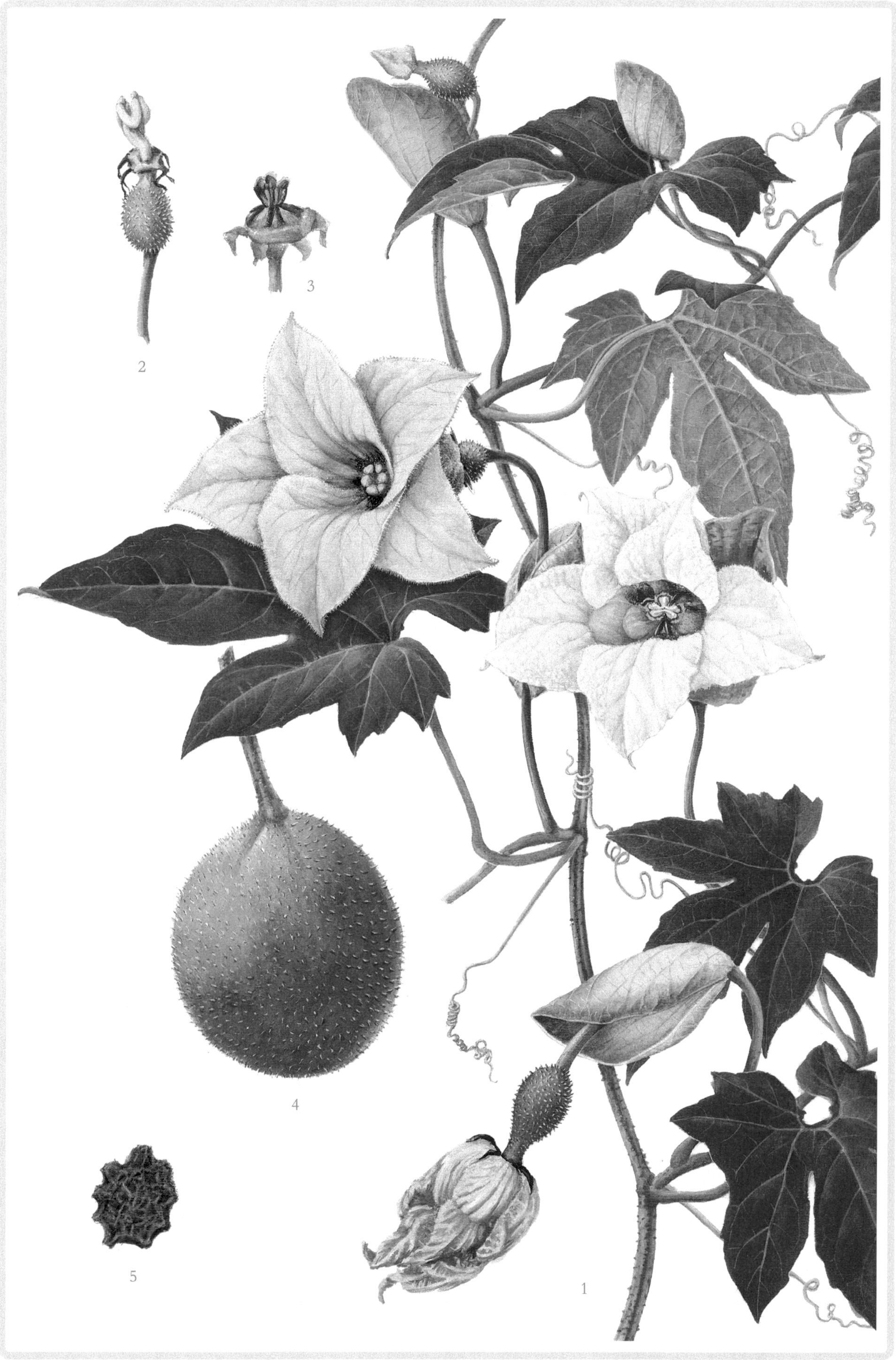

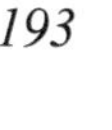

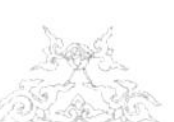

1. 花枝（flowering stem） 2. 雌蕊（pistil） 3. 雄蕊（stamen） 4. 果实（fruit） 5. 种子（seed）

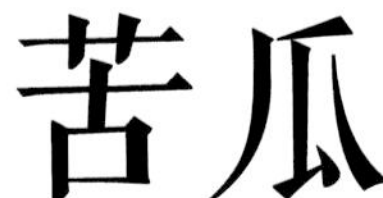

苦瓜

Kugua

Momordica charantia

基　　源　葫芦科 Cucurbitaceae 苦瓜属 *Momordica* 植物苦瓜 *Momordica charantia* L. 的干燥果实。药材名为“苦瓜”。

形态特征　一年生攀援草本。卷须不分枝。叶大，肾状圆形，通常 5-7 深裂，裂片卵状椭圆形，基部收缩，边缘具波状齿。花雌雄同株。雄花单生，有柄，中部或基部有苞片；花萼钟形，五裂；花冠黄色，五裂，裂片卵状椭圆形。雌花单生，基部有苞片。果实长椭圆形，具瘤状突起，成熟时橘黄色，自顶端 3 瓣开裂。

生境分布　全国各地均有栽培。

采收加工　秋季采收果实，切片晒干。

性味功能　寒，苦。清暑涤热，明目，解毒。

主治用法　主要用于暑热烦渴，消渴，赤眼疼痛，痢疾，疮痈肿毒。

化学成分　果实含有生物碱、皂苷、多肽、维生素和矿物质等多种成分。

备　　注　果实可供食用。

Source　It is the dried fruit of *Momordica charantia* L. (Cucurbitaceae). The medicinal materials is called as “Kugua”.

Distribution　*M. charantia* is cultivated all over China.

Indications　It is used to treat extreme thirst with summer-heat, wasting thirst, red eyes with pain, dysentery, sore, swollen welling-abscess, and toxin.

Chemical Constituents　The fruit contains alkaloids, saponins, polypeptides, vitamins and minerals, etc.

Note　The fruit is edible.

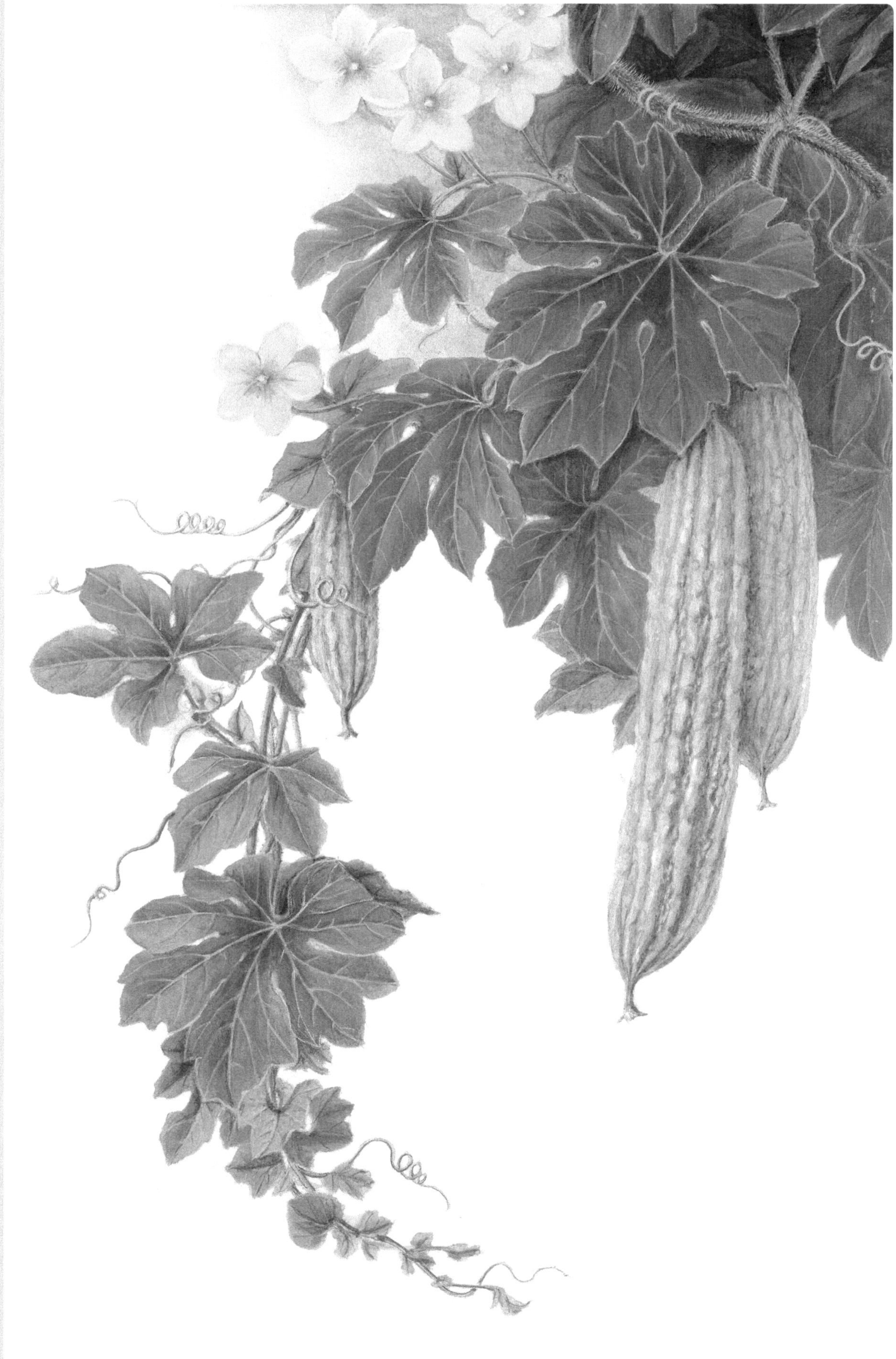

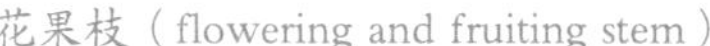

花果枝（flowering and fruiting stem）

罗汉果

Luohanguo

Siraitia grosvenorii

基　　源　葫芦科 Cucurbitaceae 罗汉果属 *Siraitia* 植物罗汉果 *Siraitia grosvenorii* (Swingle) C. Jeffrey ex Lu et Z. Y. Zhang 的干燥果实。药材名为“罗汉果”。

形态特征　攀援草本。根肥大。茎、枝粗壮，有棱沟。叶片膜质，卵形心形，先端渐尖，基部心形，弯缺半圆形，边缘微波状，有缘毛；卷须稍粗壮，2 歧，在分叉点上下同时旋卷。雌雄异株。雄花序总状；花冠黄色，被黑色腺点；雌花单生或 2-5 朵集生于总梗顶端，花萼和花冠比雄花大。果实球形，成熟时在果梗着生处残存一圈茸毛。种子多数，淡黄色，近圆形或阔卵形，扁压状。

生境分布　分布于广西、贵州、湖南南部、广东和江西。常生于海拔 400-1400 m 的山坡林下、河边湿地、灌丛。广西作为重要药用植物栽培。

采收加工　秋季果实由嫩绿色变深绿色时采收，晾数天后，低温干燥。

性味功能　凉，甘。清热润肺，利咽开音，滑肠通便。

主治用法　主要用于肺热燥咳，咽痛失音，肠燥便秘。

化学成分　主要含有罗汉果皂苷，罗汉果皂苷作为罗汉果甜味剂的主要成分。另外还含有果糖、氨基酸、黄酮等。

备　　注　本品常作为凉茶配方的主要用料。

Source　It is the dried fruit of *Siraitia grosvenorii* (Swingle) C. Jeffrey ex Lu et Z. Y. Zhang (Cucurbitaceae). The medicinal material is called as “Luohanguo”.

Distribution　*S. grosvenorii* is distributed in Guangxi, Guizhou, southern Hunan, Guangdong, and Jiangxi. It commonly grows on hillside forests, riverside wetland, and shrub at an altitude of 400–1400 m. It is an important medicinal plant which cultiated in Guangxi.

Indications　It is used to treat irritating dry cough due to lung heat, sore throat and loss of voice, intestinal dryness with constipation.

Chemical Constituents　It mainly contains mogroside, which is the main sweetening agent. It also contains fructose, amino acids, flavonoids, etc.

Note　It is often used as a main material in cool herbal tea.

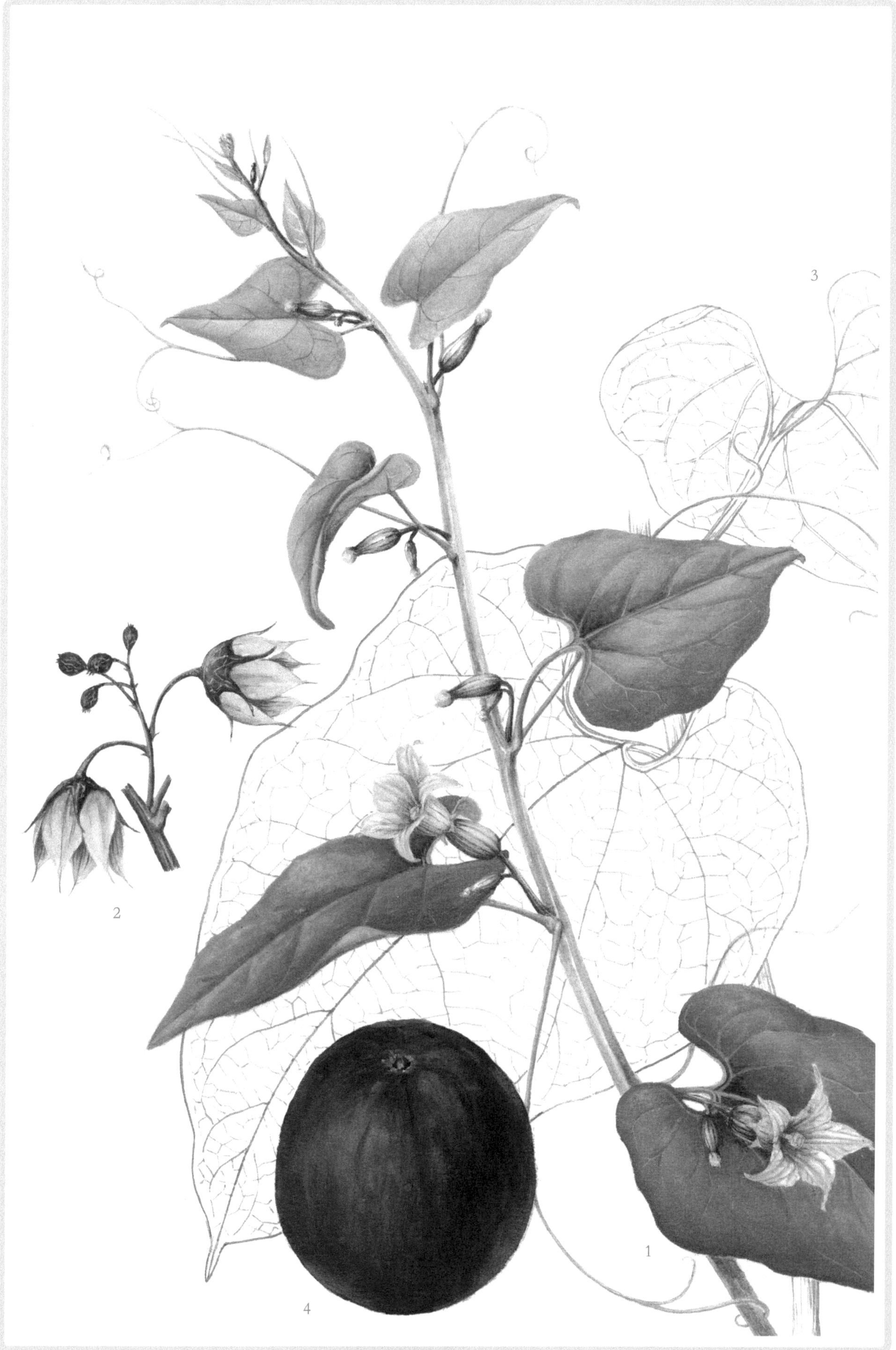

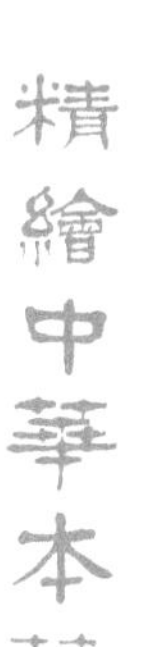

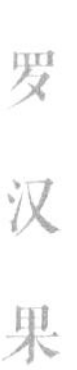

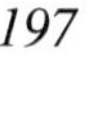

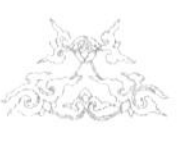

1. 花枝（flowering stem） 2. 花序（inflorescence） 3. 叶（leaf） 4. 果实（fruit）

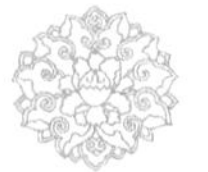

番木瓜

Fanmugua

Carica papaya

基　源　番木瓜科 Caricaceae 番木瓜属 *Carica* 植物番木瓜 *Carica papaya* L. 干燥果实。药材名为“番木瓜”。

形态特征　软木质常绿小乔木。茎具粗大的叶痕。叶大，圆形，常 5-9 深裂，裂片再为羽状分裂；叶柄中空。花乳黄色，单性异株或杂性，雄花序下垂状圆锥花序，雌花序及杂性花序为聚伞花序；雄花萼绿色，基部连合；雌蕊具短梗，萼片绿色；花瓣乳黄色，长圆形至披针形。浆果长圆形，成熟时橙黄色。种子多数，黑色。

生境分布　原产南美洲。我国南方大部分省区已广泛栽培。

采收加工　夏、秋二季采收成熟果实，鲜用或切片晒干。

性味功能　平，甘。消食下乳，除湿通络，解毒驱虫。

主治用法　用于消化不良，胃、十二指肠溃疡疼痛，乳汁稀少，风湿痹痛，肢体麻木，湿疹，烂疮，肠道寄生虫病。

化学成分　果实中含有番木瓜碱、木瓜蛋白酶、凝乳酶等；淡黄色的果实中含有隐黄素、蝴蝶梅黄素等色素；红色的果实中含有西红柿烃；种子中含有异硫氰酸苄酯、番木瓜苷等。

Source　It is the dried fruit of *Carica papaya* L. (Caricaceae). The medicinal material is called as “Fanmugua”.

Distribution　*C. papaya* is native to South America. It is widely cultivated in most provinces of southern China.

Indications　It is used to treat indigestion, gastric and duodenal ulcer pain, hypogalactia, wind–dampness impediment pain, numbness of the limbs, eczema, rotten sore, and intestinal parasitic disease.

Chemical Constituents　The fruit contains capaine, papain, chymosin, etc. The light yellow fruit contains crypotoflavine, violaxanthin and other pigments. The red fruit contains lycopene. The seed contains benzyl isothiocyanate, carposide, etc.

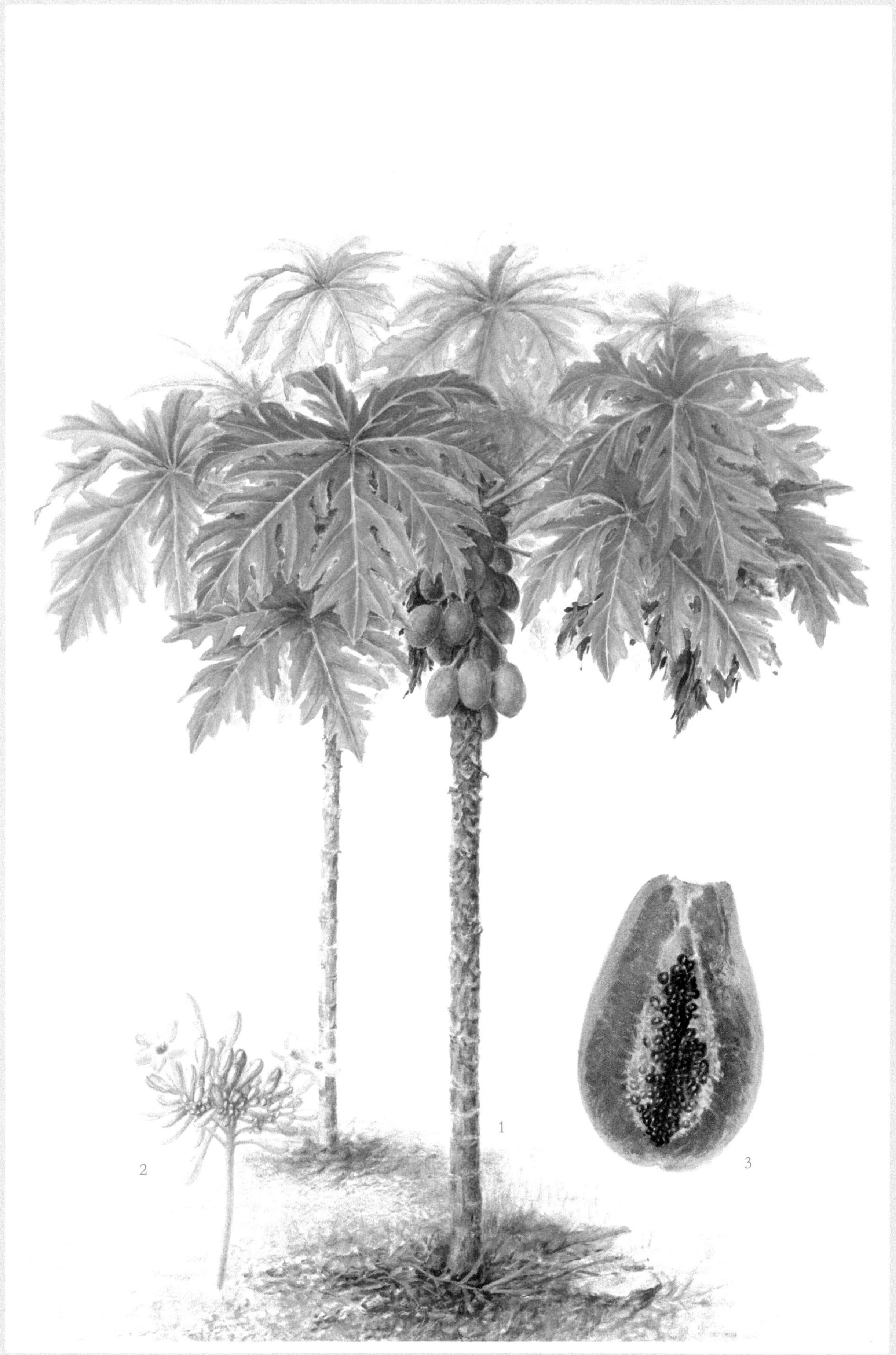

1

2

3

1. 植株（plant） 2. 花序（inflorescence） 3. 果实（fruit）

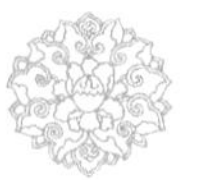

蒺藜

Jili

Tribulus terrestris

基　　源　蒺藜科 Zygophyllaceae 蒺藜属 *Tribulus* 植物蒺藜 *Tribulus terrestris* L. 的干燥成熟果实。药材名为“蒺藜”。

形态特征　一年生草本。茎平卧，无毛，被长硬毛。偶数羽状复叶；小叶对生，3-8 对，矩圆形或斜短圆形，先端锐尖或钝，基部稍偏斜，被柔毛，全缘。花腋生，花梗短于叶；花黄色，萼片 5，宿存；花瓣 5。果有分果瓣 5，硬，中部边缘有锐刺 2 枚，下部常有小锐刺 2 枚，其余部位常有小瘤体。

生境分布　分布于全国各地。常生于沙地、荒地、路旁、村落边等。

采收加工　秋季果实成熟时采割植株，晒干，打下果实，除去杂质。

性味功能　微温，辛、苦；有小毒。平肝解郁，活血祛风，明目，止痒。

主治用法　用于头痛眩晕，胸胁胀痛，乳闭乳痈，目赤翳障，风疹瘙痒。

化学成分　主要含有皂苷类，其苷元为薯蓣皂苷元、海可皂苷元和鲁期可皂甙元等。另含有蒺藜甙、山柰酚 -3- 芸香糖甙、紫云英甙和哈尔满碱等成分。

Source　It is the dried mature fruit of *Tribulus terrestris* L. (Zygophyllaceae). The medicinal material is called as “Jili”.

Distribution　*T. terrestris* is distributed all over China. It commonly grows in sandy lands, wastelands, roadsides, villages, etc.

Indications　It is used to treat headache and dizziness, distending pain in the chest and hypochondrium, duct ectasia and acute mastitis, red eye, nebula, vision obstruction, and itch due to rubella.

Chemical Constituents　It mainly contains saponins, and the aglycones are diosgenin, hecogenin, ruscogenin, etc. It also contains tribuloside, kaempferol-3-rutinoside, astragalin, harmane, etc.

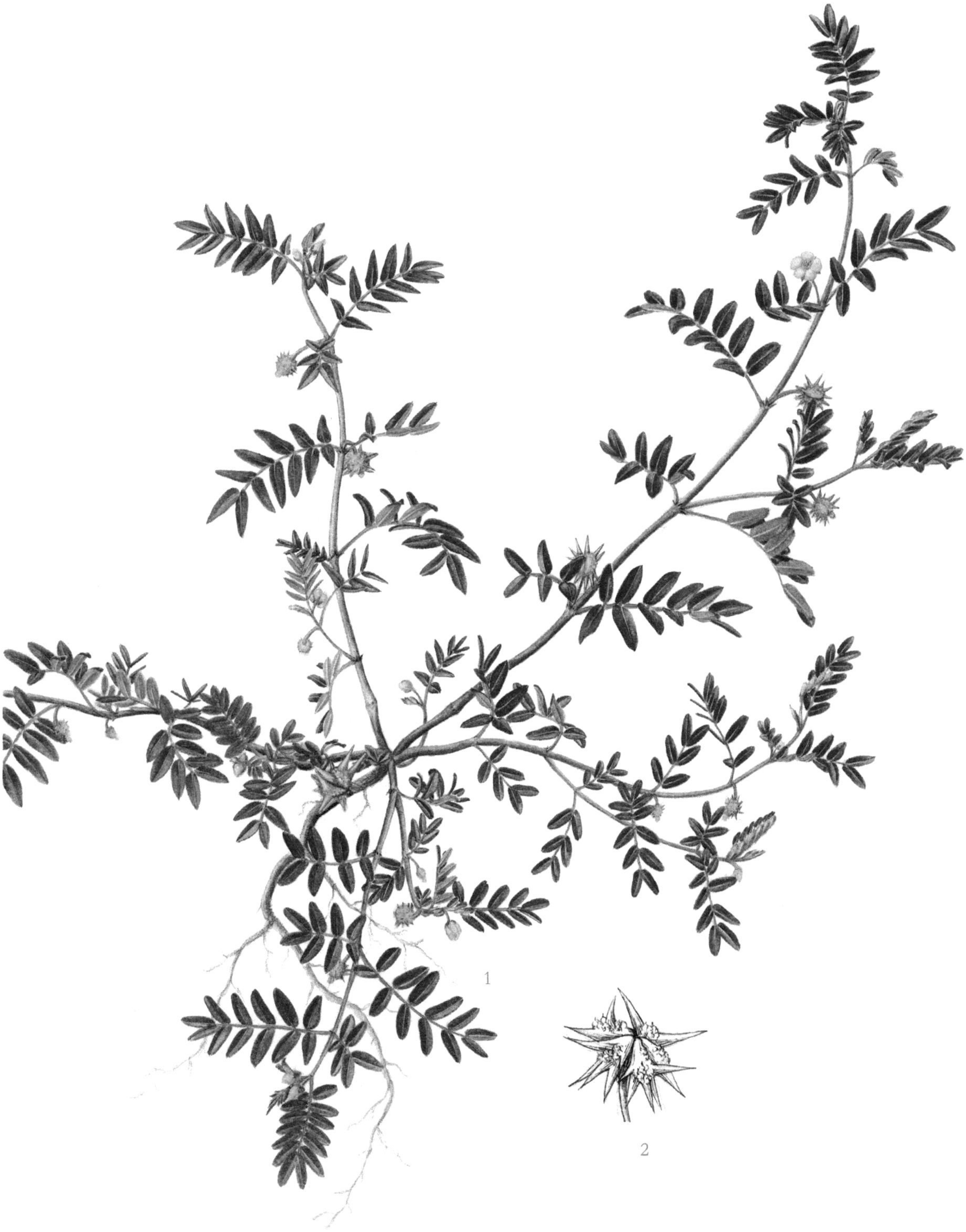

蒺藜

1. 植株（plant） 2. 果实（fruit）

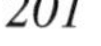

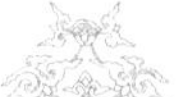

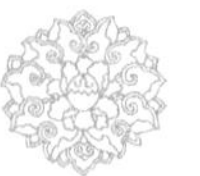

棉花

Mianhua

Gossypium hirsutum

基　源　锦葵科Malvaceae棉属*Gossypium*植物棉花*Gossypium hirsutum* L.种子上的棉毛。药材名为“棉花”。

形态特征　一年生草本。小枝疏被长毛。叶阔卵形，直径5-12cm，长、宽近相等，基部心形或心状截头形，常3浅裂，裂片宽三角状卵形。花单生于叶腋，小苞片3，分离，基部心形，被长硬毛和纤毛；花萼杯状，裂片5，三角形，具缘毛；花白色或淡黄色，后变淡红色或紫色。蒴果卵圆形；种子卵圆形，具白色长棉毛和灰白色的短棉毛。

生境分布　全国各省区均有栽培。原产墨西哥。

采收加工　秋季采收，晒干。

性味功能　温，甘。止血。

主治用法　可用于吐血，便血，血崩，出血。

化学成分　种子毛主要含纤维素、蜡、脂肪。

Source　It is the linter on seeds of *Gossypium hirsutum* L. (Malvaceae). The medicinal material is called as “Mianhua”.

Distribution　*G. hirsutum* is cultivated in many provinces of China. It is native to United Mexican States.

Indications　It is used to treat hematemesis, bloody stool, metrorrhagia, and bleeding.

Chemical Constituents　The seed hair mainly contains cellulose, wax and fat.

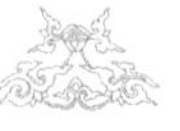

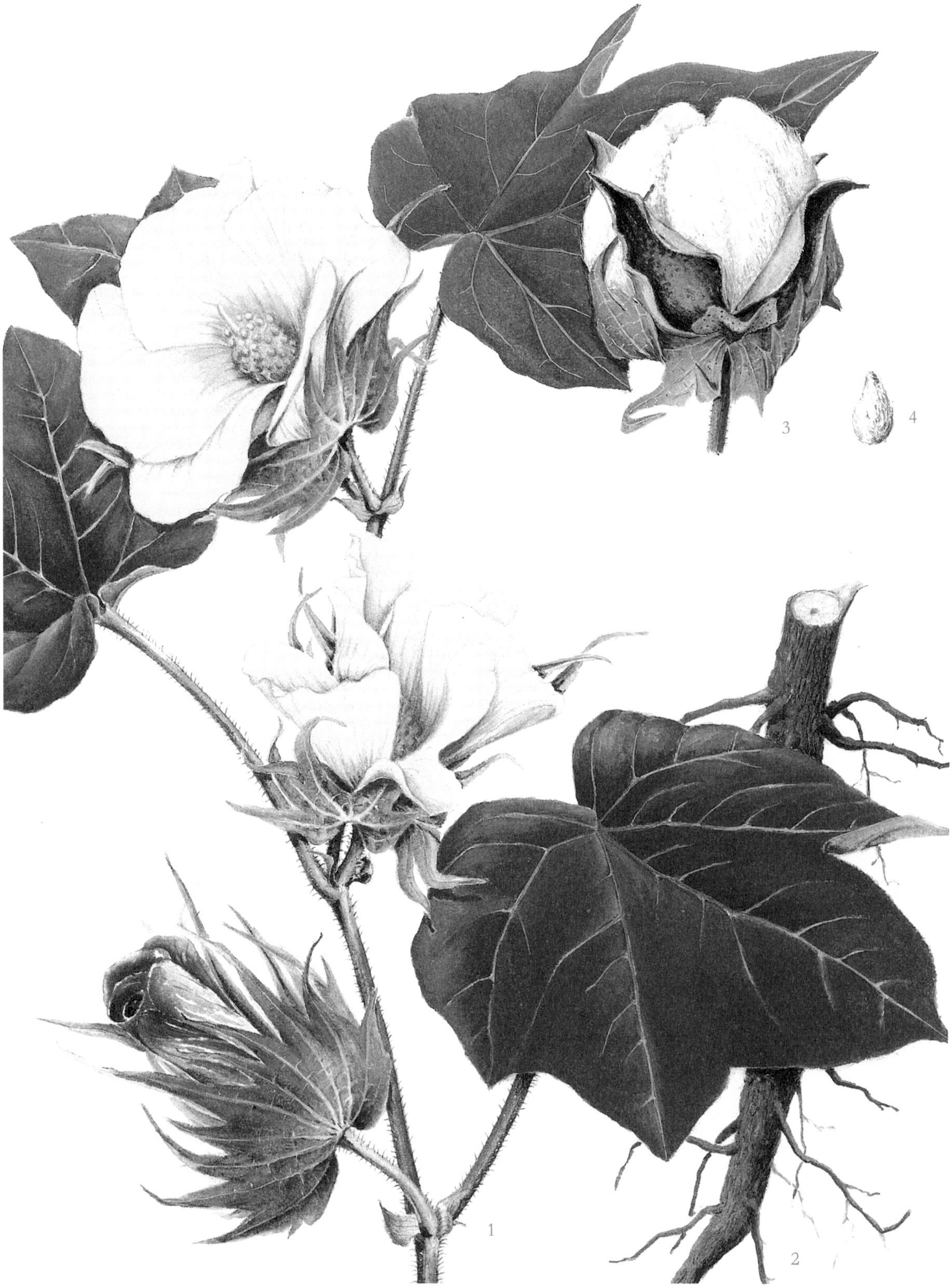

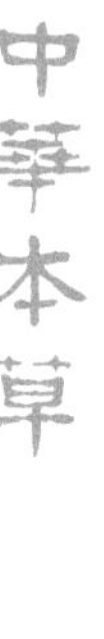

1. 花枝（flowering stem） 2. 根（root） 3. 果实（fruit） 4. 种子（seed）

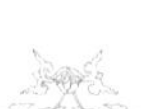

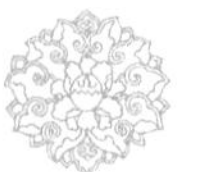

山里红

Shanlihong

Crataegus pinnatifida var. *major*

基　源　蔷薇科 Rosaceae 山楂属 *Crataegus* 植物山里红 *Crataegus pinnatifida* Bge. var. *major* N. E. Brown 的干燥成熟果实。药材名为“山楂”。

形态特征　落叶乔木。小枝圆柱形，当年生枝紫褐色。叶片宽卵形或三角状卵形，先端短渐尖，基部截形至宽楔形，通常两侧各有 3-5 羽状裂片，边缘有尖锐稀疏不规则锯齿。伞房花序具多花；花萼筒钟状，外面密被灰白色柔毛，萼片三角卵形；花瓣倒卵形或近圆形，白色。果实近球形，深红色，有浅色斑点。

生境分布　分布于华北、华东、华中各省区，常生于山坡疏林。北方各地常见栽培。

采收加工　秋季果实成熟时采收，切片，干燥。

性味功能　微温，酸、甘。消食健胃，行气散瘀，化浊降脂。

主治用法　用于肉食积滞，胃脘胀满，泻痢腹痛，瘀血经闭，产后瘀阻，心腹刺痛，胸痹心痛，疝气疼痛，高脂血症。焦山楂消食导滞作用增强。用于肉食积滞，泻痢不爽。

化学成分　果实中主要含有有机酸类，如山楂酸、柠檬酸、绿原酸等；黄酮类，如金丝桃苷、槲皮素、牡荆素等；另含有糖分、蛋白质、维生素 C 等；叶中含有槲皮素、金丝桃苷、牡荆素鼠李糖苷、盐酸乙胺、山梨醇等。

备　注　果肉酸甜可口，为常见水果。叶亦可入药，主要用于活血化瘀，理气通脉，降血脂等。

Source　It is the dried mature fruit of *Crataegus pinnatifida* Bge. var. *major* N. E. Brown. (Rosaceae). The medicinal material is called as “Shanzha”.

Distribution　*C. pinnatifida* is distributed in North, East and Central China. It commonly grows in sparse forests on the hillside. It is commonly cultivated throughout northern China.

Indications　It is used to treat meat-type food accumulation, gastic distention, diarrhea with abdominal pain, static blood and amenorrhea, postpartum stagnation of blood stasis, stabbing pain in the heart and abdomen, heart pain due to chest impediment, pain due to hernia, hyperlipidemia. Stir-baking Fructus Cratoegi to brown provides better effect on digestion and elimination of food stagnation and can be used for meat-type food stagnation and diarrhea.

Chemical Constituents　The fruit mainly contains organic acids (e.g., maslinic acid, citric acid, chlorogenic acid), flavonoids (e.g., hyperoside, quercetin, vitexin), saccharides, protein, vitamin C, etc. The leaves contain quercetin, hyperoside, vitexin rhamnoside, ethylamine hydrochloride, sorbitol, etc.

Note　The fruit is a common with sweet and sour pulp. The leaves can also be used as medicine, which have the function of activating blood and resolving stasis, regulating the flow of qi to unblock collaterals, and lowering blood lipid, etc.

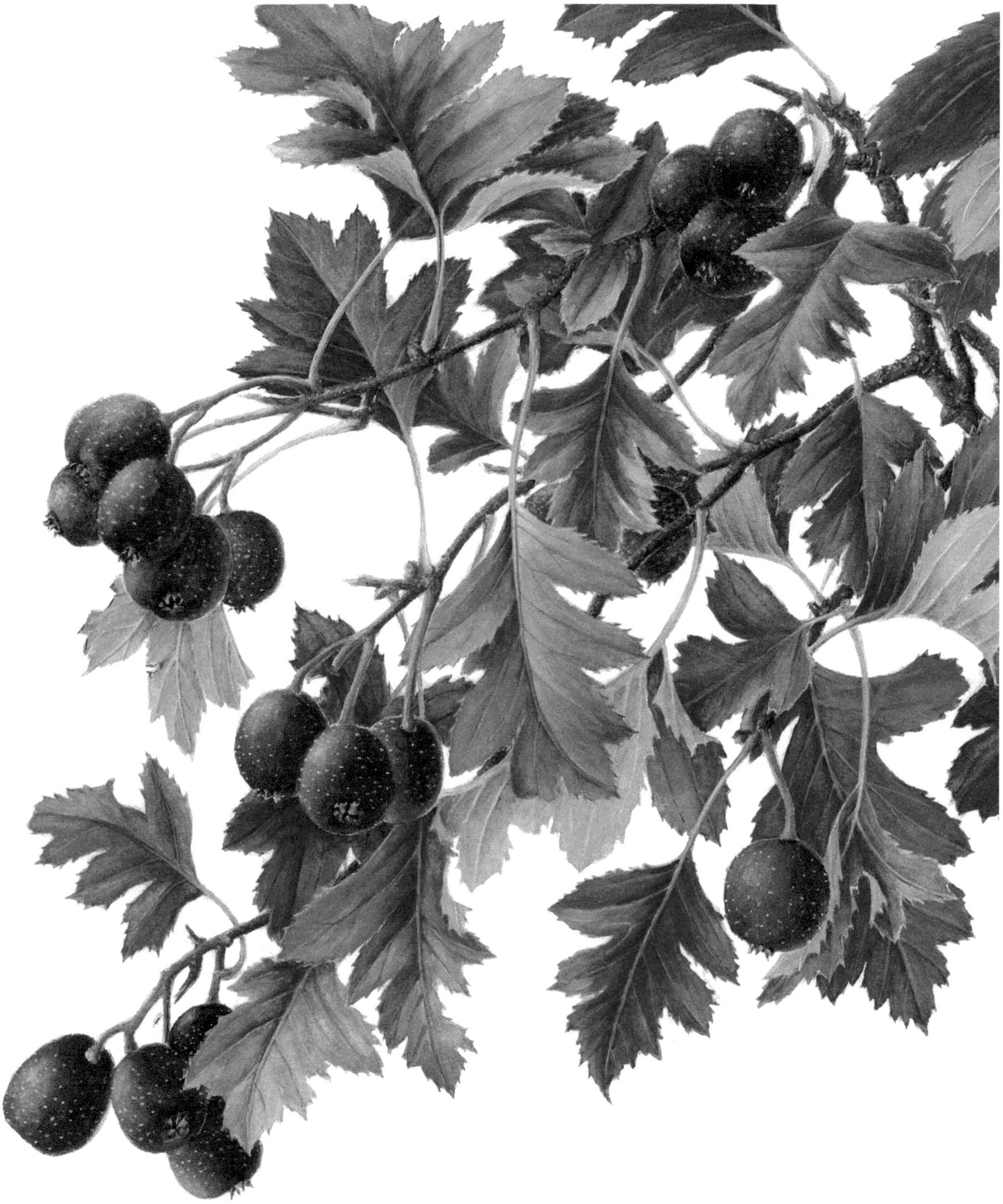

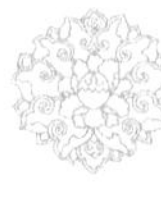

果枝（fruiting stem）

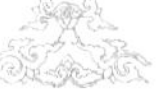

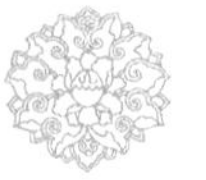

木瓜

Mugua

Chaenomeles sinensis

基　源　蔷薇科 Rosaceae 木瓜属 *Chaenomele*s 植物木瓜 *Chaenomeles sinensis* (Thouin) Koehne 的干燥近成熟果实。药材名为“光木瓜”。

形态特征　灌木或小乔木。树皮成片状脱落；小枝无刺，圆柱形。单叶互生；托叶膜质，卵状披针形，边缘具腺齿；叶片椭圆卵形或椭圆长圆形，先端急尖，基部宽楔形，边缘有刺芒状尖锐锯齿。花单生于叶腋，花梗短粗，无毛；萼筒钟状，萼片边缘有腺齿；花瓣倒卵形，淡粉红色。梨果长椭圆形，木质，芳香，果梗短。

生境分布　分布于华南、华中、华东等地。生于山坡疏林中，各地常见栽培。

采收加工　10-11 月将成熟果实摘下，纵剖为 2 块或 4 块，内表面向上晒干。

性味功能　平，酸、涩。和胃舒筋，祛风湿，消痰止咳。

主治用法　主要用于吐泻转筋，风湿痹痛，咳嗽痰多，泄泻，痢疾，跌打损伤，脚气水肿。

化学成分　含有黄酮类化合物及鞣质。

Source　It is the dried near mature fruit of *Chaenomeles sinensis* (Thouin) Koehne. (Rosaceae). The medicinal material is called as “Guangmugua”.

Distribution　*C. sinensis* is distributed in South China, Central China, and East China. It grows in sparse forests on hillsides and commonly cultivated in many regions.

Indications　It is used to treat vomiting and diarrhoea with spasm, wind–dampness impediment pain, cough with profuse sputum, diarrhea, dysentery, traumatic injury, and beriberi with edema.

Chemical Constituents　It mainly contains flavonoids and tannins.

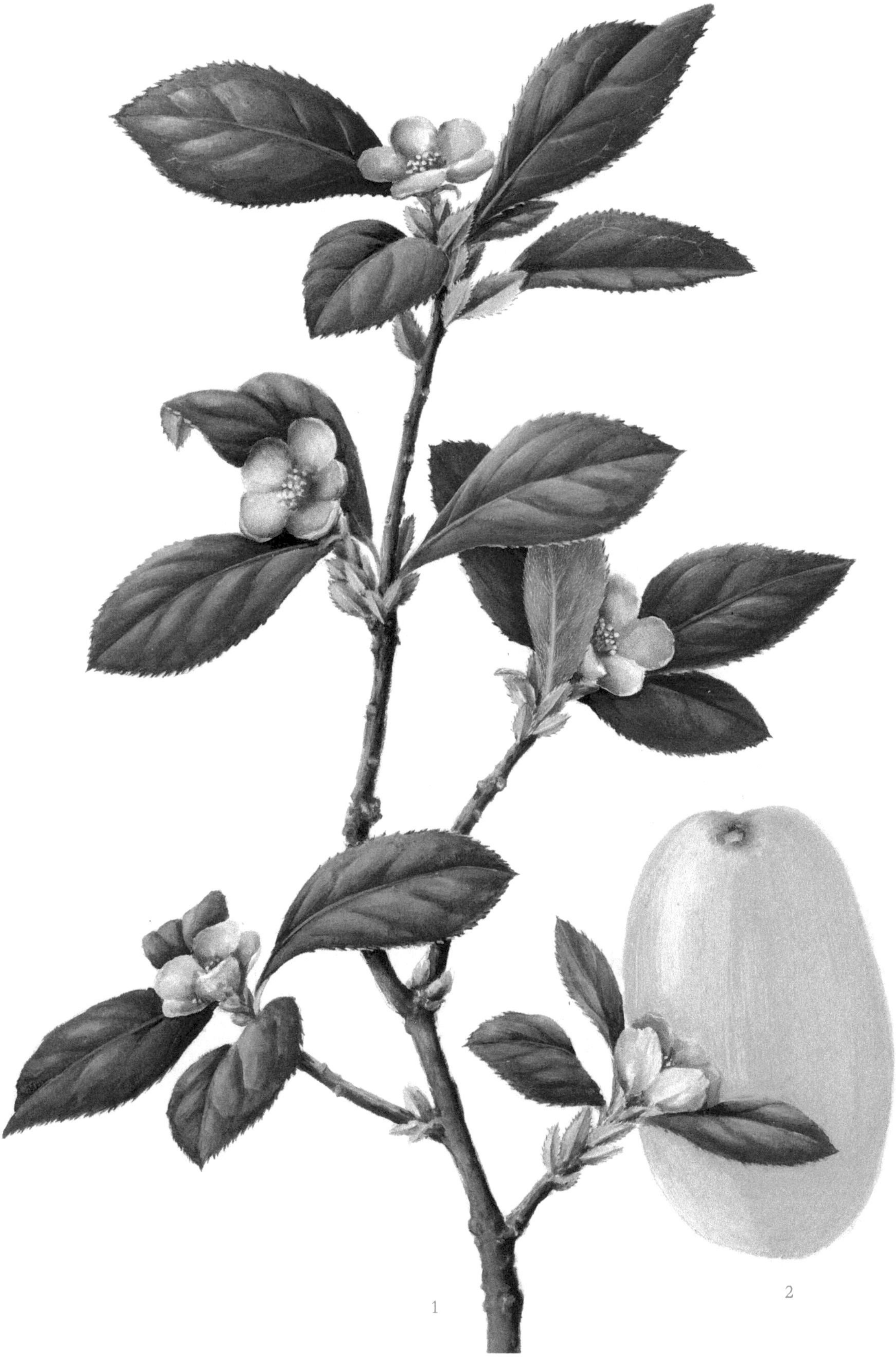

1

2

1. 花枝（flowering stem） 2. 果实（fruit）

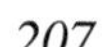

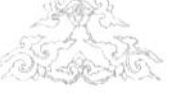

贴梗海棠

Tiegenghaitang

Chaenomeles speciosa

基　源　蔷薇科 Rosaceae 木瓜属 *Chaenomeles* 植物贴梗海棠 *Chaenomeles speciosa* (Sweet) Nakai 的干燥近成熟果实。药材名为“木瓜”。

形态特征　落叶灌木。枝条有刺；小枝圆柱形，紫褐色。叶片卵形至椭圆形，边缘有尖锐锯齿；托叶大，草质，肾形，边缘有重锯齿。花先叶开放，3-5 朵簇生于二年生老枝上；萼筒钟状，萼片直立；花瓣倒卵形或近圆形，基部延伸成短爪，猩红色至淡红色。果实卵球形，芳香，果梗短或近于无梗。

生境分布　分布于陕西、甘肃、四川、贵州等省区。各地常见栽培。道地药材产自安徽宣城。

采收加工　夏、秋二季果实绿黄时采收，置沸水中烫至外皮灰白色，对半纵剖，晒干。

性味功能　温，酸。舒筋活络，和胃化湿。

主治用法　主要用于湿痹拘挛，腰膝关节酸重疼痛，暑湿吐泻，转筋挛痛，脚气水肿。

化学成分　主要含有三萜类，如齐墩果酸、熊果酸；有机酸类，如反丁烯二酸、柠檬酸、苹果酸和酒石酸等；以及黄酮类和鞣质类成分。

Source　It is the dried near mature fruit of *Chaenomeles speciosa* (Sweet) Nakai. (Rosaceae). The medicinal material is called as “Mugua”.

Distribution　*C. speciosa* is distributed in Shaanxi, Gansu, Sichuan, Guizhou and other provinces. It is commonly cultivated all over China. Authentic medicinal materials are sourced from Xuancheng, Anhui Province.

Indications　It is used to treat damp impediment and contracture, spasm,aching pain in lower back and knee ioint, vomiting and diarrhea due to summerheat dampness, spasm and crampy pain, beriberi with edema.

Chemical Constituents　It mainly contains triterpenoids (e.g., oleanolic acid, ursolic acid), organic acids (e.g., fumaric acid, citric acid, malic acid, tartaric acid), flavonoids and tannins.

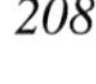

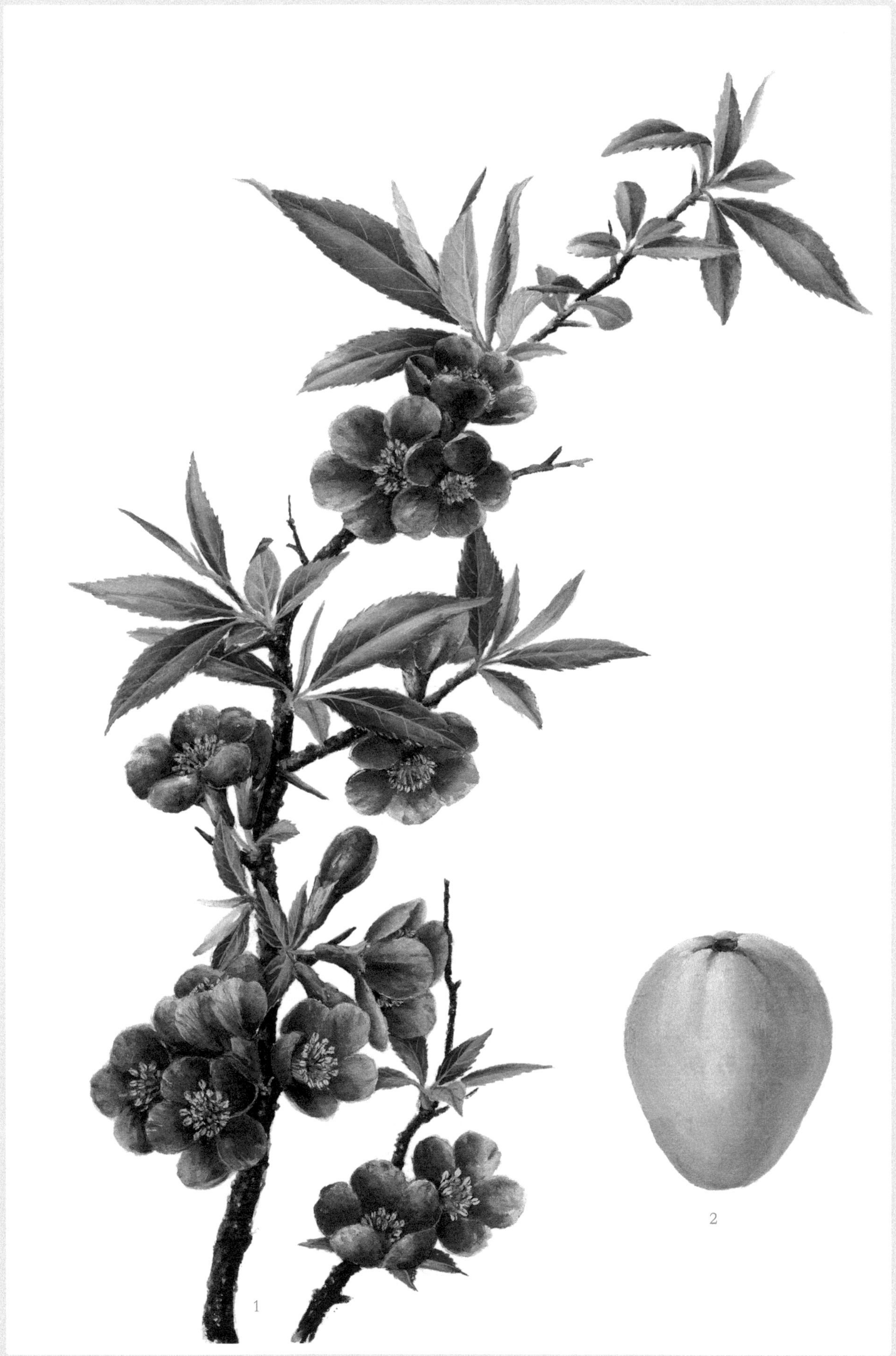

1

2

1. 花枝（flowering stem） 2. 果实（fruit）

罂粟

Yingsu

Papaver somniferum

基　　源　罂粟科 Papaveraceae 罂粟属 *Papaver* 植物罂粟 *Papaver somniferum* L. 的干燥成熟果壳。药材名为“罂粟壳”。

形态特征　一年生或二年生草本。有乳汁。茎直立，不分枝，无毛，具白粉。叶互生；茎下部叶有短柄，上部叶无柄，抱茎；叶缘具波状锯齿，被白粉。花单一，顶生，花蕾下垂，具长柄；萼片 2，早落；花瓣 4 或为重瓣，近扇形，边缘浅波状或分裂，白色、粉红色或红色等。蒴果球形，孔裂。种子多数，细小，肾形。

生境分布　原产南欧。

采收加工　秋季将成熟果实或已割取浆汁后的成熟果实摘下，破开，除去种子和枝梗，干燥。

性味功能　平，酸、涩；有毒。敛肺，涩肠，止痛。

主治用法　主要用于久咳，久泻，脱肛，脘腹疼痛。本品易成瘾，不宜常服；孕妇及儿童禁用；运动员慎用。

化学成分　主要含有生物碱类，如吗啡、罂粟碱、可待因等；另含有景天庚糖、内消旋肌醇等。

备　　注　罂粟未成熟果实中含乳汁，干后即为鸦片，其提取物是多种镇静剂、麻醉剂的原料。我国禁止非法种植。

Source　It is the dried mature fruit shell of *Papaver somniferum* L. (Papaveraceae). The medicinal material is called as “Yingsuke”.

Distribution　It is native to south European.

Indications　It is used to treat chronic cough, chronic diarrhea, prolapse of rectum, and epigastric pain. It is inappropriate for long-term use as it is highly addictive. Pregnant women and children are not allowed to use it. Athletes should use it with caution.

Chemical Constituents　It mainly contains alkaloids, e.g., morphine, papaverine, codeine, etc. It also contains sedoheptulose, meso-inositol, etc.

Note　The immature fruit of *P. somniferum* contains latex, which becomes opium after dried. Its extract is a raw material for various sedatives and anesthetics. The illegally planted *P. somniferum* is prohibited in China.

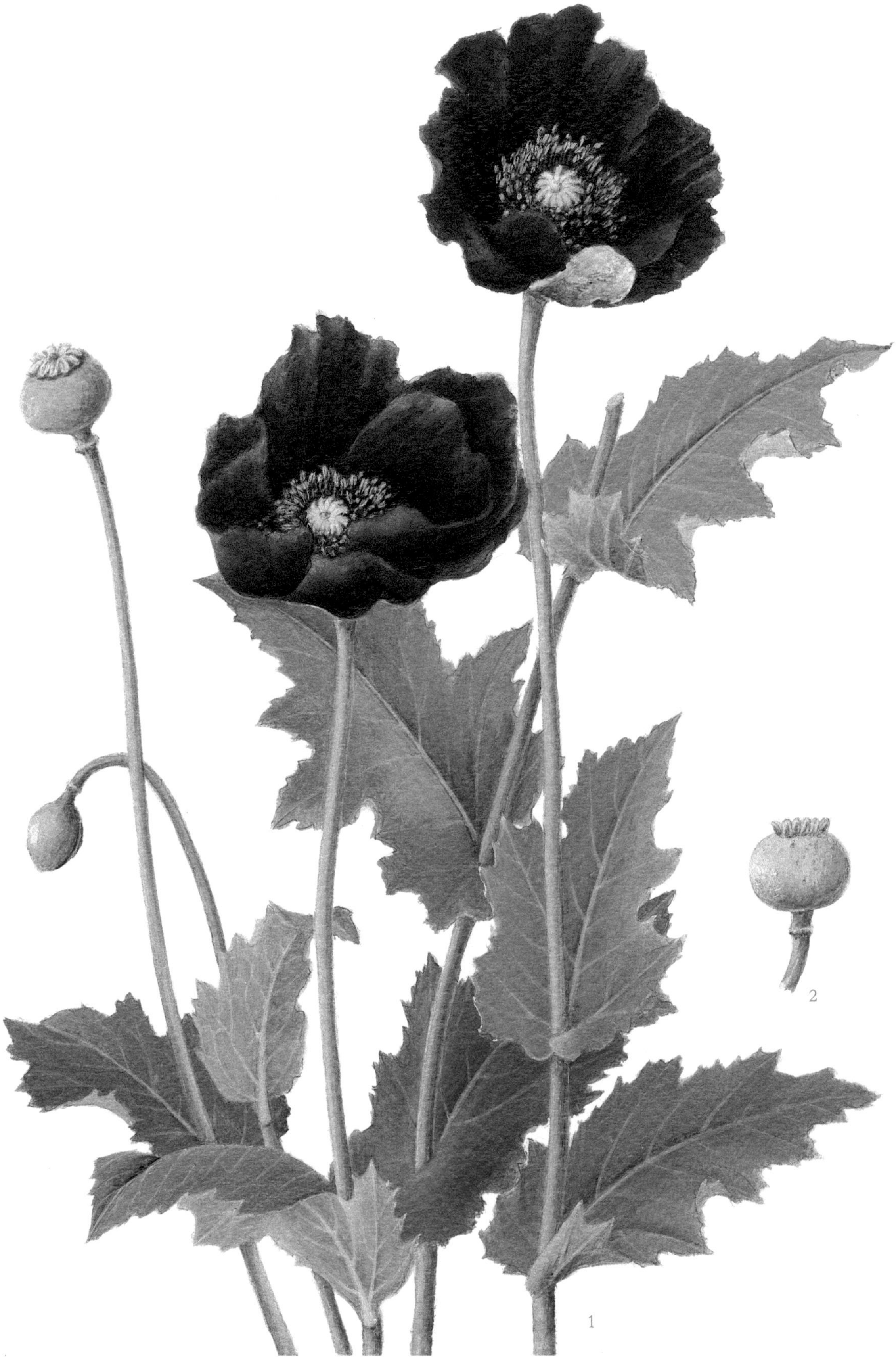

1

2

1. 植株（plant） 2. 果实（fruit）

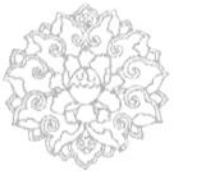

蕺菜

Jicai

Houttuynia cordata

基　源　三白草科 Saururaceae 蕺菜属 *Houttuynia* 植物蕺菜 *Houttuynia cordata* Thunb. 的新鲜全草或干燥地上部分。药材名为“鱼腥草”。

形态特征　多年生草本，有腥味。茎下部伏地，节上轮生小根，上部直立。叶互生，薄纸质，有腺点；托叶膜质，条形，下部与叶柄合生，基部扩大，略抱茎；叶片阔卵形，先端短渐尖，基部心形，全缘，上面绿色，下面紫红色。穗状花序生于茎顶；总苞片 4，倒卵形，白色；花小而密。蒴果卵圆形，具宿存花柱。

生境分布　分布于我国长江流域以南的大部分省区，以及陕西、甘肃。常生于水边湿地或潮湿的山坡。

采收加工　夏季茎叶茂盛花穗多时采割，除去杂质，晒干。

性味功能　微寒，辛。清热解毒，消痈排脓，利尿通淋。

主治用法　用于肺痈吐脓，痰热喘咳，热痢，热淋，痈肿疮毒。不宜久煎。

化学成分　主要含有挥发油类，如鱼腥草素、月桂烯、乙酸龙脑酯、芳樟醇等；黄酮类，如槲皮素、槲皮苷、金丝桃苷等；另含有机酸、氨基酸、蕺菜碱和甾醇类等。

备　注　鱼腥草亦可鲜用。鱼腥草的嫩根茎可作为食品和调味品，名为“折耳根”，深受广大西南地区群众的喜爱。

Source　It is the fresh herb or dried oerial part of *Houttuynia cordata* Thunb (Saururaceae). The medicinal material is called as “Yuxingcao”.

Distribution　*H. cordata* is distributed in most provinces to the south of the Yangtze River, and in Shaanxi and Gansu Province. It commonly grows in wetlands or hillsides with dramp environment.

Indications　It is used to treat lung abscess with pyemesis, phleqm-heat with panting and cough, heat dysentery, heat stranqury, swollen abscess, sore and toxin. It should not be decocted for a long time.

Chemical Constituents　It mainly contains essential oils (e.g., houttuynin, myrcene, bronyl acetate, linalool), flavonoids (e.g., quercetin, quercitrin, hyperin), organic acids, amino acids, cordarine and sterols, etc.

Note　*H. cordata* can also be used in fresh. The young rhizome named “zheergen”, is used as food and condiments, has high popularity in southwest of China.

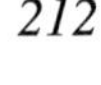

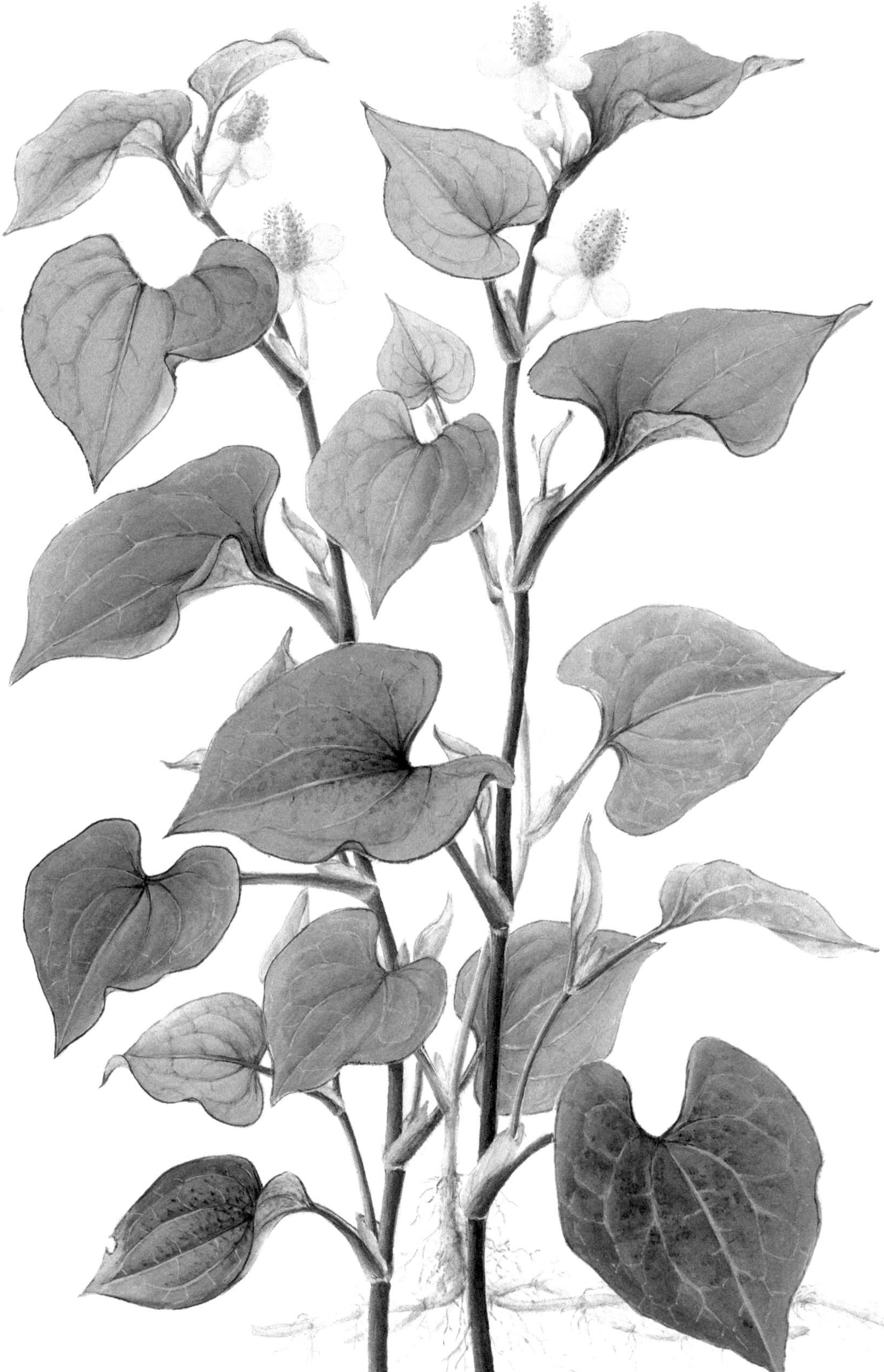

植株（plant）

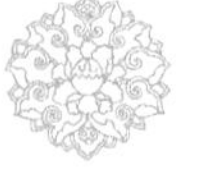

箭叶淫羊藿

Jianyeyinyanghuo

Epimedium sagittatum

基　　源　小檗科 Berberidaceae 淫羊藿属 *Epimedium* 植物箭叶淫羊藿 *Epimedium sagittatum* (Sieb. et Zucc.) Maxim. 的干燥叶。药材名为“淫羊藿”。

形态特征　多年生草本。根状茎粗短，节结状，质硬，多须根。一回三出复叶基生和茎生；小叶 3 枚，革质，卵形至卵状披针形，叶缘具刺齿；花茎具 2 枚对生叶；圆锥花序；花梗无毛；花较小，白色；萼片 2 轮，外萼片 4 枚，具紫色斑点，内萼片卵状三角形，白色；花瓣囊状，淡棕黄色。蓇果。

生境分布　主要分布于华东、华南、华中部分省区。常生于山地、密林、石缝等阴凉潮湿地。

采收加工　夏、秋二季茎叶茂盛时采收，晒干或阴干。

性味功能　温，辛、甘。补肾阳，强筋骨，祛风湿。

主治用法　用于肾阳虚衰，阳痿遗精，筋骨痿软，风湿痹痛，麻木拘挛。

化学成分　地上部分含黄酮类成分，如淫羊藿苷、槲皮素、山奈酚等；另外还含有亚麻酸、棕榈酸、生物碱类成分。

备　　注　炮制淫羊藿使用羊脂油炙。

Source　It is the dried leaf of *Epimedium sagittatum* (Sieb. et Zucc.) Maxim. (Berberidaceae). The medicinal material is called as “Yinyanghuo”.

Distribution　*E. sagittatum* is mainly distributed in some provinces of East, South and Central China. It commonly grows in shady and damp areas of mountains, dense forests, and rock crevices.

Indications　It is used to treat debilitation of kidney yang, impotence and seminal emission, flaccidity of sinews and bones, pain due to rheumatic arthralgia, numbness and contracture.

Chemical Constituents　The aerial part contains flavonoids, e.g., icariin, quercetin, kaempferol. It also contains linolenic acid, palmitic acid and alkaloids.

Note　Herba Epimedii Brevicornus is processed through stir-baking with caproin.

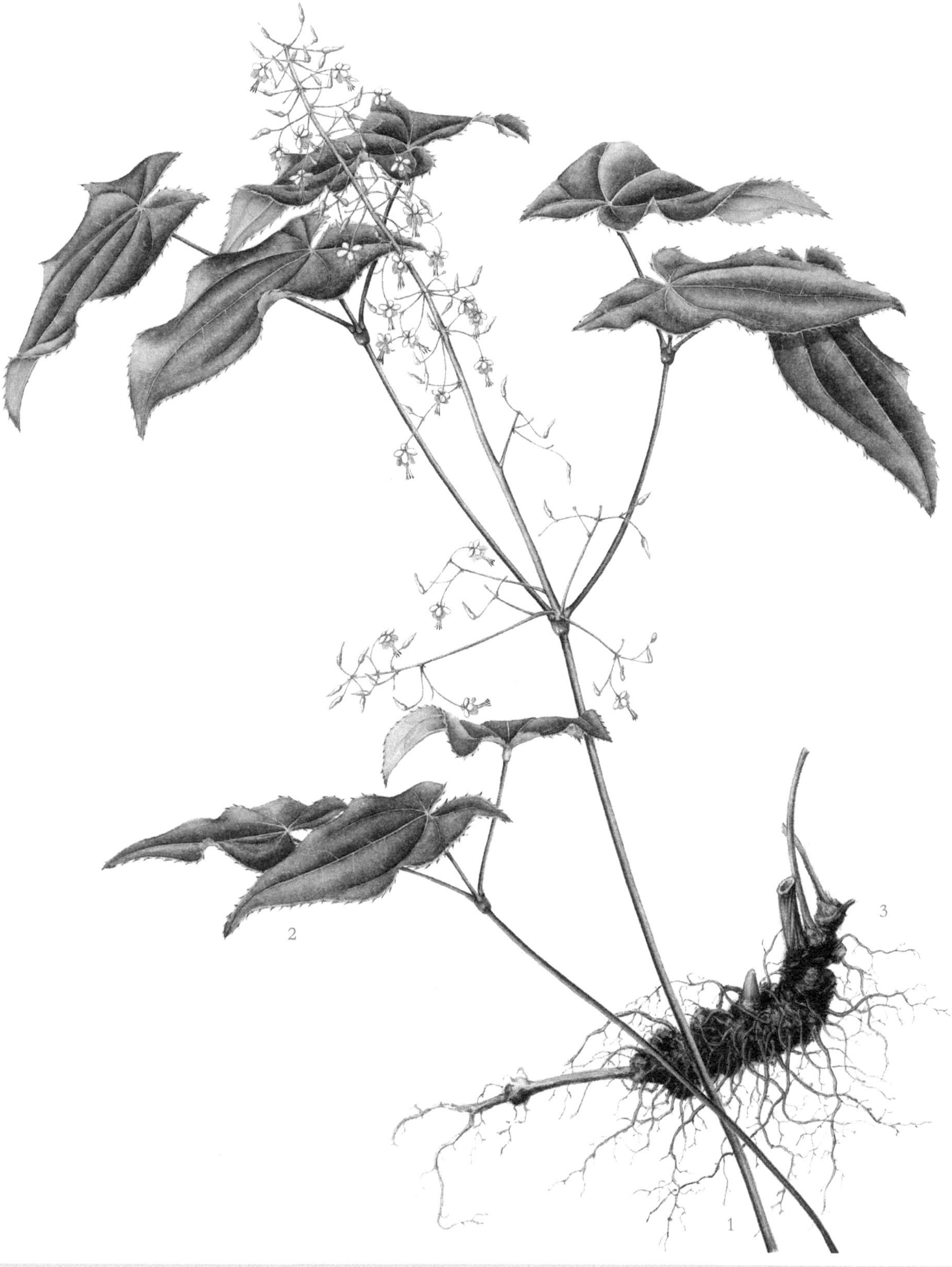

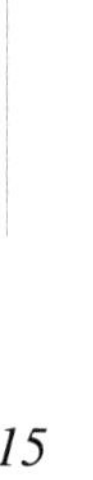

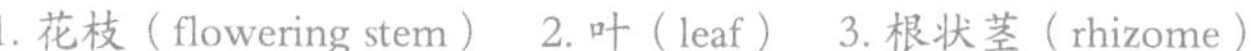

1. 花枝（flowering stem） 2. 叶（leaf） 3. 根状茎（rhizome）

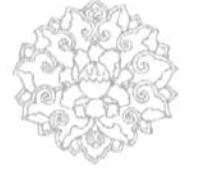

马齿苋

Machixian

Portulaca oleracea

基　　源　马齿苋科 Portulacaceae 马齿苋属 *Portulaca* 植物马齿苋 *Portulaca oleracea* L. 的干燥地上部分。药材名为“马齿苋”。

形态特征　一年生草本，全株无毛。茎伏地铺散，多分枝，圆柱形，淡绿色或带暗红色。叶互生，扁平，肥厚，倒卵形，似马齿状，顶端圆钝，有时微凹，全缘。花无梗，常 3-5 朵簇生枝端，午时盛开；萼片 2，对生，绿色；花瓣 5，黄色，倒卵形，顶端微凹，基部合生。蒴果卵球形，盖裂。种子细小，具疣状凸起。

生境分布　分布于我国南北各地。生于田边、路旁，为常见的农田杂草。

采收加工　夏、秋二季采收，除去残根和杂质，洗净，略蒸或烫后晒干。

性味功能　寒，酸。清热解毒，凉血止血，止痢。

主治用法　用于热毒血痢，痈肿疔疮，湿疹，丹毒，蛇虫咬伤，便血，痔血，崩漏下血。

化学成分　主要含有马齿苋素；另外还含有儿茶酚酸类、甾体类、香豆素类、黄酮类和蒽醌类化合物等。

备　　注　嫩茎可供食用。

Source　It is the dried aerial part of *Portulaca oleracea* L. (Portulacaceae). The medicinal material is called as “Machixian”.

Distribution　*P. oleracea* is distributed all over China. It grows near fields and roadsides. which is a common weed in farmland.

Indications　It is used to treat hematodiarrhoea caused by heat toxin, swollen abscess, furuncle, sore, eczema, erysipelas, snake and insect bites, bloody stool, hemorrhoidal bleeding, and metrorrhagia and metrostaxis with blood.

Chemical Constituents　It mainly contains bacoside. It also contains catecholates, steroids, coumarins, flavonoids, anthraquinones, etc.

Note　The immature stem is edible.

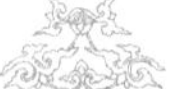

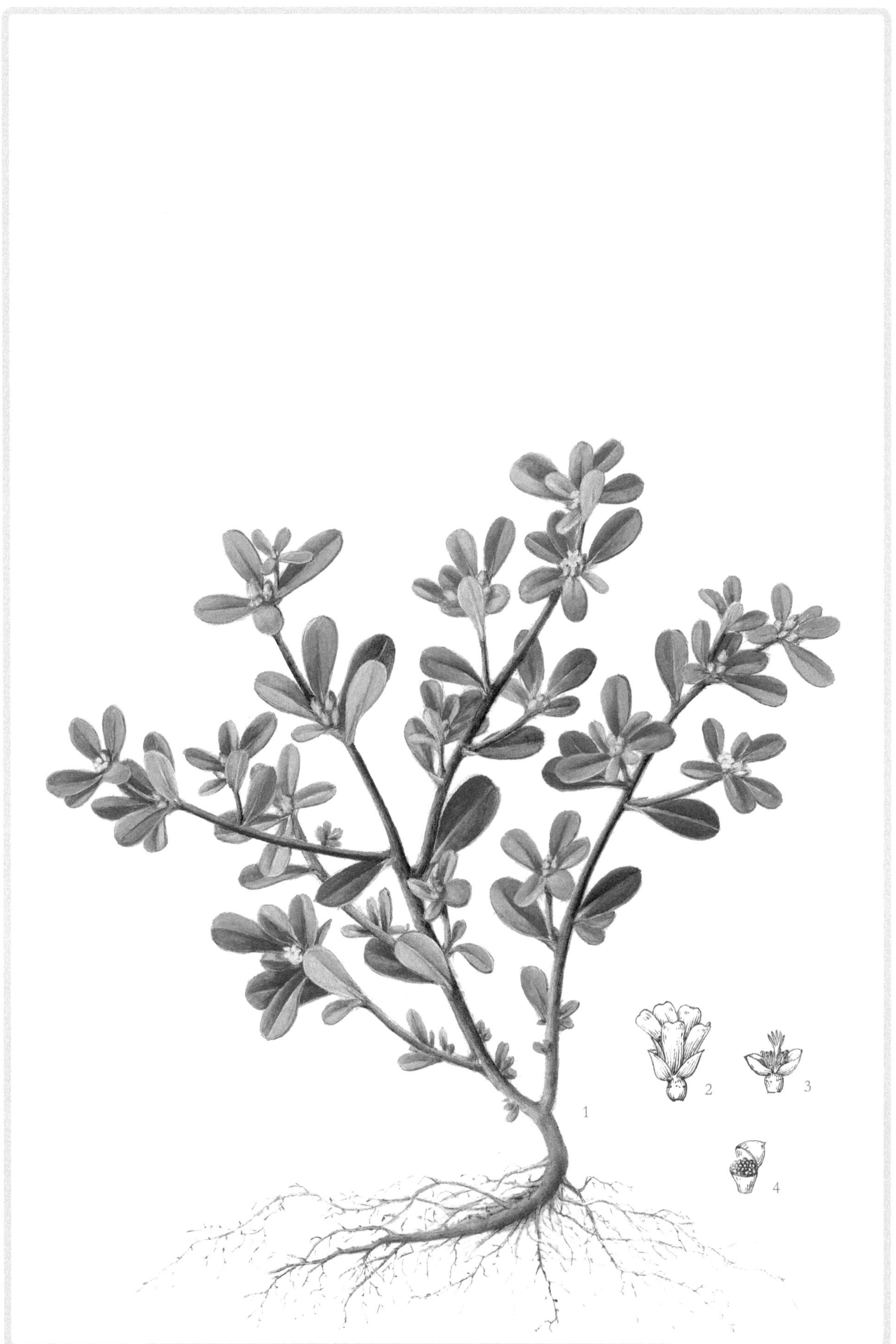

1. 植株（plant） 2. 花（flower） 3. 雄蕊及雌蕊（stamen and pistil） 4. 果实及种子（fruit and seed）

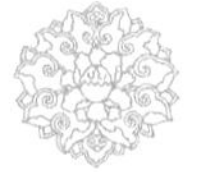

冰凉花

Bingliānghua
Adonis amurensis

基　　源　毛茛科 Ranunculaceae 侧金盏花属 *Adonis* 植物冰凉花 *Adonis amurensis* Regel et Radde 的干燥带根全草。药材名为“冰凉花”。

形态特征　多年生草本。茎无毛或顶部有稀疏短柔毛，基部有数个膜质鳞片；茎下部叶有长柄，无毛。叶片正三角形，三全裂，全裂片有长柄，二至三回细裂。花两性，单朵顶生，萼片约 9，淡灰紫色；花瓣约 10，黄色，倒卵状长圆形或狭倒卵形，无毛。瘦果倒卵球形，被短柔毛，有短宿存花柱。

生境分布　分布于我国东北及山东、江苏北部。常生于山坡草地和林下潮湿肥沃处。

采收加工　早春采集，洗净，晒干。

性味功能　平，苦；有大毒。强心，利尿，镇静。

主治用法　主要用于治疗急性和慢性心功能不全，充血性心力衰竭，心房纤维颤动，心脏性水肿等。

化学成分　根中含有强心苷及其苷元（索马林、黄麻苷、侧金盏花毒苷等）、香豆素和黄酮苷类成分；地上部分中含有毒毛旋花子苷元、洋地黄毒苷元等强心苷元和厚果酮、异热马酮、夜来香素等非强心苷元成分，以及伞形花内酯及东莨菪素等香豆素类成分。

Source　It is the dried herb with root of *Adonis amurensis* Regel et Radde. (Ranunculaceae). The medicinal material is called as “Bingliānghua”.

Distribution　*A. amurensis* is distributed in Northeast China, Shandong and northern Jiangsu. It commonly grows on grasslands on hillsides, and floor of forests with damp and fertile environment.

Indications　It is used to treat acute and chron cardial insufficiency, congestive heart failure, atrial fibrillation, cardiac edema, etc.

Chemical Constituents　The root contains cardiac glycoside and its aglycone (e.g., somalin, corchoroside, adonitoxin), coumarins, and flavonoids. The aerial parts contain cardiac aglycones (e.g., strophanthidin, digitoxigenin), non-cardiac aglycones (e.g., lineolone, isoramanone, pergularin), and coumarins (e.g., umbelliferone, scopoletin).

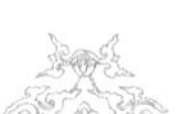

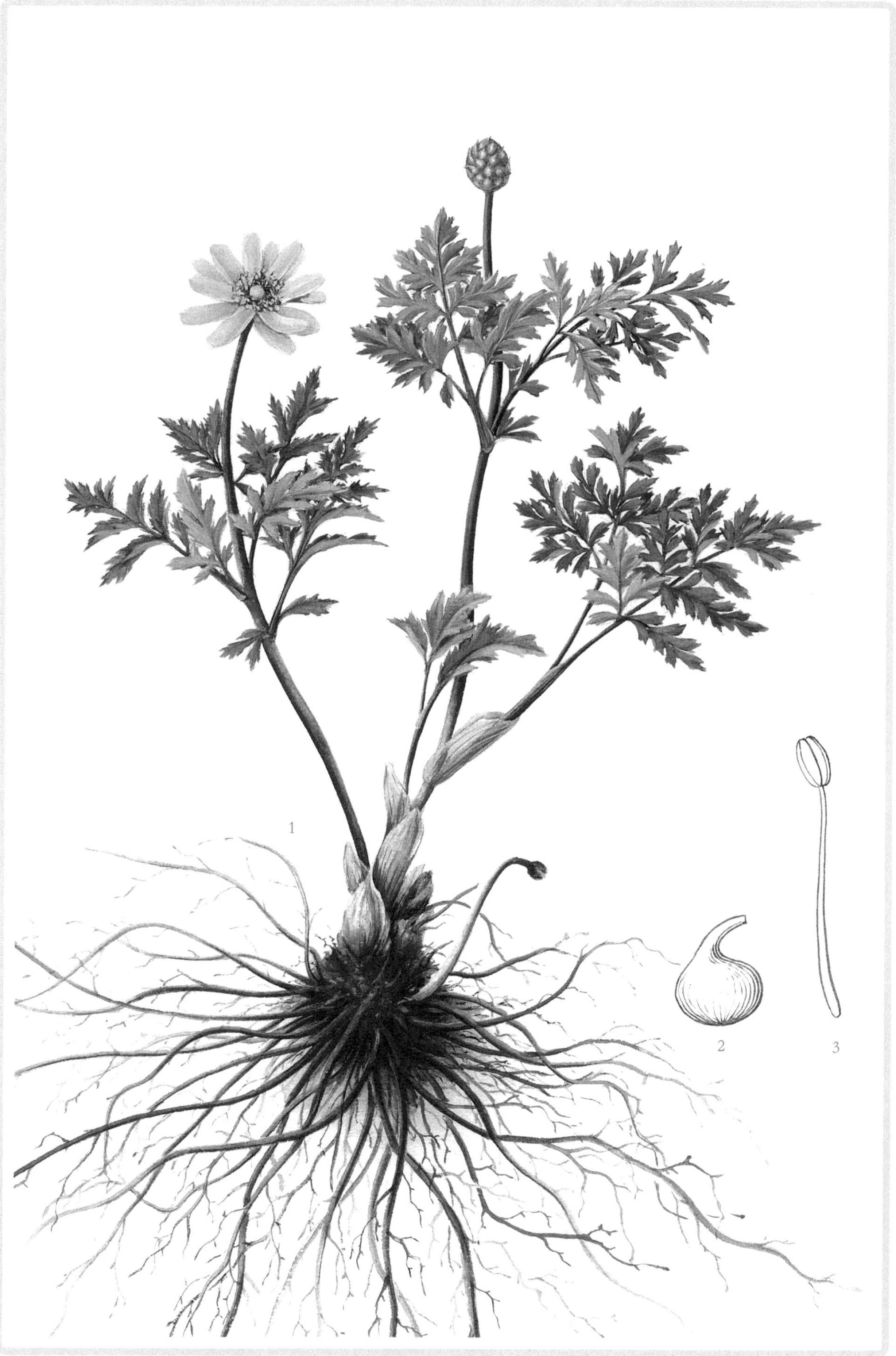

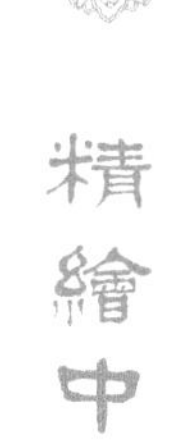

1. 植株（plant）　2. 心皮（carpel）　3. 雄蕊（stamen）

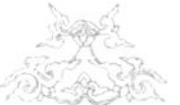

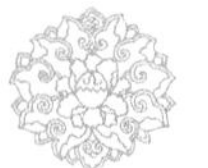

打破碗花花

Dapowanhuahua

Anemone hupehensis

基　　源　毛茛科 Ranunculaceae 银莲花属 *Anemone* 植物打破碗花花 *Anemone hupehensis* Lem. 的干燥根或全草。药材名为“打破碗花花”。

形态特征　多年生草本。基生叶 3-5，有长柄，叶柄疏被柔毛，基部有短鞘；通常为三出复叶，小叶片卵形，不分裂或三至五浅裂，边缘有锯齿，两面有疏糙毛。花葶直立，疏被柔毛；聚伞花序有分枝；苞片 3，为三出复叶；花梗有毛；萼片 5，紫红色或粉红色，倒卵形，外面有短绒毛。聚合果球形；瘦果有细柄，密被绵毛。

生境分布　分布于我国中部大部分省区，常生于海拔 400-1800 m 的低山、丘陵草地或路边。

采收加工　6-8 月花未开放前采挖，除去须根及泥土，晒干。

性味功能　平，苦、辛；有小毒。清热利湿，解毒杀虫，消肿散瘀。

主治用法　痢疾，泄泻，疟疾，蛔虫病，疮疖痈肿，瘰疬，跌打损伤。孕妇慎服；肾炎及肾功能不全者禁服。

化学成分　全草含白头翁素、齐墩果酸等成分。

Source　It is the root or herb of *Anemone hupehensis* Lem. (Ranunculaceae). The medicinal material is called as “Dapowanhuahua”.

Distribution　*A. hupehensis* is distributed in most provinces and regions in the central China, and commonly grows in low mountains, hilly grasslands and roadsides at an altitude of 400–1800 m.

Indications　It is used to treat dysentery, diarrhea, malaria, ascariasis, sore, boil, swollen abscess, scrofula, and traumatic injury. Pregnant women should take it with caution. People with nephritis and renal insufficiency are prohibited to take it.

Chemical Constituents　The herb contains anemonin, oleanolic acid, etc.

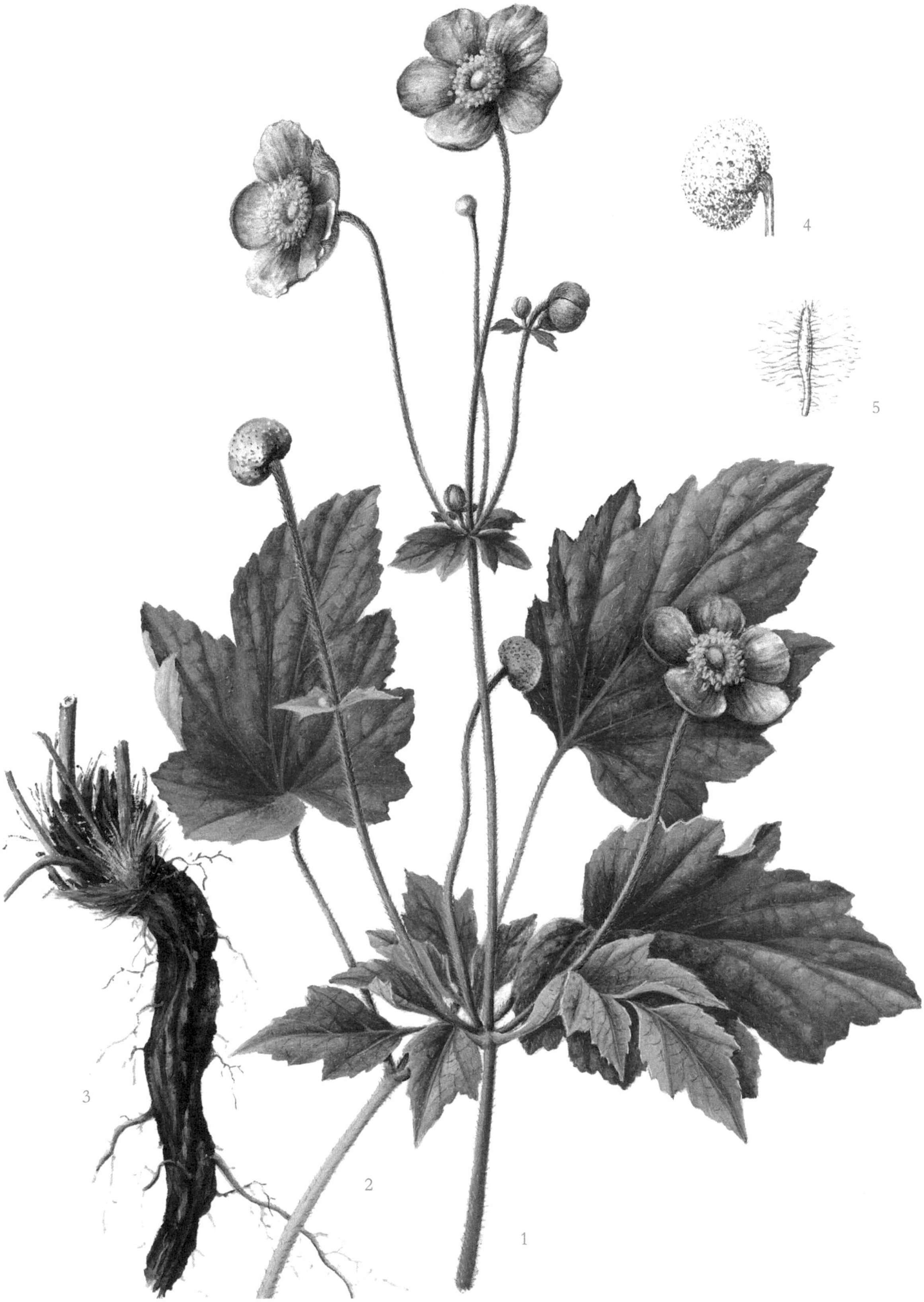

1. 花枝（flowering stem） 2. 叶（leaf） 3. 根（root） 4. 果实（fruit） 5. 种子（seed）

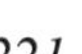

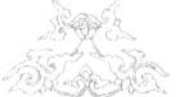

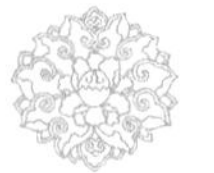

肉苁蓉

Roucongrong

Cistanche deserticola

基　　源　列当科 Orobanchaceae 肉苁蓉属 *Cistanche* 植物肉苁蓉 *Cistanche deserticola* Y. C. Ma 的干燥带鳞叶的肉质茎。药材名为“肉苁蓉”。

形态特征　多年生寄生草本。茎肉质肥厚。被多数肉质鳞片状叶，黄色至褐黄色，覆瓦状排列，卵形至长圆状披针形；茎下部叶较短，排列紧密，上部较长，排列稀疏。穗状花序圆柱形，花多数而密集；花萼钟形，淡黄色或白色，五浅裂；花冠管状钟形，5 浅裂，裂片近圆形，紫色或淡紫色，管部白色。蒴果椭圆形。种子多数。

生境分布　分布于内蒙古、宁夏、甘肃、新疆。生于有梭梭分布的荒漠地区。

采收加工　春季苗刚出土时或秋季冻土之前采挖，除去茎尖。切段，晒干。

性味功能　温，甘、咸。补肾阳，益精血，润肠通便。

主治用法　用于肾阳不足，精血亏虚，阳痿不孕，腰膝酸软，筋骨无力，肠燥便秘。

化学成分　主要含有松果菊苷、毛蕊花糖苷，以及甜菜碱、甘露醇、氨基酸、多糖等。

备　　注　肉苁蓉寄生于梭梭 *Haloxylon ammodendron* (C. A. Mey.) Bunge. 等植物的根部，以吸取水分和养分。

Source　It is the dried succulent stem with scaly leaf of *Cistanche deserticola* Y. C. Ma (Orobanchaceae). The medicinal is called as “Roucongrong”.

Distribution　*C. deserticola* is distributed in Inner Mongolia, Ningxia, Gansu and Xinjiang. It grows on dunes in deserts with Sacsaoul distributed.

Indications　It is used to treat insufficiency of kidney yang, depletion of blood and essence, impotence and infertility, soreness and weakness of waist and knees, weakness of sinews and bones, and intestinal dryness with constipation.

Chemical Constituents　It mainly contains echinacoside, acteoside, betaine, mannitol, amino acids, polysaccharides, etc.

Note　*C. deserticola* is parasitic on the roots of plants, e.g., *Haloxylon ammodendron* (C. A. Mey.) Bge., to absorb water and nutrients.

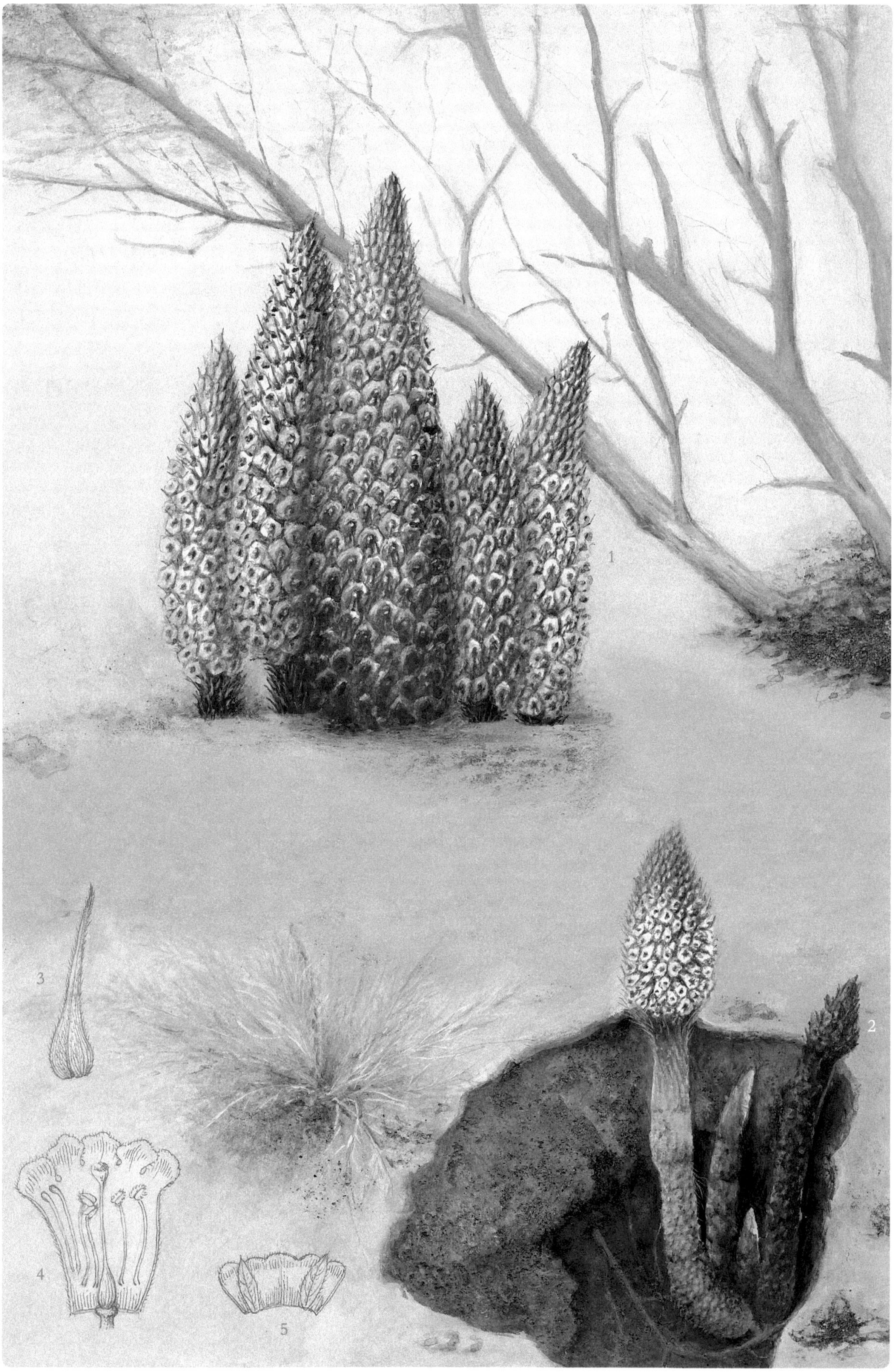

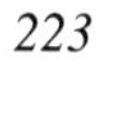

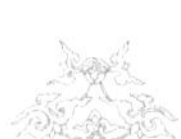

1、2 植株及生境（plant and habitat） 3. 苞片（bract） 4. 雄蕊及雌蕊（stamen and pistil） 5. 小苞片（bractlet）

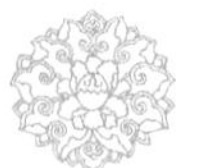

含羞草

Hanxiucao

Mimosa pudica

基　　源　豆科Fabaceae含羞草属*Mimosa*植物含羞草*Mimosa pudica* L.的干燥全草。药材名为“含羞草”。

形态特征　亚灌木状草本。茎圆柱状，具分枝，有散生、下弯的钩刺及倒生刺毛。托叶披针形；羽片和小叶触之即闭合下垂；羽片通常2对；小叶10-20对，线状长圆形，先端急尖，边缘具刚毛。头状花序圆球形，具长总花梗，单生或2-3个生于叶腋；花小，淡红色，多数。荚果长圆形，扁平，稍弯曲。种子卵形。

生境分布　原产南美洲。现广为栽培。

采收加工　夏季采收全草，除去泥沙，洗净，晒干；或扎成把，晒干。

性味功能　微寒，苦、涩、微苦；有小毒。凉血解毒，清热利湿，镇静安神。

主治用法　主要用于感冒，小儿高热，支气管炎，肝炎，肠炎，结膜炎，泌尿系结石，水肿，劳伤咳血，鼻衄，血尿，神经衰弱，失眠，疮疡肿毒，带状疱疹，跌打损伤。

化学成分　叶含有收缩性蛋白质、三磷腺苷、三磷腺苷酶、含羞草碱等；种子含有油脂类成分，其中的脂肪酸主要有亚麻酸、亚油酸、油酸、棕榈酸、硬脂酸。

Source　It is the dried herb of *Mimosa pudica* L. (Fabaceae). The medicinal material is called as “Hanxiucao”.

Distribution　*M. pudica* is native to South America and is widely cultivated at present.

Indications　It is used to treat cold, pediatric high fever, bronchitis, hepatitis, enteritis, conjunctivitis, urinary calculi, edema, hemoptysis due to impairment caused by overstrain, epistaxis, hematuria, neurasthenia, insomnia, sore, ulcer, pyogenic toxin, herpes zoster, and traumatic injury.

Chemical Constituents　The leaves contain contractile proteins, adenosine triphosphate, adenosine triphosphatase, mimosine, etc. The seed contains lipids, in which the main fatty acids are linolenic acid, linoleic acid, oleic acid, palmitic acid, and stearic acid.

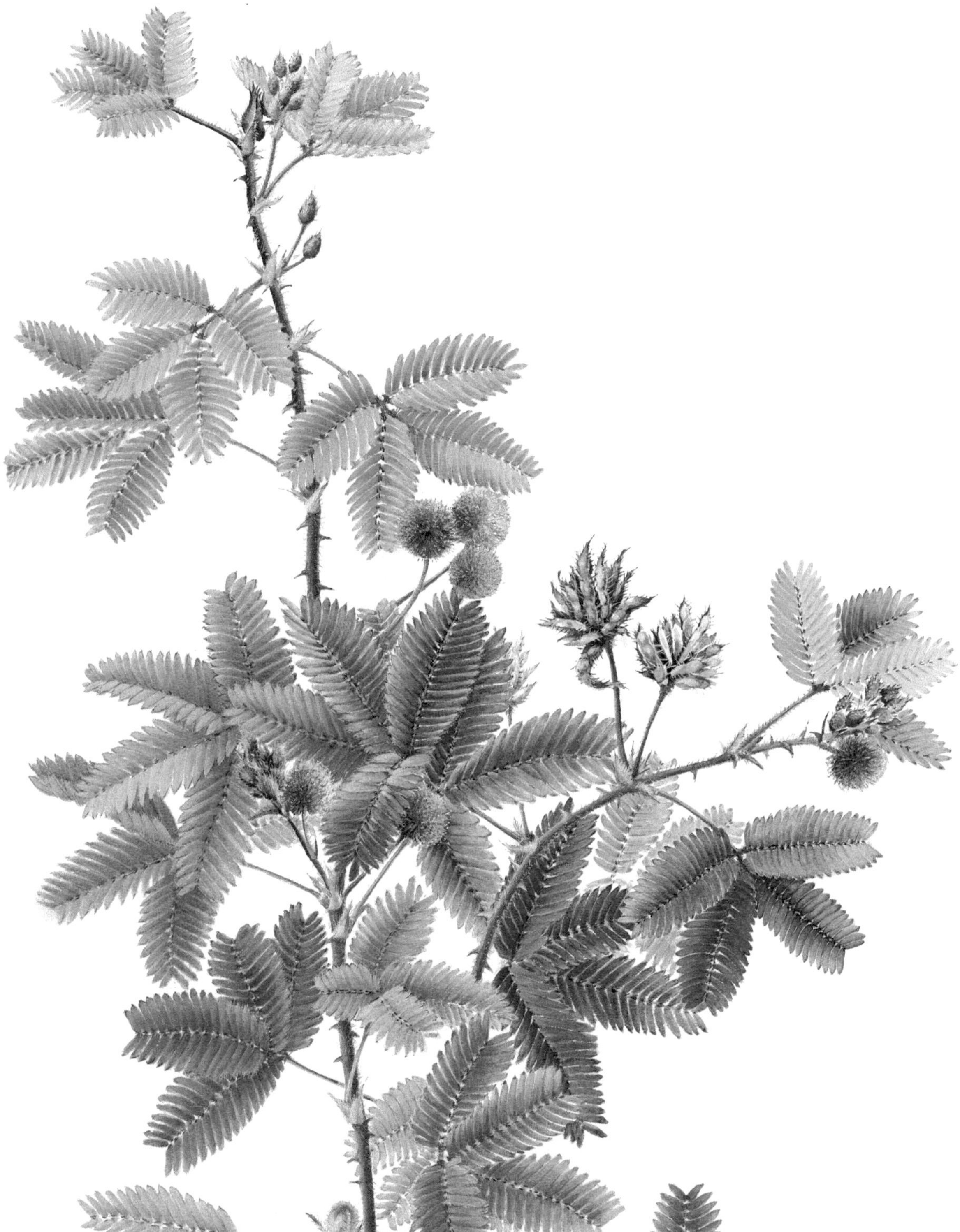

花果枝（flowering and fruiting stem）

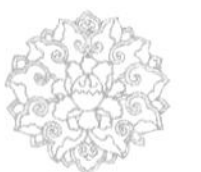

铁扫帚

Tiesaozhou

Lespedeza juncea var. *sericea*

基　源　豆科Fabaceae胡枝子属*Lespedeza*植物铁扫帚*Lespedeza juncea* (L. f.) Pers. var. *sericea* (Thunb.) Maxim 的干燥全草。药材名为“夜关门”。

形态特征　直立小灌木。上部有细长的分枝。叶互生，三出复叶；叶片倒披针形，先端截形或微凹，有短尖，基都狭楔形，上面有少数短毛，下面密被白色柔毛。花单生，或2-4朵丛生叶腋，几无花梗；花萼浅杯状；花冠碟形，白色，有紫斑，旗瓣中央紫红色，倒卵形，翼瓣斜长椭圆形，龙骨瓣顶端钝而偏斜，一侧基部下延成耳，均具爪。荚果斜卵圆形，表面有白色绢毛或近无毛。种子肾圆形。

生境分布　分布于华东、中南、西南、陕西等地。生于低山坡路边、空旷地杂草丛中。

采收加工　结果盛期时，齐地割起，拣去杂质，晒干，或洗净鲜用。

性味功能　凉，苦、涩。补肾涩精，健脾利湿，祛痰止咳，清热解毒。

主治用法　可用于肾虚，遗精，遗尿，尿频，白浊，带下，泄泻，痢疾，水肿，小儿疳积，咳嗽气喘，跌打损伤，目赤肿痛，痈疮肿毒，毒虫咬伤。咳嗽兼表寒者慎服。

化学成分　种子中含儿茶素、表儿茶素、黎豆胺；茎含木质素、多聚酚类、缩合鞣质；叶中含木质素、鞣质、β-谷甾醇、琥珀酸、槲皮素、山柰酚、松醇、胡桃甙、三叶豆甙、异牡荆素、多聚酚类、缩合鞣质等。

Source　It is the dried herbor root of *Lespedeza juncea* (L. f.) Pers. var. *sericea* (Thunb.) Maxim. The medicinal material is called as “Yeguanmen”.

Distribution　*L. juncea* is distributed in East, Central South and Southwest China, Shaanxi, etc. It grows by the roadside of low-altitude hillside and weeds in open area.

Indications　It is used to treat kidney deficiency, seminal emission, enuresis, frequent urination, gonorrhea, leukorrhea, diarrhea, dysentery, edema, infantile malnutrition, coughing and panting, traumatic injury, red eyes with pain and swelling, abscess and sore with pyogenic toxin, and poisonous insect bites. Patients with cough and exterior cold should take it with caution.

Chemical Constituents　The seed contains catechin, epicatechin, and stizolamine. The stem contains lignin, polyphenols and condensed tannins. The leaves contain lignin, tannins, β-sitosterol, succinic acid, quercetin, kaempferol, pinitol, juglanin, trifolin, isovitexin, polyphenols, condensed tannins, etc.

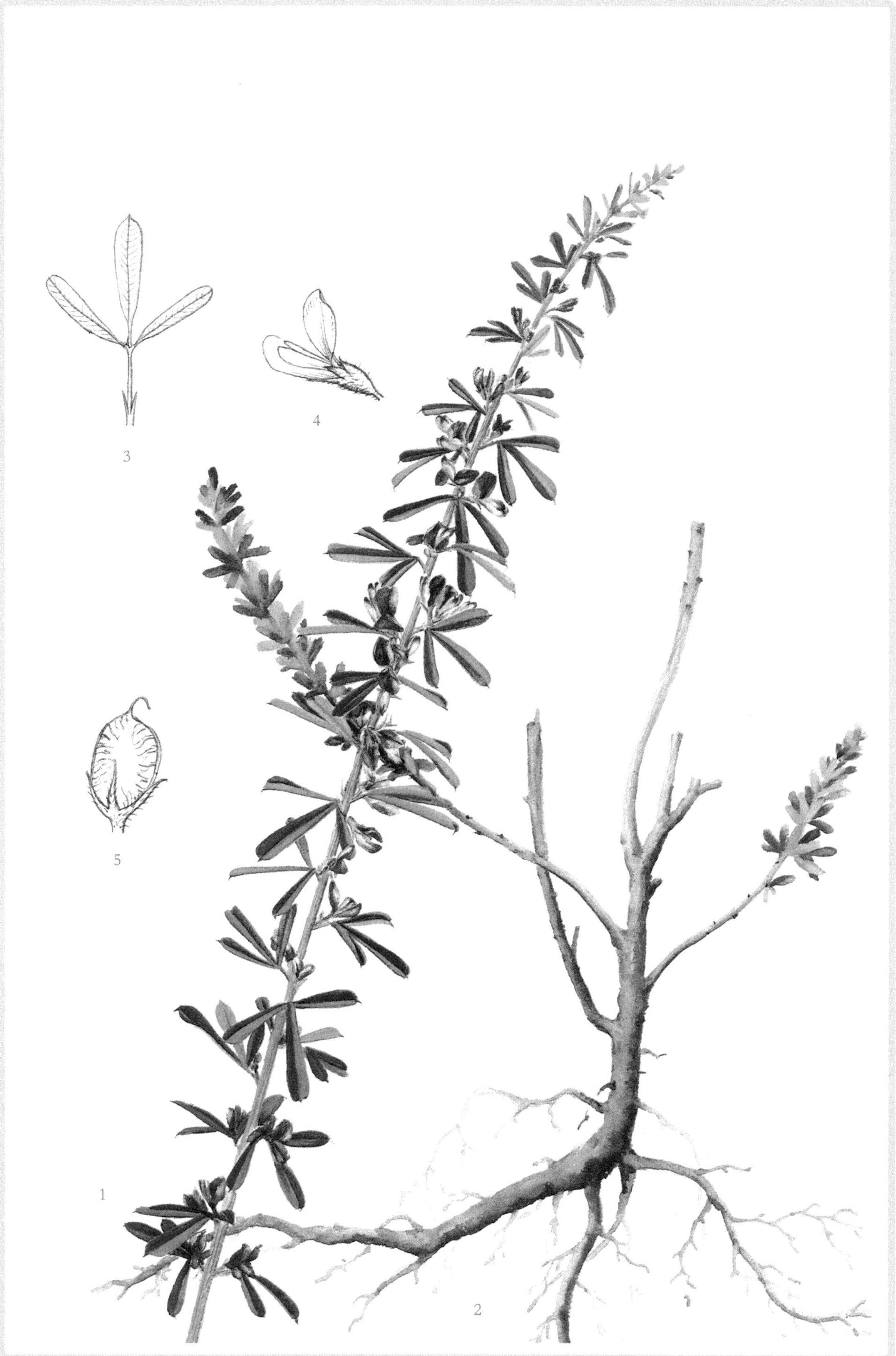

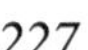

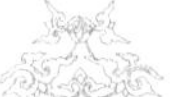

1. 花枝（flowering stem） 2. 根（root） 3. 叶（leaf） 4. 花（flower） 5. 果实（fruit）

草珊瑚

Caoshanhu

Sarcandra glabra

基　　源　金粟兰科 Chloranthaceae 草珊瑚属 Sarcandra 植物草珊瑚 *Sarcandra glabra* (Thunb.) Nakai 的干燥全草。药材名为“肿节风”。

形态特征　常绿半灌木；茎与枝节膨大。叶革质，椭圆形、卵形至卵状披针形，顶端渐尖，基部尖或楔形，边缘具粗锐锯齿，齿尖有一腺体，两面均无毛；叶柄部合生成鞘状。穗状花序顶生，通常分枝，多少成圆锥花序状；花黄绿色；雄蕊 1 枚，肉质。核果球形，熟时红色。

生境分布　分布于我国长江以南各省区，生于海拔 400-1500 m 的山坡、沟谷林下荫湿处。

采收加工　夏、秋二季采收，除去杂质，晒干。

性味功能　苦、辛，平。清热凉血，活血消斑，祛风通络。

主治用法　主要用于血热发斑发疹，风湿痹痛，跌打损伤。

化学成分　主要含有左旋类没药素甲，异秦皮定，延胡索酸，琥珀酸，黄酮苷，香豆精衍生物及挥发油等。

Source　It is the dried herb of *Sarcandra glabra* (Thunb.) Nakai (Chloranthaceae). The medicinal material is called as “Zhongjiefeng”.

Distribution　*S. glabra* is distributed in the south of the Yangtze River. It often grows on the floors of shady and damp forests on mountain slopes, in valleys at an altitude of 400–1500 m.

Indications　It is commonly used to heat in blood, eruption, rubella, and wind–dampness impediment pain, traumatic injury.

Chemical Constituents　It mainly contains istanbulin A, isofraxiden, fumaric acid, succinic acid, favone glycosides, coumarin derivatives, and volatile oil, etc.

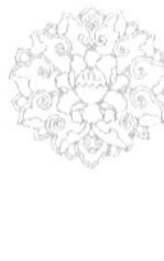

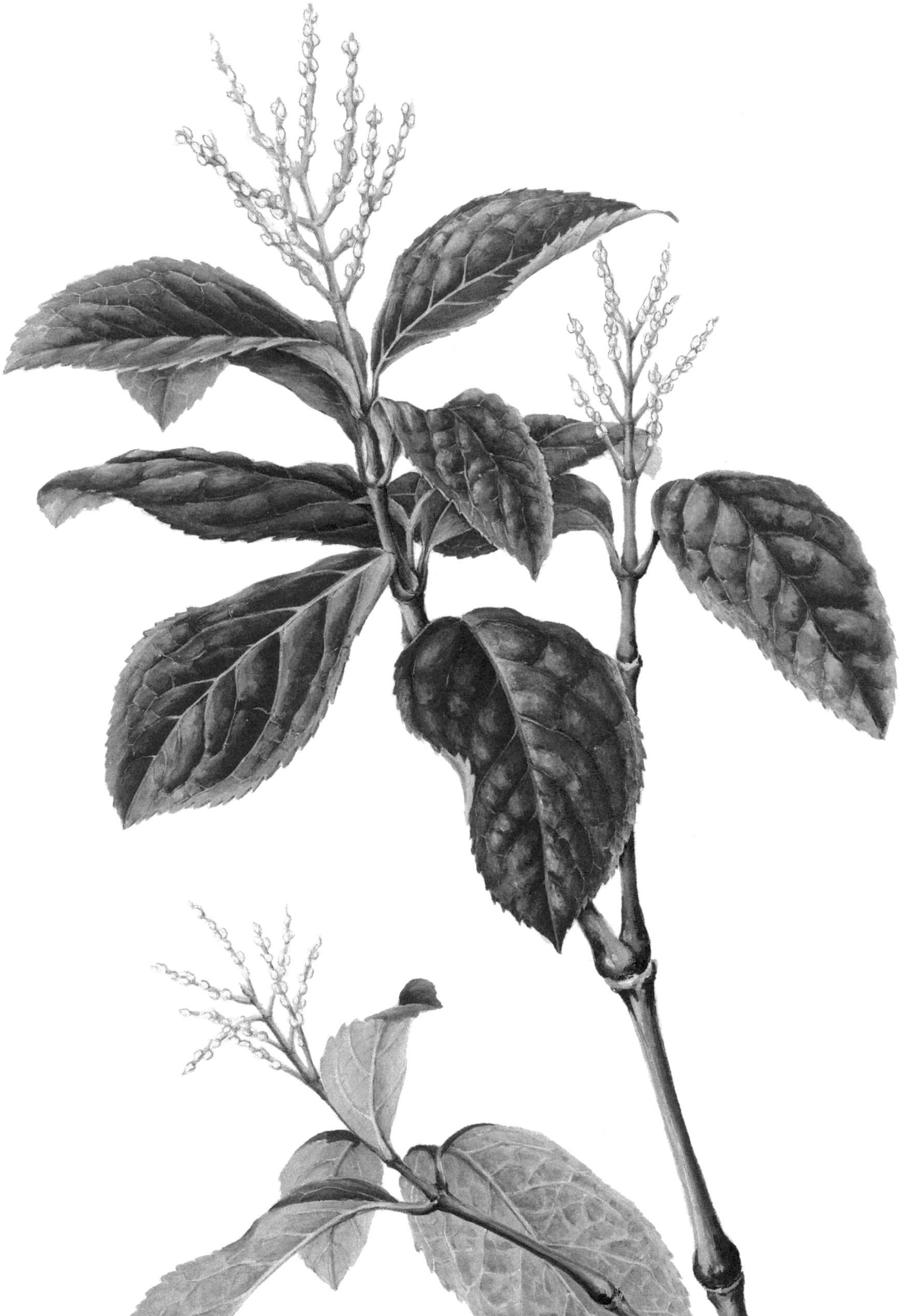

草珊瑚

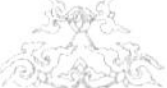

花枝（flowering stem）

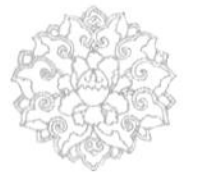

肾茶

Shencha

Clerodendranthus spicatus

基　源　唇形科 Lamiaceae 肾茶属 *Clerodendranthus* 植物肾茶 *Clerodendranthus spicatus* (Thunb.) C. Y. Wu ex H. W. Li 的干燥全草。药材名为“猫须草”。

形态特征　多年生草本。茎直立，四棱。叶卵形或卵状长圆形，边缘具粗牙齿，纸质，被短柔毛及腺点。轮伞花序具 6 朵花，枝顶成总状花序。花萼二唇形，果时增大；花冠浅紫或白色，外面被微柔毛，上唇上疏布锈色腺点，冠檐大，二唇形，上唇大，外反；雄蕊 4 枚，超出花冠，前对略长；花柱伸出花冠较长。小坚果卵形。

生境分布　分布于华南大部分省区。常生于林下潮湿处，多为栽培。

采收加工　一般每年可采收 2-3 次，每次在现蕾开花前采收为佳，割下茎叶，晒至七成干后，于清晨捆扎成把，再曝晒至全干。

性味功能　凉，甘、淡、微苦。清热利湿，通淋排石。

主治用法　主要用于急慢性肾炎，膀胱炎，尿路结石，胆结石，风湿性关节炎等。

化学成分　全草含有三萜类、甾醇类、黄酮类、挥发油类等。三萜类主要含有 α- 香树脂醇、熊果酸；甾醇类主要含有 β- 谷甾醇、胡萝卜苷；黄酮类主要含有三裂鼠尾草素、异甜橙素等；挥发油类主要含有柠檬烯、龙脑等。

Source　It is the dried herb of *Clerodendranthus spicatus* (Thunb.) C. Y. Wu ex H. W. Li (Lamiaceae). The medicinal material is called as “Maoxucao”.

Distribution　*C. spicatus* is distributed in most provinces of South China. It commonly grows in the damp ground in the forest. and mostly cultivated.

Indications　It is used to treat acute and chronic nephritis, cystitis, lithangiuria, gallstone, rheumatic arthritis, etc.

Chemical Constituents　The herb contains triterpenoids (e.g., α-amyrin, ursolic acid), sterols (e.g., β-sitosterol, daucosterol), flavonoids (e.g., salvigenin, isosinensetin), and volatile oils (e.g., limonene, borneol), etc.

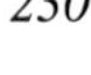

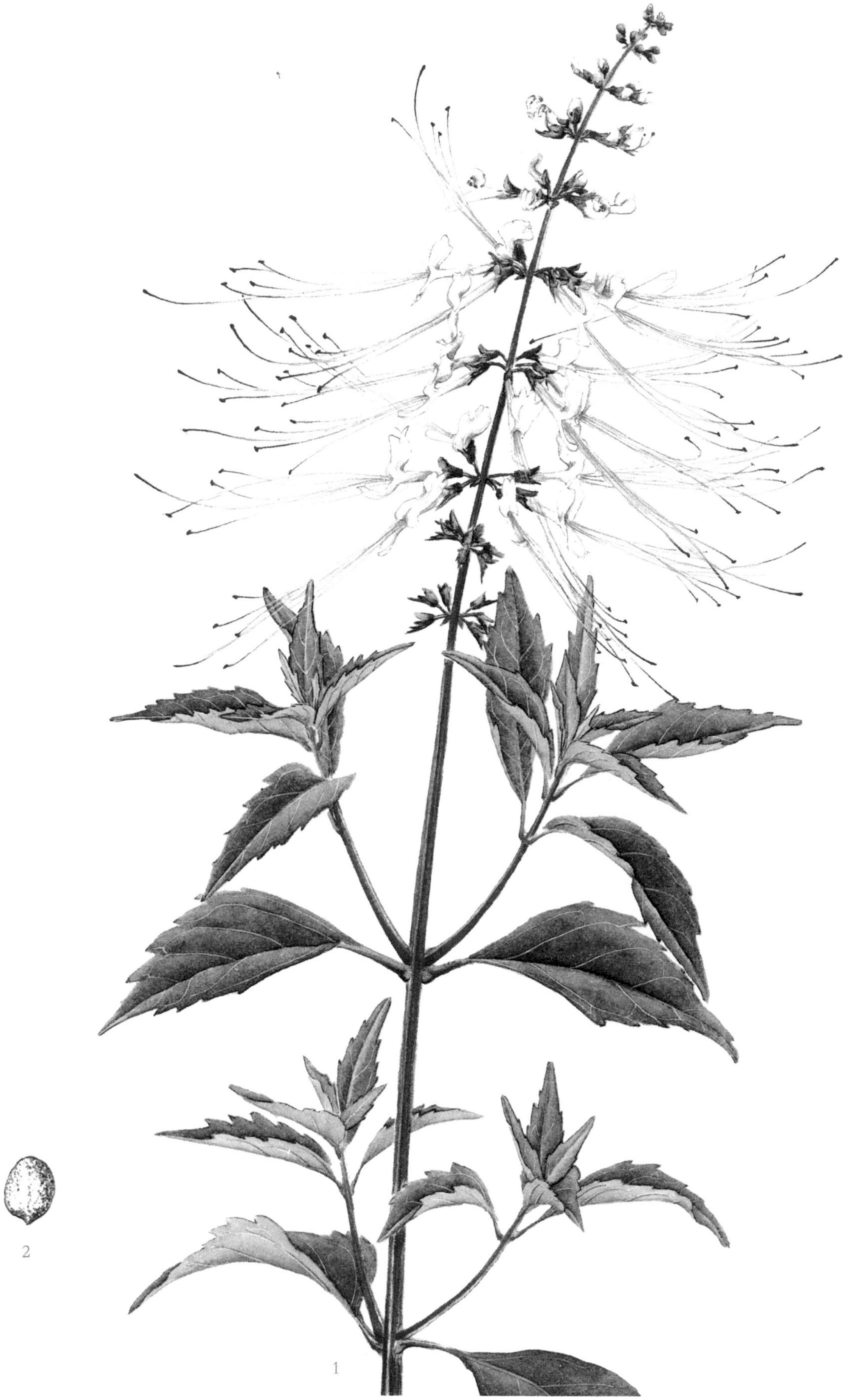

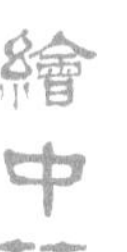

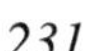

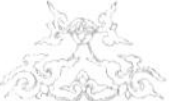

1. 花枝（flowering stem） 2. 种子（seed）

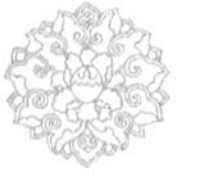

鸭跖草

Yazhicao

Commelina communis

基　　源　鸭跖草科 Commelinaceae 鸭跖草属 *Commelina* 植物鸭跖草 *Commelina communis* L. 的全草。药材名为“鸭跖草”。

形态特征　一年生披散草本。茎匍匐生根，多分枝。叶披针形至卵状披针形。总苞片佛焰苞状，与叶对生，折叠状，展开后为心形，边缘常有硬毛。聚伞花序，下面一枝具不育花 1 朵；上面一枝具花 3-4 朵，具短梗；萼片膜质；花瓣蓝色；内面 2 枚具爪。蒴果椭圆形，种子 4 粒。种子棕黄色，有不规则窝孔。

生境分布　分布于我国华东、华中、华南的大部分省区。常见生于潮湿的路旁、山坡、田边等。

采收加工　夏、秋二季采收，晒干。

性味功能　寒，甘、淡。清热泻火，解毒，利水消肿。

主治用法　用于感冒发热，热病烦渴，咽喉肿痛，水肿尿少，热淋涩痛，痈肿疔毒。

化学成分　鲜品中含有蓝鸭跖草苷、黄鸭跖草苷等。

Source　It is the dried herb of *Commelina communis* L. (Commelinaceae). The medicinal material is called as “Yazhicao”.

Distribution　*C. communis* is distributed in most provinces of East China, Central China, and South China. It commonly grows by the wet roadsides, on hillsides, in the fields, etc.

Indications　It is used to treat cold and fever, extreme thirst caused by febrile disease, sore swollen throat, edema with oliguria, unsmooth and painful urination seen in heat strang, swollen abscess boils and toxin.

Chemical Constituents　The fresh herb contains commelinin, favocommelin, etc.

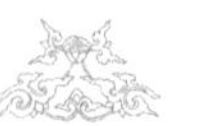

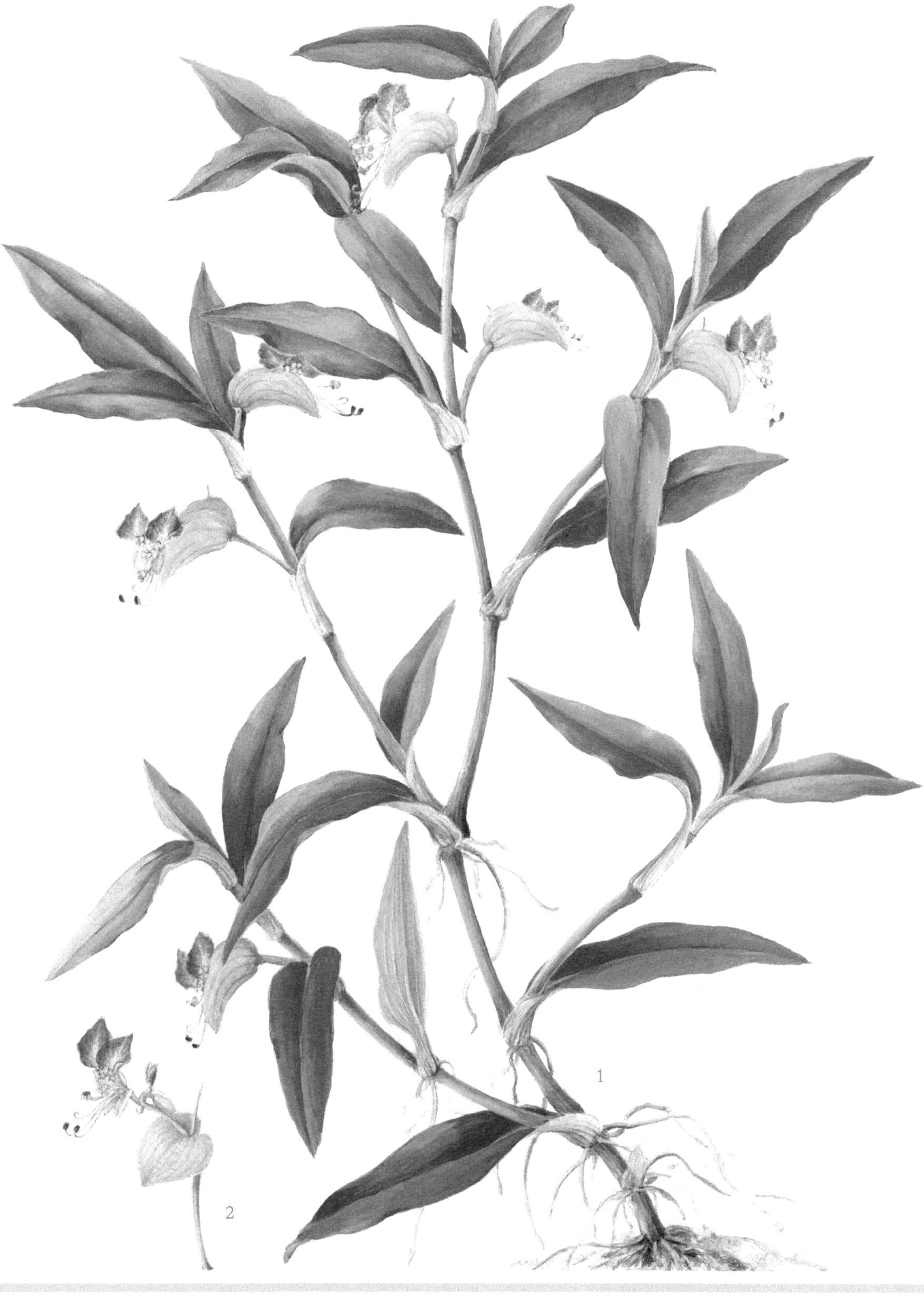

鸭跖草

1. 植株（plant） 2. 花枝（flowering stem）

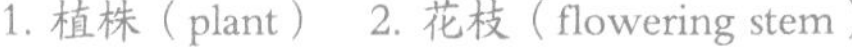

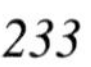

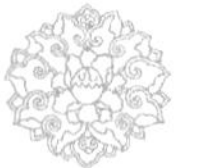

天山雪莲

Tianshanxuelian
Saussurea involucrata

基　　源　菊科 Asteraceae 风毛菊属 *Saussurea* 植物天山雪莲 *Saussurea involucrata* (Kar. et Kir.) Sch.-Bip. 的干燥地上部分。药材名为“天山雪莲”。

形态特征　多年生草本。根状茎粗壮，颈部被多数褐色的叶残迹；茎粗壮，无毛。叶密集，无柄，叶片椭圆形，边缘有尖齿；最上部叶苞叶状，膜质，黄白色，宽卵形，包围总花序，边缘有尖齿。头状花序 10-20 个，茎顶密集成球形的总花序；小花紫色。瘦果长圆形；冠毛污白色，2 层，外层小，糙毛状，内层长，羽毛状。

生境分布　分布于新疆。生于海拔 2400 m 以上的石缝中或草甸上。

采收加工　夏、秋二季花开时采收，阴干。

性味功能　温，微苦。温肾助阳，祛风胜湿，通经活血。

主治用法　主要用于风寒湿痹痛，类风湿性关节炎，小腹冷痛，月经不调。水煎服或酒浸服。

化学成分　主要含有大苞雪莲碱、金合欢素、槲皮素、紫丁香苷、绿原酸、蛇床子内酯、佛手内酯、大苞雪莲内酯、雪莲内酯、胡萝卜苷、琥珀酸、原儿茶酸、β-谷甾醇等。

备　　注　天山雪莲为常用维药。

Source　It is the dried aerial part of *Saussurea involucrata* (Kar. et Kir.) Sch.-Bip. (Asteraceae). The medicinal material is called as “Tianshanxuelian”.

Distribution　*S. involucrata* is distributed in Xinjiang Province. It grows in rock crevices or meadows at an altitude of over 2400 m.

Indications　It is used to treat the pain of wind–cold–dampness impediment, rheumatoid arthritis, cold pain in the lower abdomen, and menstrual irregularities. It should be taken after decotted with water or soak ed with wine.

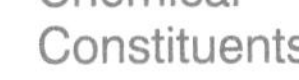

Chemical Constituents　It mainly contains involucratine, acacetin, quercetin, syringin, chlorogenic acid, cnidium lactone, bergapten, involucratolactone, xuelianlactone, daucosterol, succinic acid, protocatechuic acid, β-sitosterol, etc.

Note　It is a commonly-used medicinal material in Uyghurs.

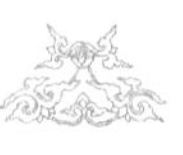
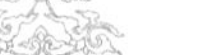

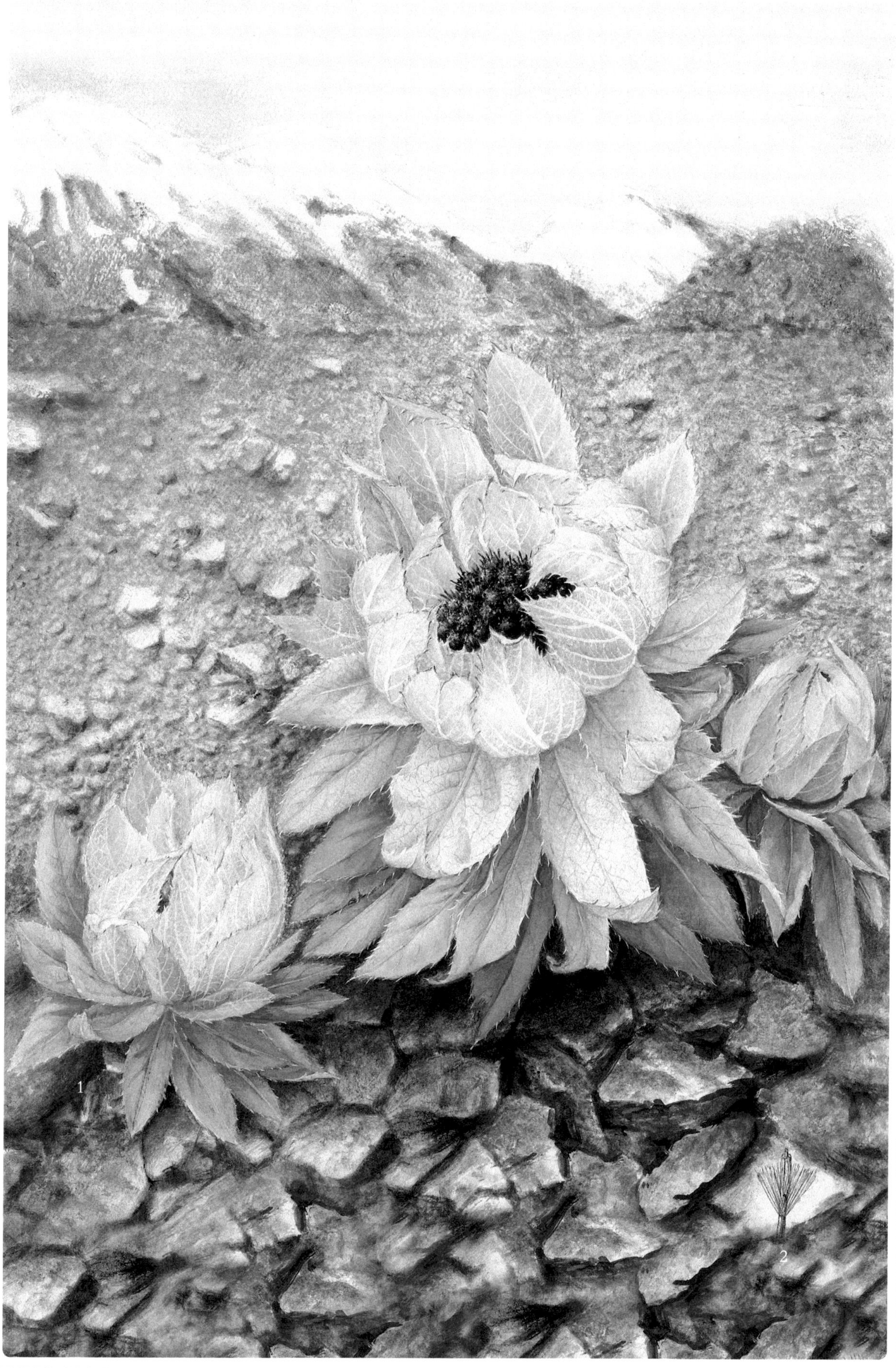

1

2

1. 植株及生境（plant and habitat） 2. 花（flower）

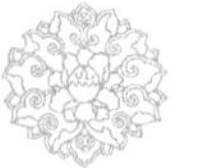

水母雪兔子

Shuimuxuetuzi

Saussurea medusa

基　源　菊科 Asteraceae 风毛菊属 *Saussurea* 植物水母雪兔子 *Saussurea medusa* Maxim 的带根全草。药材名为“雪莲花”。

形态特征　多年生多次结实草本。根状茎细长，上部发出数个莲座状叶丛；茎直立，密被白色棉毛。叶密集，两面灰绿色，被白色长棉毛。头状花序多数，在茎端密集成半球形；总苞狭圆柱状；总苞片 3 层，外层长椭圆形，紫色，外面被白色或褐色棉毛，中层倒披针形，内层披针形；小花蓝紫色。瘦果纺锤形；冠毛白色，2 层，外层短，糙毛状，内层长，羽毛状。

生境分布　主要分布于横断山区以及云南、西藏、甘肃等地。生于海拔 4000 m 以上多砾石的高山山坡或流石滩上。

采收加工　6-7 月间，开花时拔取全株，除去泥土，晾干。

性味功能　温，甘、微苦。温肾壮阳，调经止血。

主治用法　主要用于阳痿，腰膝酸软，女子带下，月经不调，风湿痹症，外伤出血。

化学成分　地上部分含有生物碱、黄酮类、苯丙素类、倍半萜类、挥发油、多糖类等多种化学成分。

Source　It is the dried herb with root of *Saussurea medusa* Maxim. (Asteraceae). The medicinal material is called as “Xuelianhua”.

Distribution　*S. medusa* is mainly distributed in Hengduan Mountains, Yunnan, Tibet, Gansu and other regions. It grows on mountain slopes with loose stones or screes at an altitude of over 4000 m.

Indications　It is used to treat impotence, soreness and weakness of waist and knees, vaginal discharge, menstrual irregularities, rheumatic arthralgia, bleeding due to external injury.

Chemical Constituents　The aerial parts of *S. medusa* contains alkaloids, flavonoids, phenylpropanoids, sesquiterpenoids, volatile oils, polysaccharides, etc.

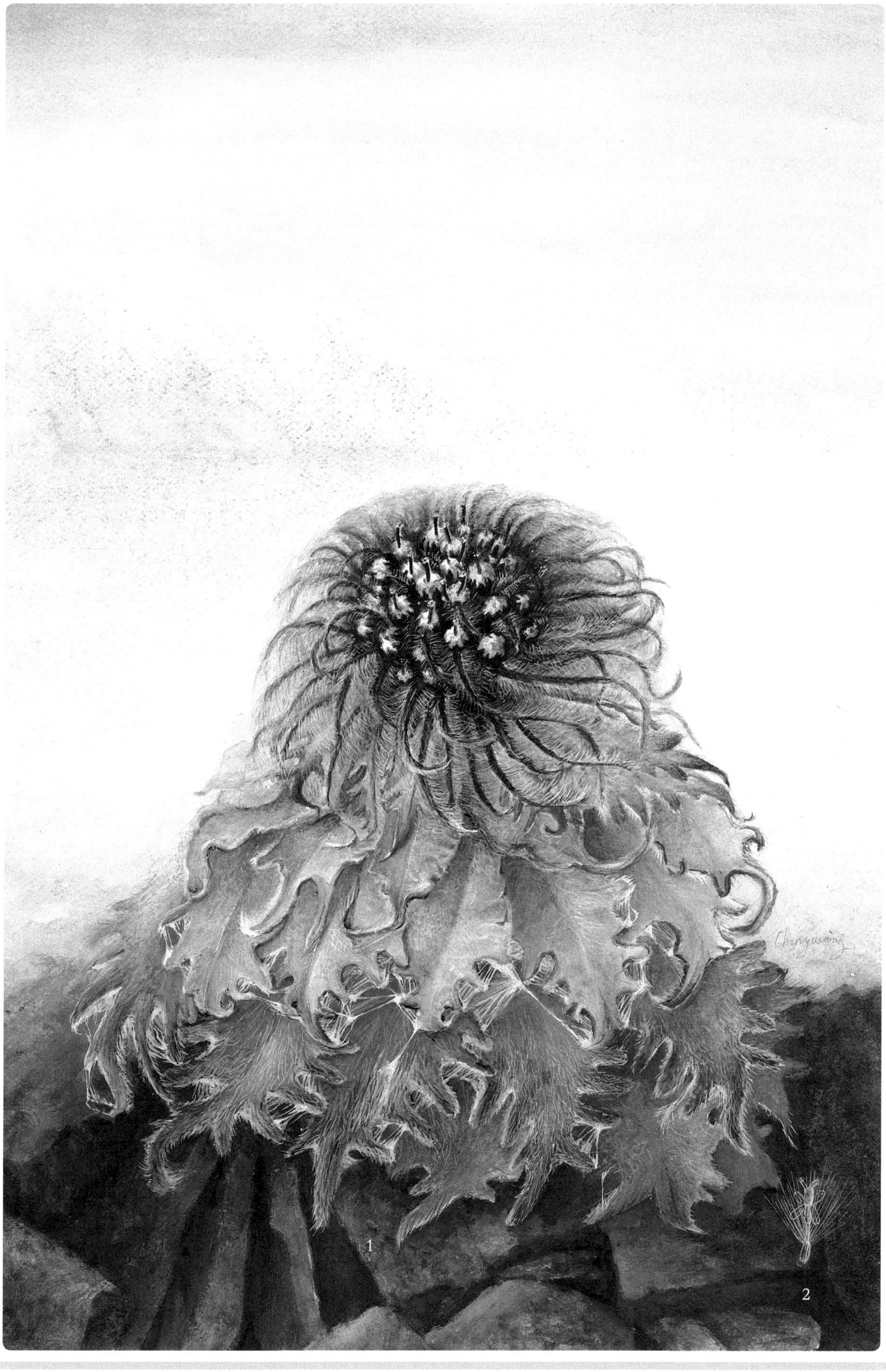

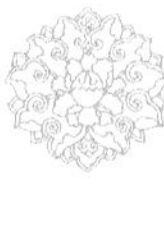

水母雪兔子

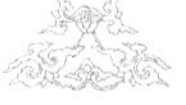

1. 植株及生境（plant and habitat） 2. 花（flower）

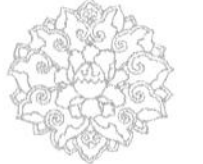

绵头雪兔子

Miantouxuetuzi

Saussurea laniceps

基　　源　菊科 Asteraceae 风毛菊属 *Saussurea* 植物绵头雪兔子 *Saussurea laniceps* Hand.-Mazz. 的带根全草。药材名为“雪莲花”。

形态特征　多年生一次结实草本。茎上部密被白色或淡褐色的棉毛，基部有褐色残存的叶柄。叶极密集，倒披针形或长椭圆形，上面密被蛛丝状棉毛，后脱毛，下面密被褐色绒毛。头状花序多数，在茎端密集成圆锥状穗状花序。总苞宽钟状；总苞片 3-4 层，外面被白色或褐色棉毛；小花白色。瘦果圆柱状；冠毛鼠灰色，2 层，外层短，糙毛状，内层长，羽毛状。

生境分布　主要分布于我国四川西部、西藏东部、云南。生于海拔 4000 m 以上的高山流石滩上。

采收加工　6-7 月，开花时拔取全株，除去泥土，晾干。

性味功能　温，甘、微苦。温肾壮阳，调经止血。

主治用法　主要用于阳痿，腰膝酸软，女子带下，月经不调，风湿痹症，外伤出血。

化学成分　全草含东莨菪素、伞形花内酯、对羟基苯乙酮、大黄素甲醚、β - 谷甾醇等。

Source　It is the dried herb with root of *Saussurea laniceps* Hand.-Mazz. (Asteraceae). The medicinal material is called as “Xuelianhua”.

Distribution　It is mainly distributed in western Sichuan, eastern Tibet and Yunnan. It grows on the alpine rocky beaches at an altitude of more than 4000 m.

Indications　It is used to treat impotence, soreness and weakness of waist and knees, leukorrhea, menstrual irregularities, rheumatic arthralgia, bleeding due to external injury.

Chemical Constituents　The herb contains scopoletin, umbelliferone, *p*-hydroxyacetophenone, physcion, β-sitosterol, etc.

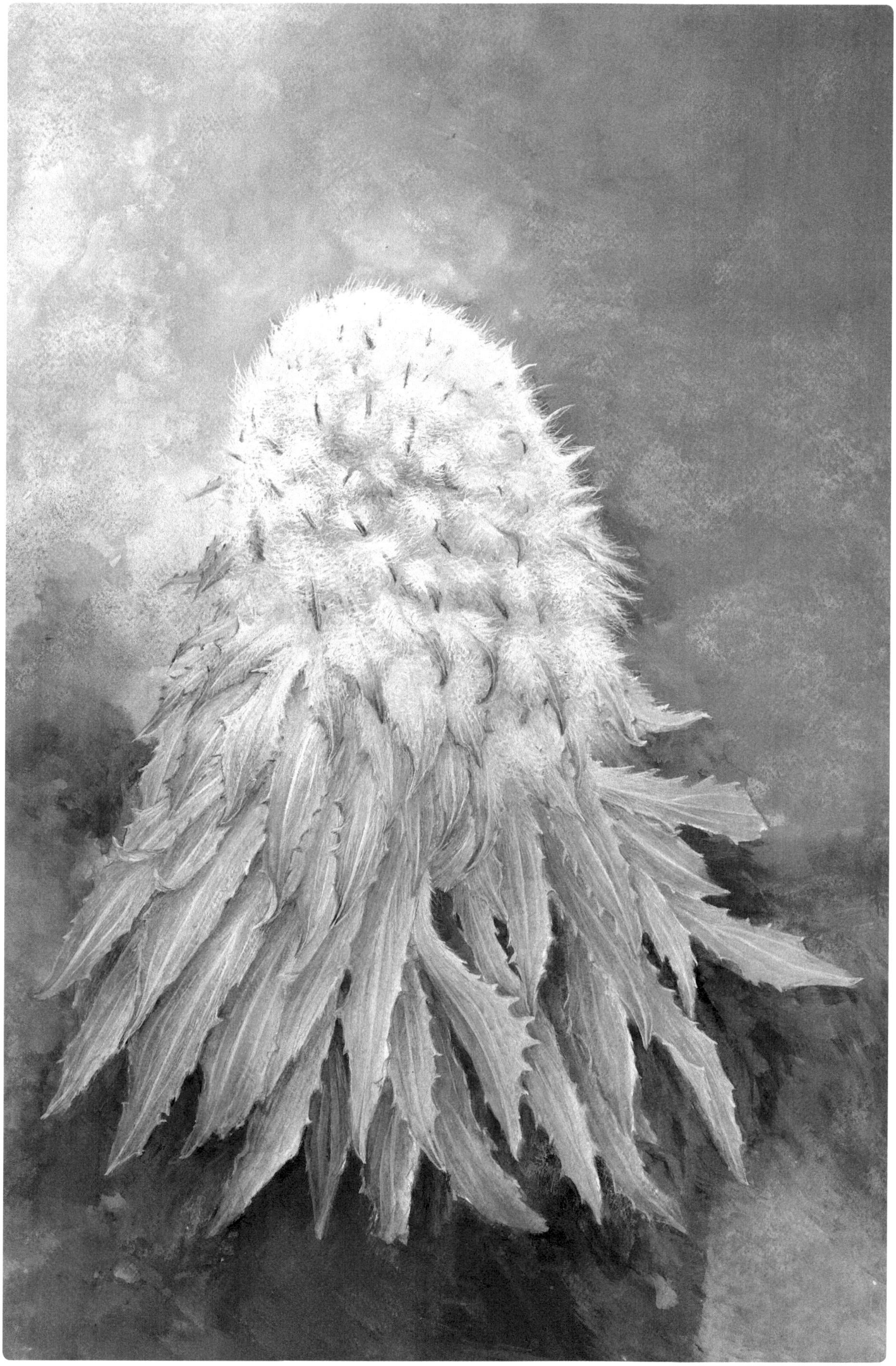

植株及生境（plant and habitat）

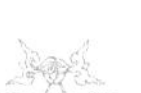

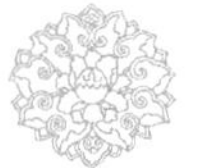

黄花蒿

Huanghuahao

Artemisia annua

基　　源　菊科 Asteraceae 蒿属 *Artemisia* 植物黄花蒿 *Artemisia annua* L. 的干燥地上部分。药材名为“青蒿”。

形态特征　一年生草本。全株具较强气味。茎直立，具纵条纹，多分枝。基生叶平铺地面，开花时凋谢；茎生叶互生，幼时绿色，老时变为黄褐色；叶片三回羽状全裂，裂片短细；叶轴两侧具窄翅。头状花序细小，球形，具细软短梗，组成圆锥状；花全为管状花，黄色，外围为雌花，中央为两性花。瘦果椭圆形。

生境分布　分布于我国南北各地，生于山坡、荒地、田埂边等。

采收加工　秋季花盛开时采割，除去老茎，阴干。

性味功能　寒，苦、辛。清虚热，除骨蒸，解暑热，截疟，退黄。

主治用法　用于温邪伤阴，夜热早凉，阴虚发热，骨蒸劳热，暑邪发热，疟疾寒热，湿热黄疸。后下。

化学成分　主要含有青蒿素、青蒿甲素、青蒿乙素等倍半萜类，以及黄酮类、香豆素类和挥发油类成分。

备　　注　屠呦呦致力于中医药研究实践，从黄花蒿中发现了青蒿素，解决了抗疟治疗失效难题，荣获国家最高科学技术奖、诺贝尔生理学或医学奖等称号。

Source　It is the dried aerial part of *Artemisia annua* L. (Asteraceae). The medicinal material is called as “Qinghao”.

Distribution　*A. annua* is distributed all over China. It grows on hillsides, wastelands, field footpaths, etc.

Indications　It is used to treat pathogenic warmth damaging yin, night fever abating at dawn, yin-deficiency heat, bone-steaming with hectic fever, fever due to summer-heat pathogen, chills and fever due to malaria, jaundice due to dampness–heat. It should be decocted later.

Chemical Constituents　It mainly contains sesquiterpenes (e.g., artemisinin, arteannuin A, arteannuin B), flavonoids, coumarins, and volatile oils.

Note　Youyou TU is committed to the research and practice of TCM and discovered Artemisinin in *A. annua*, which has solved the failure of antimalarial therapy. She has won the State Preeminent Science and Technology Award of China and the Nobel Prize in Physiology or Medicine.

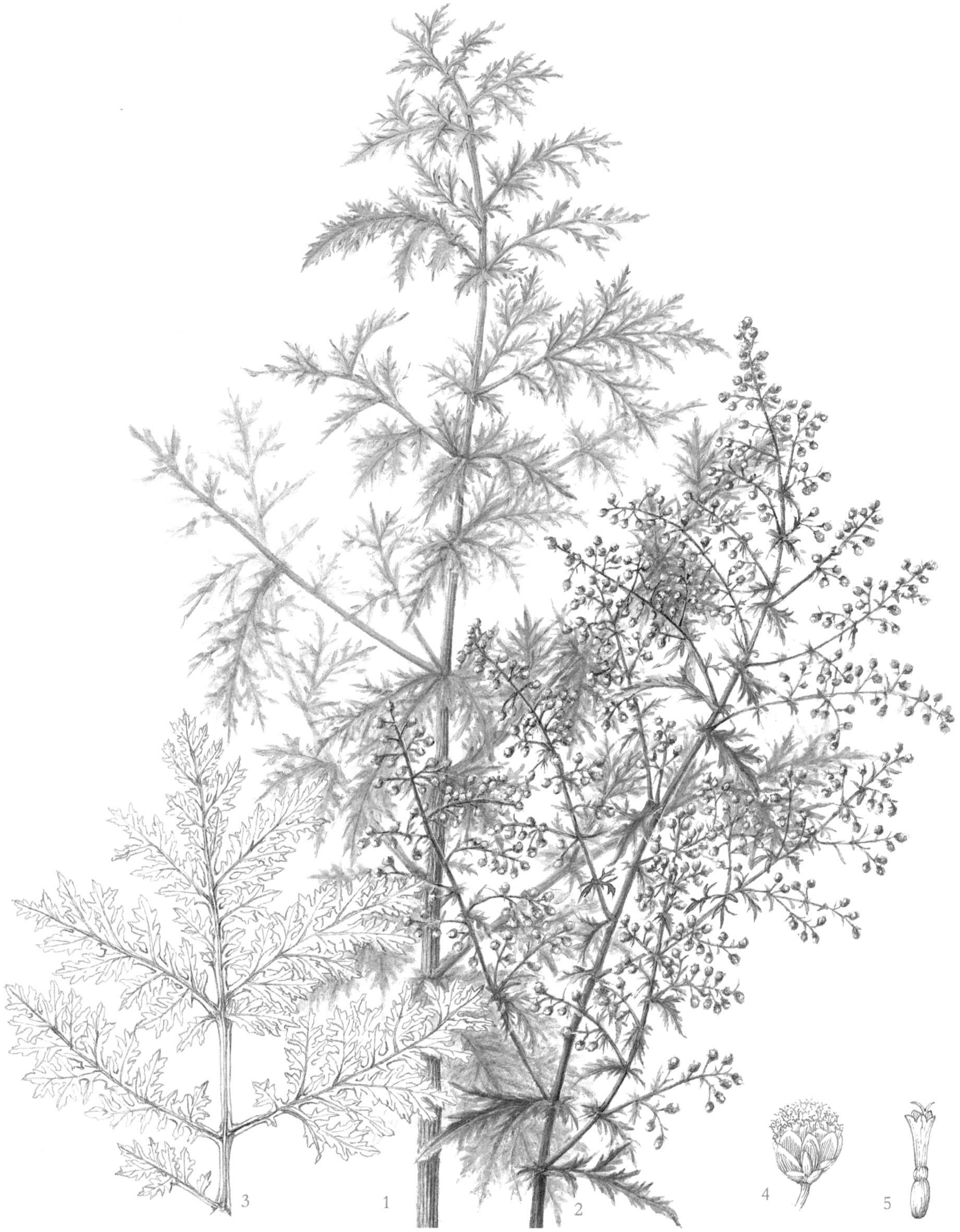

1. 植株（plant） 2. 花枝（flowering stem） 3. 叶（leaf） 4. 花序（inflorescence） 5. 花（flower）

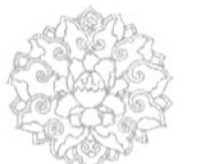

蒲公英

Pugongying

Taraxacum mongolicum

基　　源　菊科 Asteraceae 蒲公英属 *Taraxacum* 植物蒲公英 *Taraxacum mongolicum* Hand.-Mazz. 的干燥全草。药材名为“蒲公英”。

形态特征　多年生草本。全株含白色乳汁，被白色疏软毛。根外皮黄棕色。叶排列呈莲座状；具叶柄，基部两侧扩大呈鞘状；叶片倒披针形或倒卵形，基部狭窄，下延，边缘不规则羽状分裂，绿色或淡紫色，被白色蛛丝状毛。头状花序单一，顶生，全为舌状花，两性；花冠黄色。瘦果倒披针形，有刺状突起；冠毛白色。

生境分布　分布于我国大部分省区。广泛生于中、低海拔地区的山坡、草地、路边、田野等环境中。

采收加工　春至秋季花初开时采挖，除去杂质，洗净，晒干。

性味功能　寒，苦、甘。清热解毒，消肿散结，利尿通淋。

主治用法　用于疔疮肿毒，乳痈，瘰疬，目赤，咽痛，肺痈，肠痈，湿热黄疸，热淋涩痛。

化学成分　主要含有蒲公英甾醇、蒲公英赛醇、蒲公英醇、β-谷甾醇、肌醇、苦味质、胆碱、菊糖、叶黄素、蝴蝶梅黄素等。

备　　注　蒲公英幼嫩的全株可供食用。

Source　It is the dried herb of *Taraxacum mongolicum* Hand.-Mazz. (Asteraceae). The medicinal material is called as “Pugongying”.

Distribution　*T. mongolicum* is distributed in most provinces in China. It grows widely on hillsides, grasslands, roadsides, fields and other environments in middle and low altitude areas.

Indications　It is used to treat furuncle, sore, pyrogenic toxin, acute mastitis, scrofula, red eyes, sore throat, lung abscess, interstinal abscess, jaundice due to dampness–heat, and unsmooth and painful urination seen in heat strangury.

Chemical Constituents　It mainly contains taraxasterol, taraxerol, taraxol, β-sitosterol, inositol, mergosin, choline, inulin, lutein, violaxanthin, etc.

Note　The young herb of *T. mongolicum* is edible.

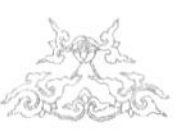

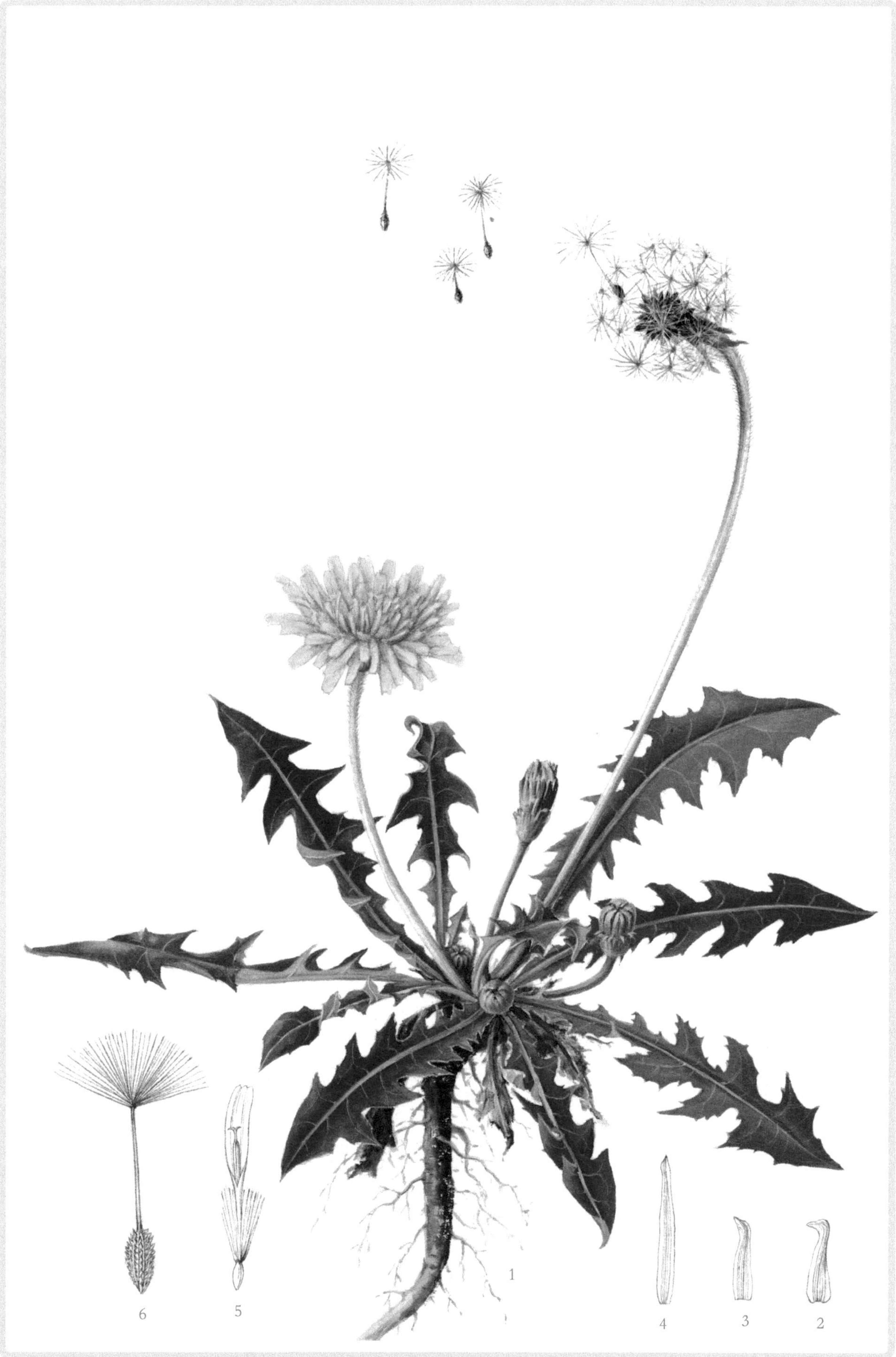

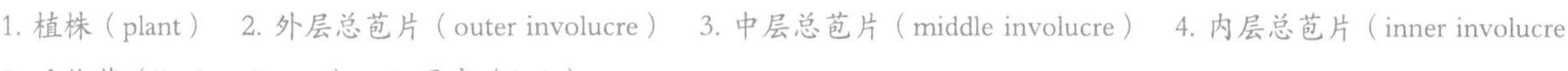

1. 植株（plant） 2. 外层总苞片（outer involucre） 3. 中层总苞片（middle involucre） 4. 内层总苞片（inner involucre）
5. 舌状花（ligulate flower） 6. 果实（fruit）

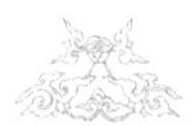

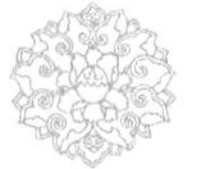

草麻黄

Caomahuang

Ephedra sinica

基　　源　麻黄科 Ephedraceae 麻黄属 *Ephedra* 植物草麻黄 *Ephedra sinica* Stapf 的干燥草质茎。药材名为“麻黄”。

形态特征　草本状灌木。小枝直伸或微曲，表面细纵槽纹不明显。节上有膜质鳞叶，叶二裂，裂片锐三角形，先端灰白色，反曲，基部联合呈筒状，红棕色。雄球花多呈复穗状；雌球花单生，在幼枝上顶生，在老枝上腋生。果实成熟时肉质红色，矩圆状卵圆形或近球形。种子通常 2 粒，表面具细皱纹。

生境分布　分布于华北、东北、西北等部分省区。生于干旱的荒地、草原、枯竭河滩附近，常成片丛生。

采收加工　秋季采割绿色的草质茎，晒干。

性味功能　温，辛、微苦。发汗散寒，宣肺平喘，利水消肿。

主治用法　主要用于风寒感冒，胸闷喘咳，风水浮肿。蜜麻黄润肺止咳。多用于表证已解，气喘咳嗽。

化学成分　主要含有麻黄碱、伪麻黄碱、去甲麻黄碱等生物碱类成分；还含有挥发油类、黄酮类和有机酸类等成分。

备　　注　麻黄根亦可入药，可固表止汗，用于自汗，盗汗。

Source　It is the dried herbaceous stem of *Ephedra sinica* Stapf. (Ephedraceae). The medicinal material is called as “Mahuang”.

Distribution　*E. sinica* is distributed in provinces of North, Northeast and Northwest China. It grows in clusters in dry wastelands, grasslands, and near dry river beach.

Indications　It is used to treat wind–cold common cold, oppression in chest, dyspnea with cough, and wind edema. Herba Ephedrae Sinicae stir-frying with honey has the function of moistening lung and relieving cough, which is commonly used to treat asthma and cough without exterior syndrome.

Chemical Constituents　It mainly contains alkaloids (e.g., ephedrine, pseudoephedrine, norephedrine), volatile oils, flavonoids, organic acids, etc.

Note　Radix Epbedrae Sinicae can also be used as the medicine, which has the function of consolidating exterior and stopping sweating. It is used to treat spontaneous sweating and night sweating.

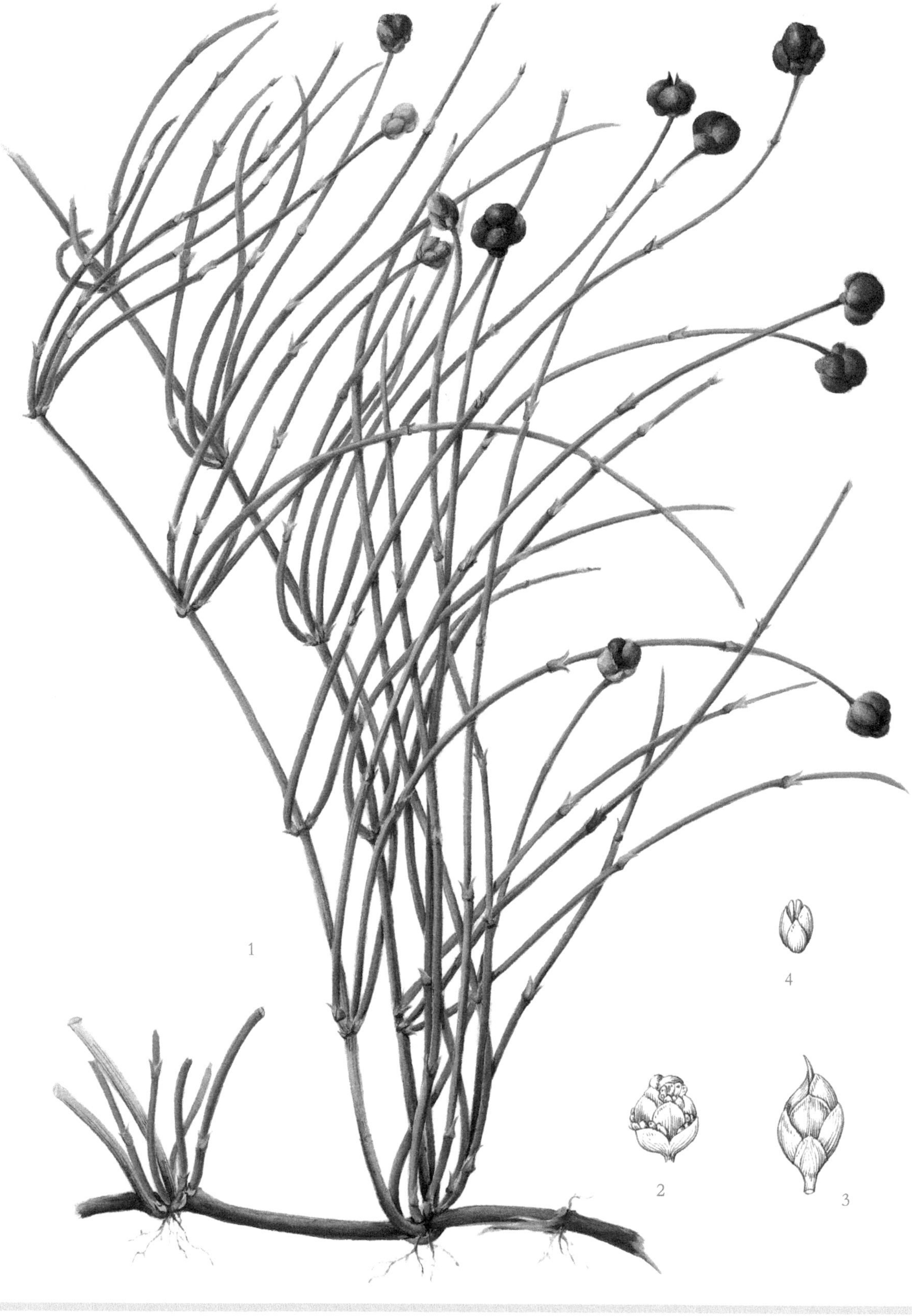

1

4

2

3

1. 植株（plant） 2. 雄球花（male cone） 3. 雌球花（female cone） 4. 种子（seed）

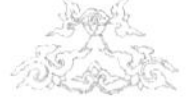

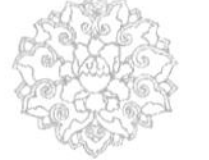

唐古红景天

Tangguhongjingtian

Rhodiola tangutica

基　源　景天科 Crassulaceae 红景天属 *Rhodiola* 植物唐古红景天 *Rhodiola tangutica* (Maxim.) S. H. Fu 的全草。药材名为“小花红景天”。

形态特征　多年生草本。主根粗长。花茎多数，丛生；花茎上的叶互生，无柄；叶片线形。花序紧密，伞房状，雌雄异株；雄株花序下有苞叶，萼片 5；雌株心皮发育成 5 枚蓇葖果，紫红色，直立或稍外弯。种子多数，有网纹，具翅，淡褐色。

生境分布　主要分布于我国四川、青海、甘肃、宁夏。生于海拔 2000-4700 m 的高山石缝中或近水边。

采收加工　春、秋二季均可采收，以秋季为好，除去地上枯萎茎叶，挖掘全株，除去泥土，晒干。

性味功能　寒，甘、涩。补气清肺，益智养心，收涩止血，散瘀消肿。

主治用法　主要用于治疗气虚体弱，病后畏寒，气短乏力，肺热咳嗽，咯血，白带腹泻，跌打损伤，烫火伤，神经症，高原反应。

化学成分　主要含有黄酮类，如红景天苷。另还含有有机酸类和挥发油等成分。

备　注　唐古红景天为藏药常用药。

Source　The herb of *Rhodiola tangutica* (Maxim.) S. H. Fu (Crassulaceae). The medicinal material is called as “Xiaohuahongjingtian”.

Distribution　*R. tangutica* is mainly distributed in Sichuan, Qinghai, Gansu, and Ningxia. It grows in the high mountain crevices or near to water source at an altitude of 2000–4700 m.

Indications　It is used to treat qi deficiency and weak health, fear of cold after illness, shortness of breath and lack of strength, cough with lung heat, hemoptysis, leucorrhea and diarrhea, traumatic injury, burns and scalds, neurosis, and high altitude reaction.

Chemical Constituents　It mainly contains flavonoids (e.g., rhodioloside), organic acids, volatile oils, etc.

Note　It is a commonly-used medicinal material in Tibetan medicine.

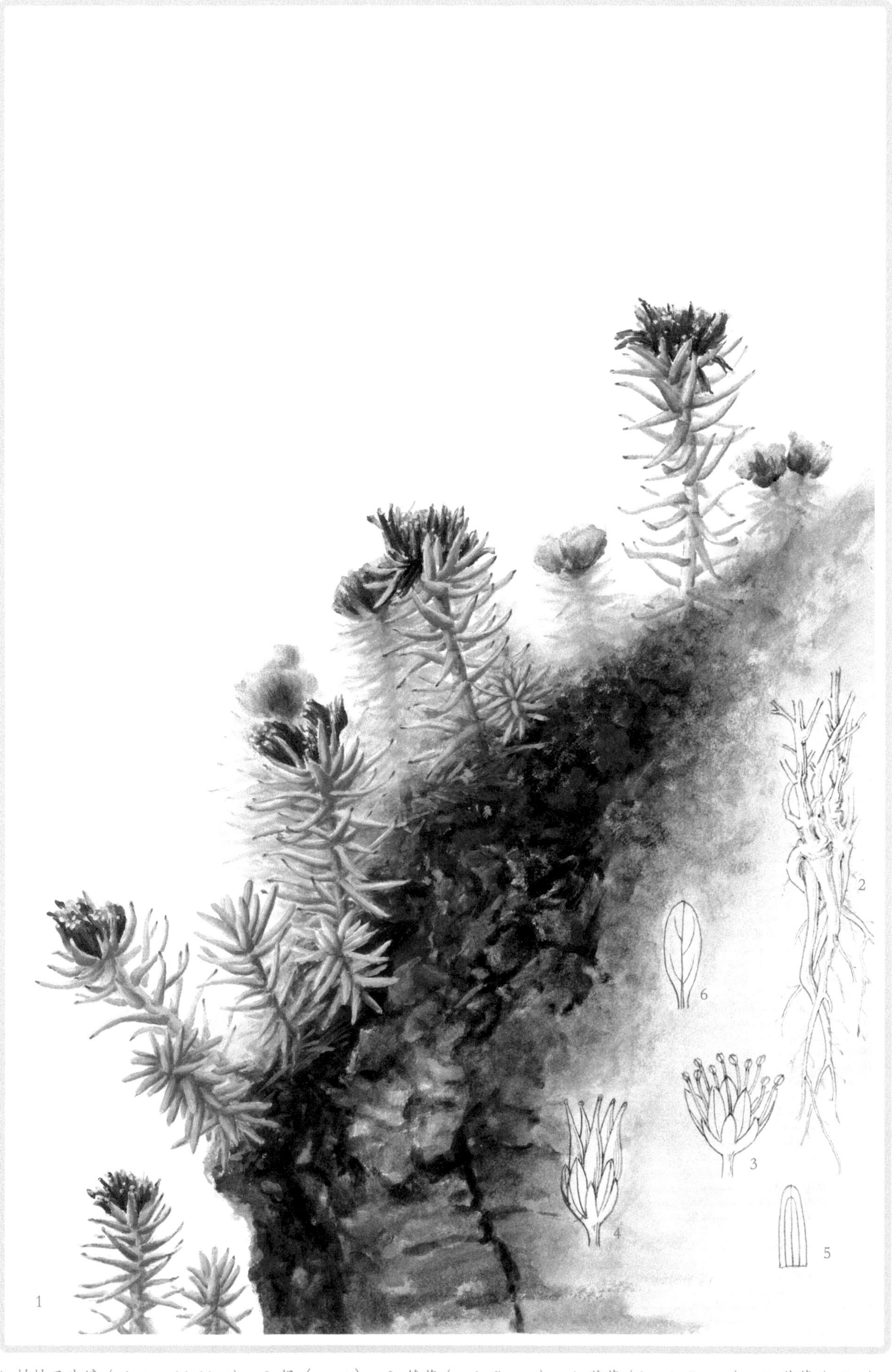

1. 植株及生境（plant and habitat） 2. 根（root） 3. 雄花（male flower） 4. 雌花（female flower） 5. 花萼（calyx）
6. 花瓣（petal）

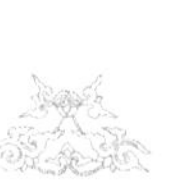

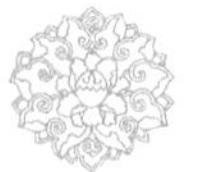

白屈菜

Baiqucai

Chelidonium majus

基　源　罂粟科 Papaveraceae 白屈菜属 *Chelidonium* 植物白屈菜 *Chelidonium majus* L. 的干燥全草。药材名为“白屈菜”。

形态特征　多年生草本。具黄色汁液。茎多分枝，分枝常被短柔毛。基生叶少，早凋落；叶柄基部扩大成鞘；叶倒卵状长圆形，羽状全裂，全裂片 2-4 对，表面绿色背面具白粉，疏被短柔毛。伞形花序；花梗纤细；萼片卵圆形，早落；花瓣倒卵形，全缘，黄色。蒴果狭圆柱形。种子卵形，暗褐色，具光泽及蜂窝状小格。

生境分布　我国大部分省区均有分布。常生于海拔 500-2000 m 的山坡路旁或干燥石缝中。

采收加工　夏、秋二季采挖，除去泥沙，阴干或晒干。

性味功能　凉，苦；有毒。解痉止痛，止咳平喘。

主治用法　主要用于胃脘挛痛，咳嗽气喘，百日咳。

化学成分　主要含有生物碱类成分，如白屈菜碱、原阿片碱等。

Source　It is the dried herb of *Chelidonium majus* L. (Papaveraceae). The medicinal material is called as “Baiqucai”.

Distribution　*C. majus* is distributed in most provinces of China, and commonly grows by the roadside of hills or in dry rocky crevices at an altitude of 500–2000 m.

Indications　It is used to treat crampy pain in stomach, coughing and panting, and whooping cough.

Chemical Constituents　It mainly contains alkaloids, e.g., chelidonine, protopine, etc.

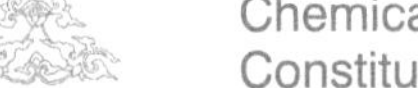

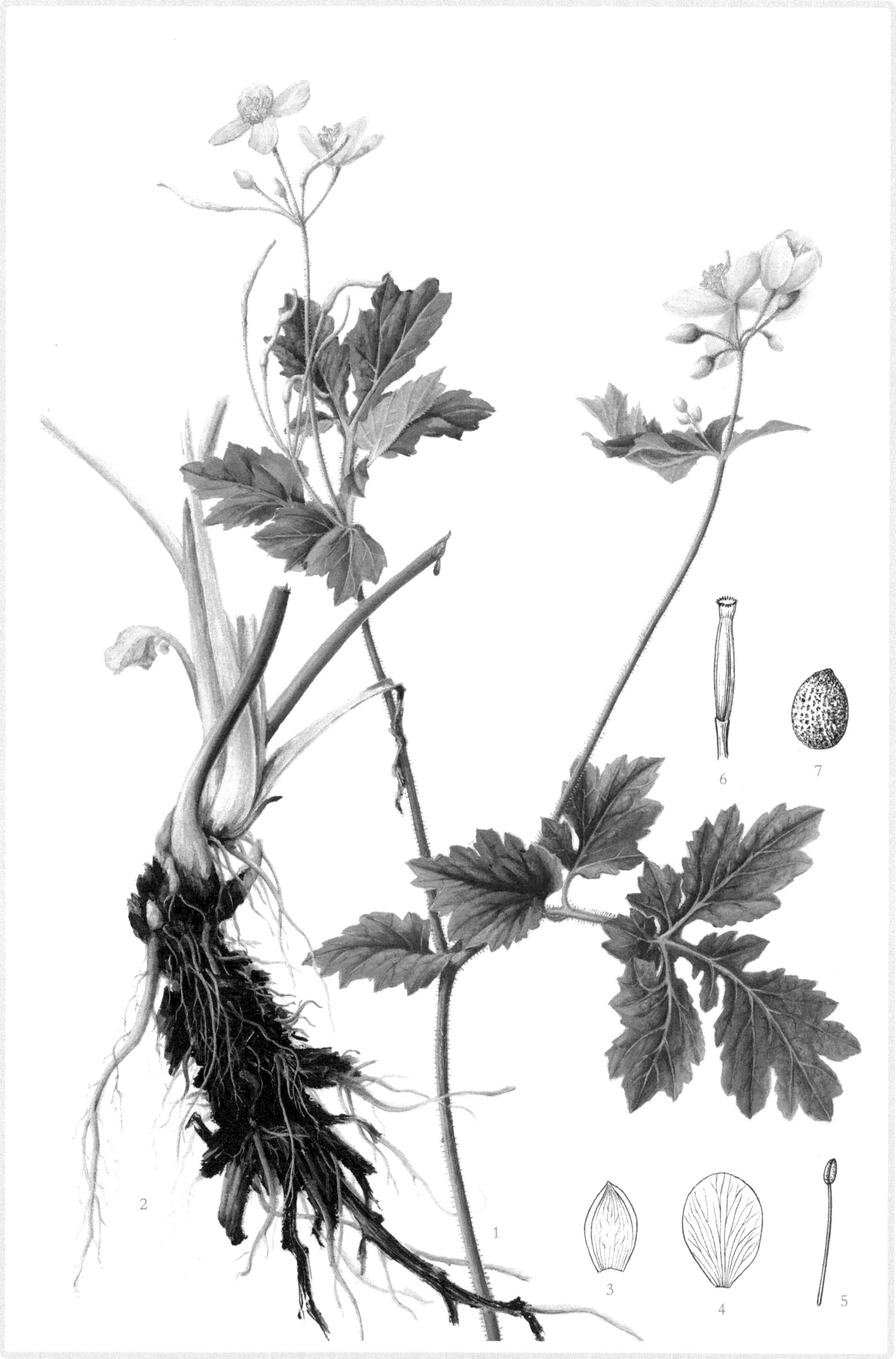

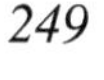

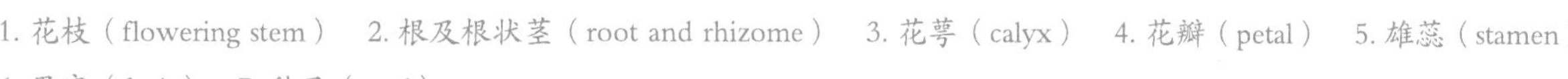

1. 花枝（flowering stem） 2. 根及根状茎（root and rhizome） 3. 花萼（calyx） 4. 花瓣（petal） 5. 雄蕊（stamen）
6. 果实（fruit） 7. 种子（seed）

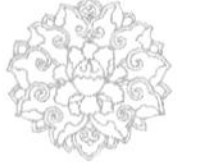

毛瓣绿绒蒿

Maobanlvronghao

Meconopsis torquata

基　　源　罂粟科 Papaveraceae 绿绒蒿属 *Meconopsis* 植物毛瓣绿绒蒿 *Meconopsis torquata* Prain 的干燥全草。药材名为“毛瓣绿绒蒿”。

形态特征　一年生草本。茎直立，基部残存叶基，密被刚毛。基生叶多数，呈莲座状，倒披针形，全缘，两面被黄褐色刚毛，叶柄基部具鞘，密被刚毛；茎生叶较小，边缘为不规则的圆裂，无柄。花茎粗壮，密被绣色刚毛。花多数，紧密排列；花瓣 4 或更多，倒卵形，淡红色，外面疏被刚毛。蒴果倒卵形，明显具肋。

生境分布　分布于西藏南部，生于海拔 4000 m 的石滩上。

采收加工　7-8 月采收全草，洗净，阴干。

性味功能　寒，苦、涩；有小毒。止咳，利水消肿。

主治用法　主要用于咳嗽，水肿。

化学成分　主要含有芹菜素、木樨草素、5,7- 二羟基色原酮、5,7,4′ - 三羟基二氢黄酮、乌苏酸等成分。

备　　注　藏医用药。

Source　It is the dried herb of *Meconopsis torquata* Prain (Papaveraceae). The medicinal material is called as “Maobanlvronghao”.

Distribution　*M. torquata* is distributed in southern Tibet. It grows on rocky beaches at an altitude of 4000 m.

Indications　It is used to treat cough and edema.

Chemical Constituents　It contains apigenin, luteolin, 5,7-dihydroxychromone, 5,7,4′-trihydroxy flavonone, ursolic acid, etc.

Note　It is used in Tibetan medicine.

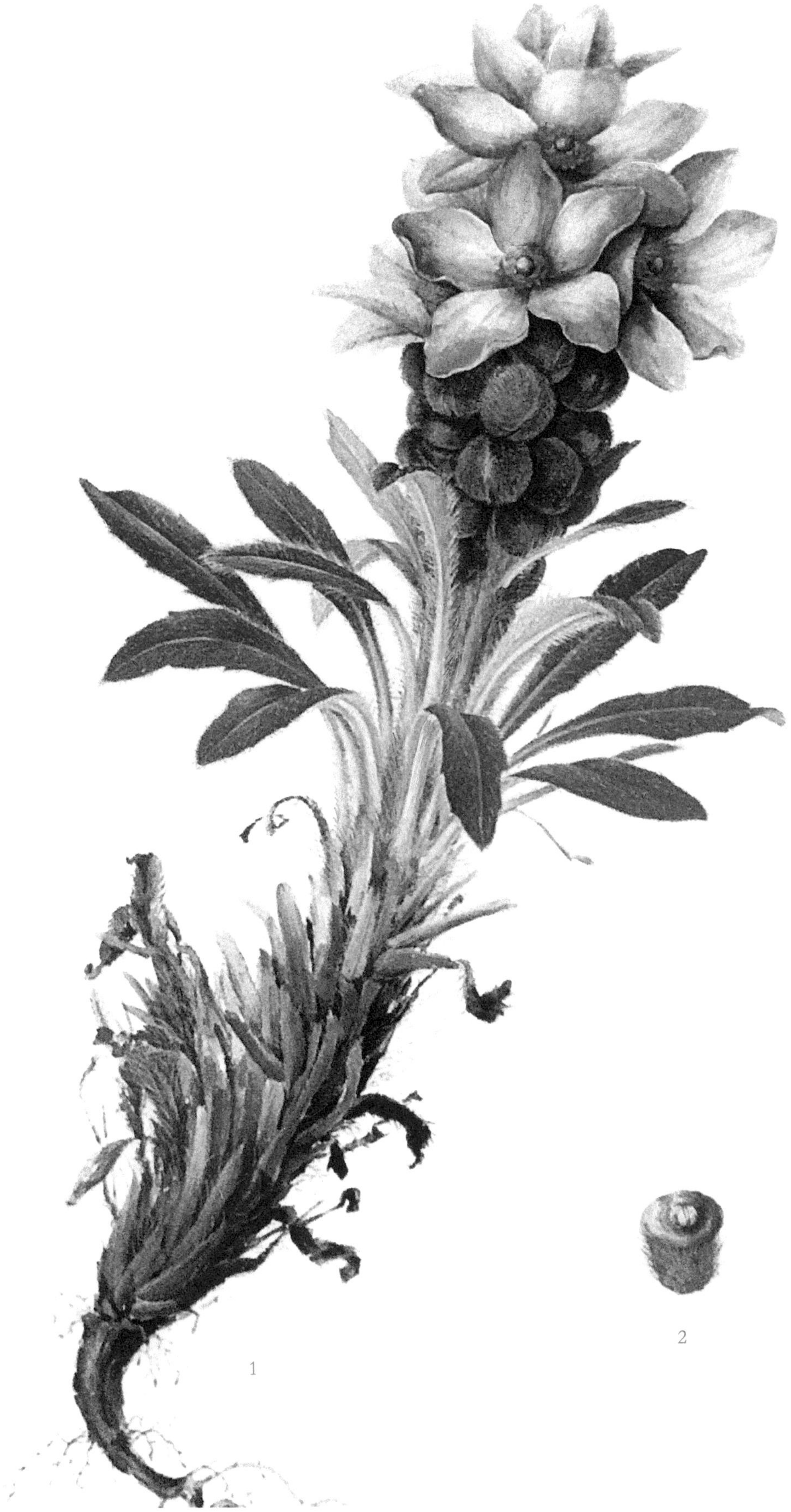

1. 植株（plant）　2. 果实（fruit）

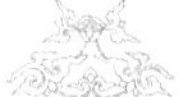

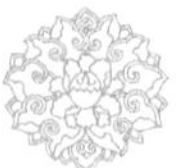

全缘叶绿绒蒿

Quanyuanyelvronghao

Meconopsis integrifolia

基　　源　罂粟科 Papaveraceae 绿绒蒿属 *Meconopsis* 植物全缘叶绿绒蒿 *Meconopsis integrifolia* (Maxim.) Franch. 的干燥全草。药材名为“全缘叶绿绒蒿”。

形态特征　一年生至多年生草本。全株被锈色和金黄色平展或反曲、多短分枝的长柔毛。茎粗壮，不分枝。基生叶莲座状，叶片倒披针形、倒卵形或匙形；茎生叶互生。花通常 4-5 朵，生于茎生叶叶腋内；花瓣 6-8，黄色，近圆形。蒴果。

生境分布　分布于喜马拉雅山区及横断山区高原。生于海拔 3800-5000 m 的高山灌丛、山坡、草甸。

采收加工　7-8 月采收全草，洗净，阴干。

性味功能　寒，苦、涩；有小毒。清热利湿，止咳。

主治用法　主要用于肺炎咳嗽，湿热黄疸，水肿，创伤久不愈合。

化学成分　全草含有机酸、强心苷、挥发油、鞣质、生物碱等成分。

备　　注　常用藏药。

Source　It is the dried herb of *Meconopsis integrifolia* (Maxim.) Franch. (Papaveraceae). The medicinal material is called as “Quanyuanyelvronghao”.

Distribution　*M. integrifolia* is distributed in the Himalayas and Hengduan Mountain plateau. It grows in the shrubs, hillsides and meadows on the mountains at an altitude of 3800–5000 m.

Indications　It is used to treat cough caused by pneumonitis, jaundice due to dampness–heat, edema, and wounds that do not heal for a long time.

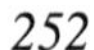

Chemical Constituents　The herb contains organic acids, cardiac glycosides, volatile oils, tannins, alkaloids, etc.

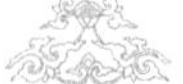

Note　It is a used as Tibetan medicine.

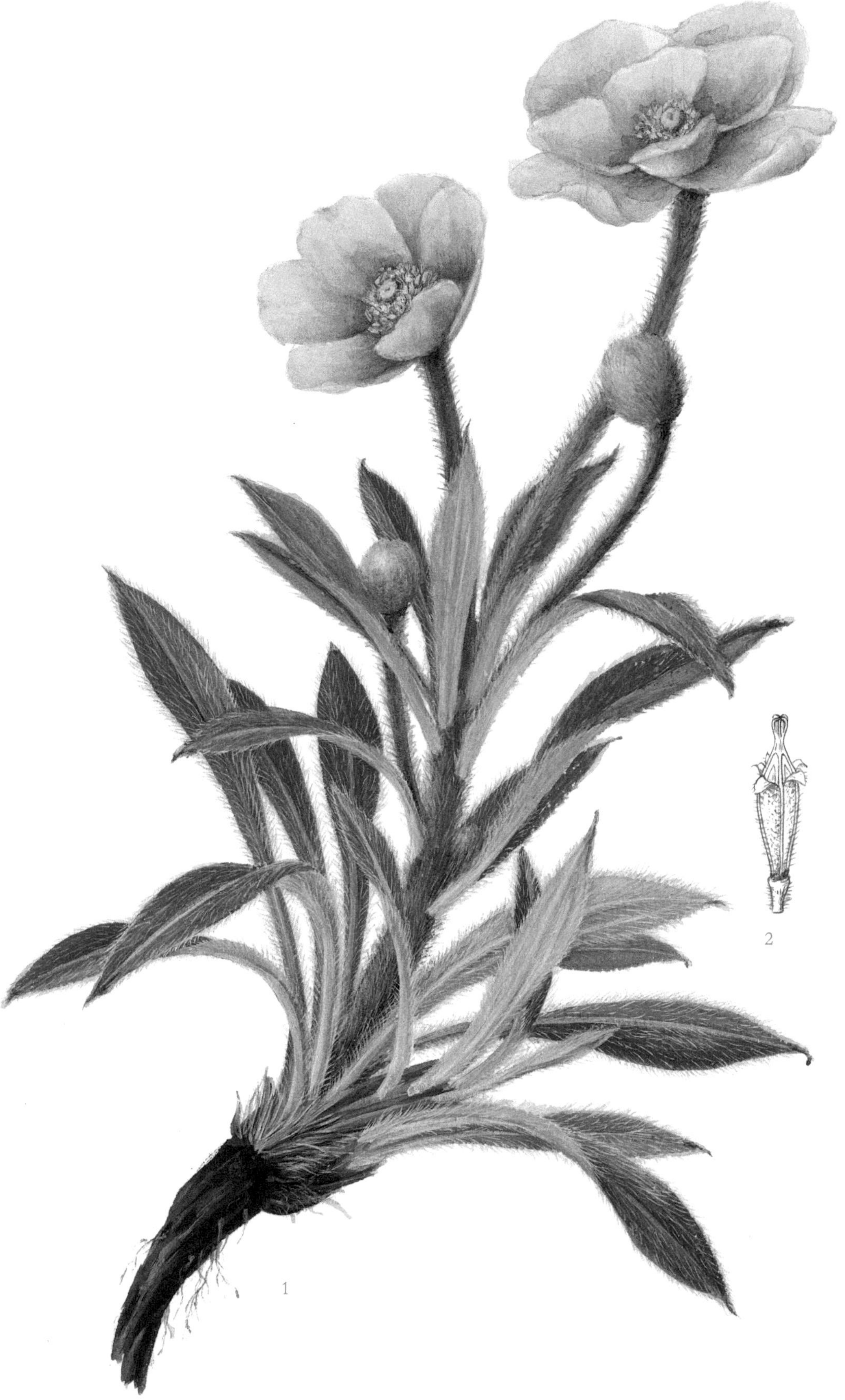

全缘叶绿绒蒿

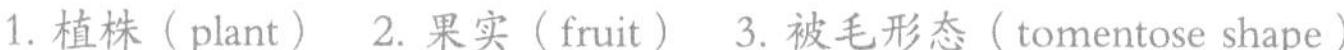

1. 植株（plant） 2. 果实（fruit） 3. 被毛形态（tomentose shape）

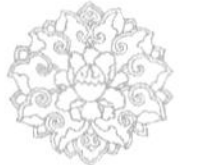

多刺绿绒蒿

Duocilvronghao

Meconopsis horridula

基　　源　罂粟科 Papaveraceae 绿绒蒿属 *Meconopsis* 植物多刺绿绒蒿 *Meconopsis horridula* Hook. f. et Thoms. 的干燥全草。药材名为“多刺绿绒蒿”。

形态特征　一年生草本。全株被黄褐色的毛状刺。叶基生，披针形，全缘或波状，两面被黄褐色平展的刺。花葶坚硬，通常 5-12；花单生于花葶上，半下垂，萼片 2，具淡黄色毛状刺，绿色，早落；花瓣 4-8，蓝紫色，宽倒卵形。蒴果卵形或长圆形，被锈色或黄褐色平展或反曲的刺。

生境分布　分布于喜马拉雅山区及横断山区高原。生于海拔 4000 m 以上的石滩、草地中。

采收加工　夏季采收，除去泥土和杂质，切段，阴干。

性味功能　寒，苦；有小毒。活血化瘀，清热解毒。

主治用法　主要用于跌打损伤，骨折，胸背疼痛，风热头痛，关节肿痛。

化学成分　全草含有生物碱，如原阿片碱、黄连碱、别隐品碱、黑水罂粟碱甲醚、罂粟红碱等成分。

备　　注　常用藏药。

Source　It is the dried herb of *Meconopsis horridula* Hook. f. et Thoms. (Papaveraceae). The medicinal material is called as “Duocilvronghao”.

Distribution　*M. horridula* is distributed in the Himalayas and the Hengduan Mountain plateau. It grows on the rocky beaches and grasslands at an altitude of more than 4000 m.

Indications　It is used to treat traumatic injury, fracture, chest and back pain, wind–heat headache, and joint pain and swelling.

Chemical Constituents　The herb contains alkaloids, e.g., protopine, coptisine, allocryptopine, amurensinine, papaverrubine, etc.

Note　It is a commonly-used medicinal material in Tibetan medicine.

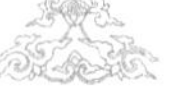

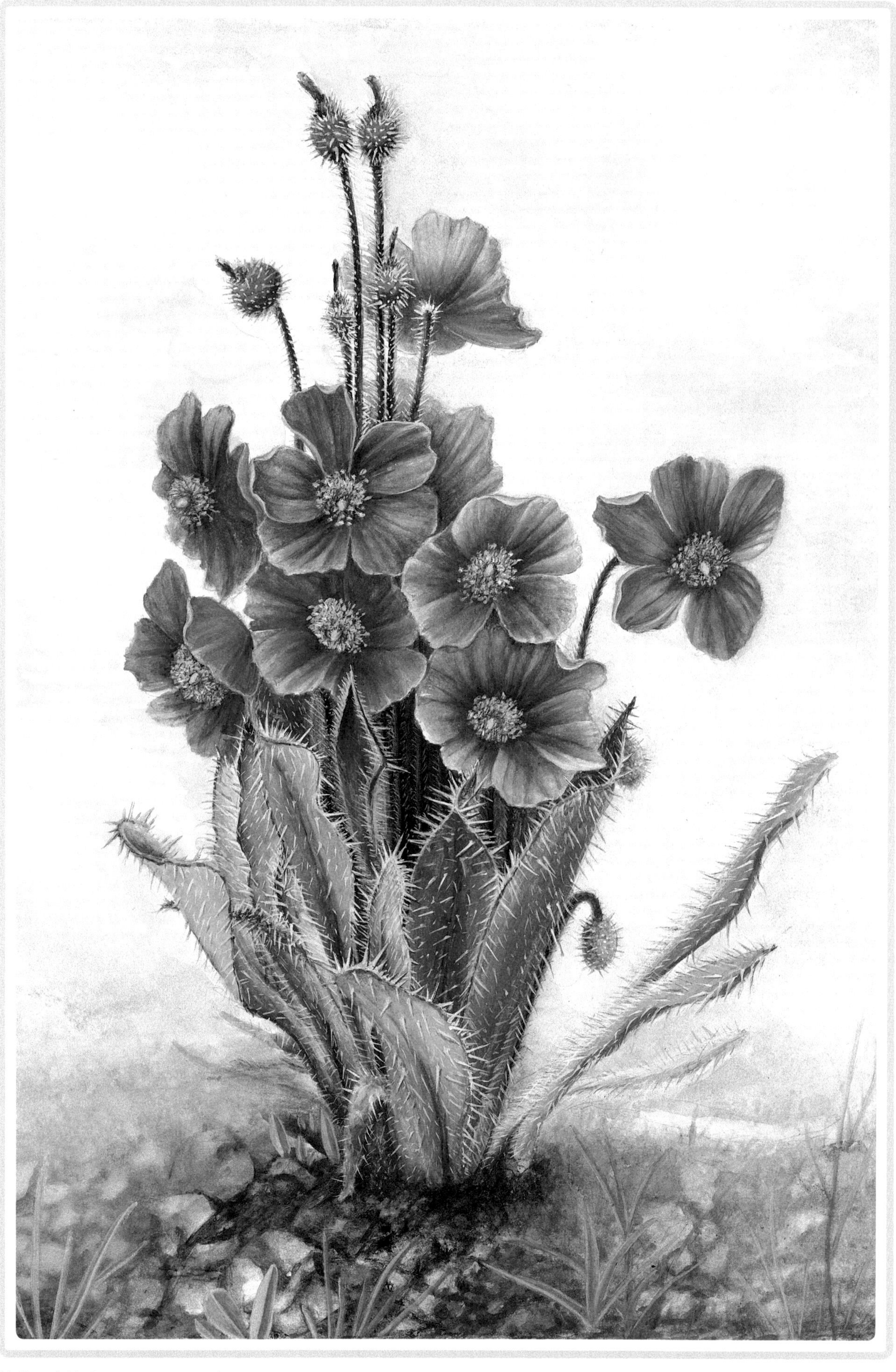

植株及生境（plant and habitat）

红花绿绒蒿

Honghualvronghao

Meconopsis punicea

基　源　罂粟科 Papaveraceae 绿绒蒿属 *Meconopsis* 植物红花绿绒蒿 *Meconopsis punicea* Maxim. 的干燥带花全草。药材名为“红花绿绒蒿”。

形态特征　多年生草本。须根纤维状。叶全部基生，莲座状，叶片倒披针形或狭倒卵形，两面密被淡黄色或棕褐色的刚毛；叶柄基部略扩大成鞘。花葶 1-6，从莲座叶丛中生出；花单生于花葶上，下垂；萼片卵形；花瓣多为 4，椭圆形，深红色。蒴果椭圆状长圆形，被淡黄色，具分枝的刚毛；种子密具乳突。

生境分布　分布于四川西北部、西藏东北部、青海东南部和甘肃西南部，生于海拔 2800-4300 m 的山坡草地。

采收加工　花盛开期采收全草，晒干。

性味功能　寒，苦。清热解毒，利湿，止痛。

主治用法　用于高热，肺结核，肺炎，肝炎，痛经，湿热水肿，头痛，高血压等。

化学成分　主要含有香草酸、肉桂酸、香豆酸、异鼠李素、威尔士绿绒蒿定碱、阿包碱等。

Source　It is the dried herb with flowers of *Meconopsis punicea* Maxim.(Papaveraceae). The medicinal material is called as “Honghualvronghao”.

Distribution　*M. punicea* is distributed in northwest Sichuan, northeast Tibet, southeast Qinghai, and southwest Gansu. It grows on grassland on hillside at an altitude of 2800–4300 m.

Indications　It is used to treat high fever, pulmonary tuberculosis, pneumonia, hepatitis, dysmenorrhea, edema due to dampness–heat, headache, hypertension, etc.

Chemical Constituents　It mainly contains vanillic acid, cinnamic acid, coumaric acid, isorhamnetin, mecambridine, alborine, etc.

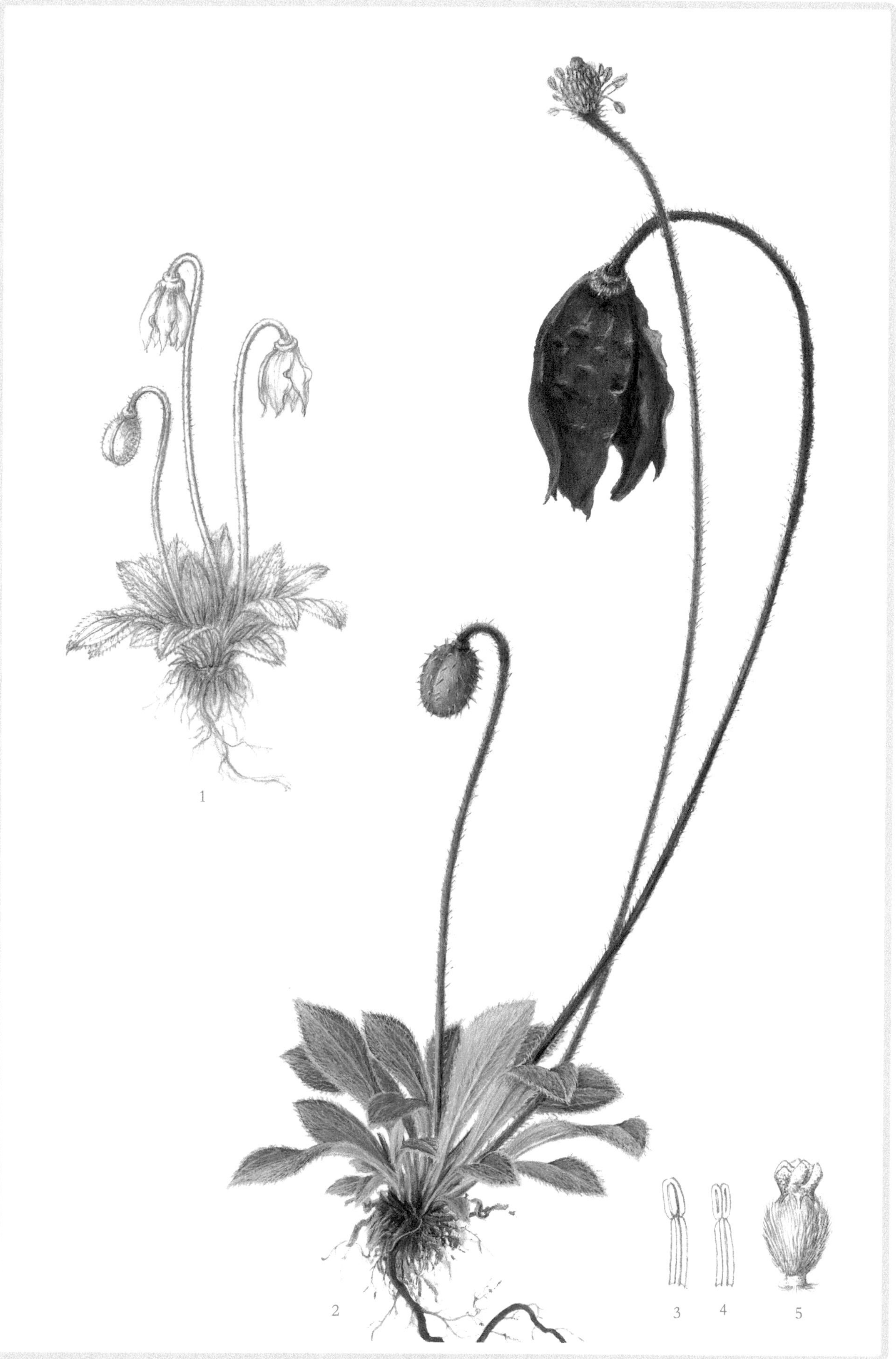

1
2
3
4
5

1~2. 植株（plant） 3~4. 雄蕊（stamen） 5. 果实（fruit）

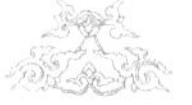

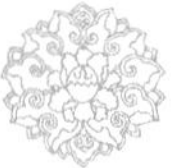

冬虫夏草

Dongchongxiacao
Cordyceps sinensis

基　　源　麦角菌科 Clavicipitaceae 虫草属 *Cordyceps* 真菌冬虫夏草菌 *Cordyceps sinensis* (Berk.) Sacc. 寄生在蝙蝠蛾科昆虫幼虫上的子座和幼虫尸体的干燥复合体。药材名为“冬虫夏草”。

形态特征　虫体与从虫头部长出的真菌子座相连而成。虫体似蚕，表面深黄色至黄棕色，有环纹20-30个，近头部的环纹较细；头部红棕色，足8对，中部4对较明显。子座细长圆柱形；表面深棕色至棕褐色，有细纵皱纹，上部稍膨大。

生境分布　分布于四川西部、青海、西藏等地。生于海拔4000 m以上的具有积雪、排水良好的高寒草甸。

采收加工　夏初子座出土、孢子未发散时挖取，晒至六七成干，除去似纤维状的附着物及杂质，晒干或低温干燥。

性味功能　平，甘。补肾益肺，止血化痰。

主治用法　主要用于肾虚精亏，阳痿遗精，腰膝酸痛，久咳虚喘，劳嗽咯血。

化学成分　冬虫夏草全体中主要含有虫草酸、糖类、蛋白质、麦角脂醇、生物碱等。

备　　注　冬虫夏草不可药食两用，也不能作为保健品的原料。

Source　It is the complex of stroma of *Cordyceps sinensis* (Berk.) Sacc. (Clavicipitaceae) parasitizing on larval corpse from Hepialidate family. The medicinal material is called as “Dongchongxiacao”.

Distribution　It is mainly distributed in western Sichuan, Qinghai, Tibet, etc. It grows in well drained and snowy alpine meadows at an altitude of over 4000 m.

Indications　It is used to treat kidney deficiency and essence depletion, impotence and seminal emission, soreness and pain of the lower back and knee, chronic cough with deficiency-type dyspnea, overstrain cough with hemoptysis.

Chemical Constituents　Cordyceps mainly contains cordycepic acid, saccharides, protein, ergosterol, alkaloids, etc.

Note　Cordyceps is not considered as medicine and food and cannot be used as a raw ingredient for health products.

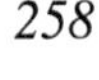

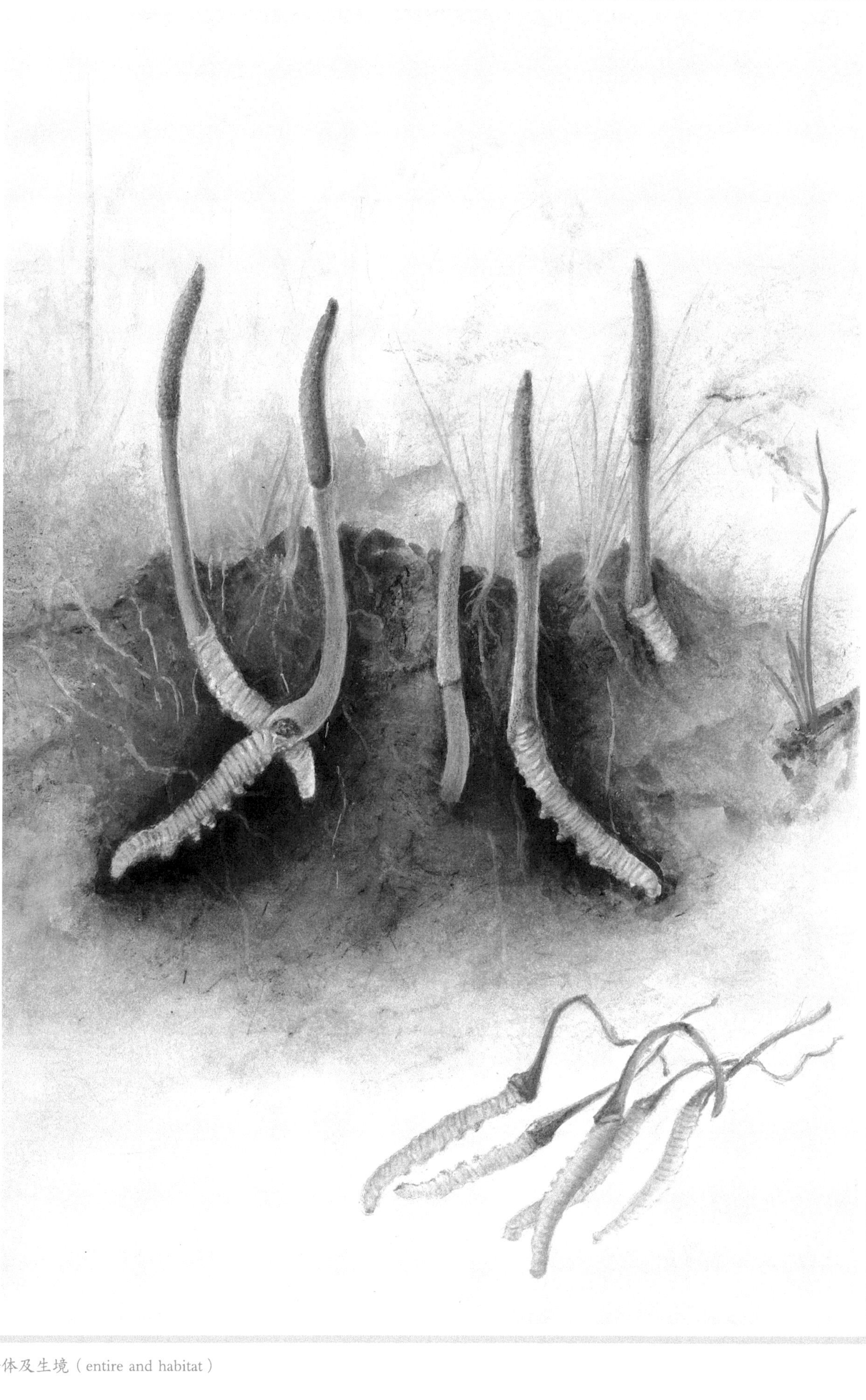

全体及生境（entire and habitat）

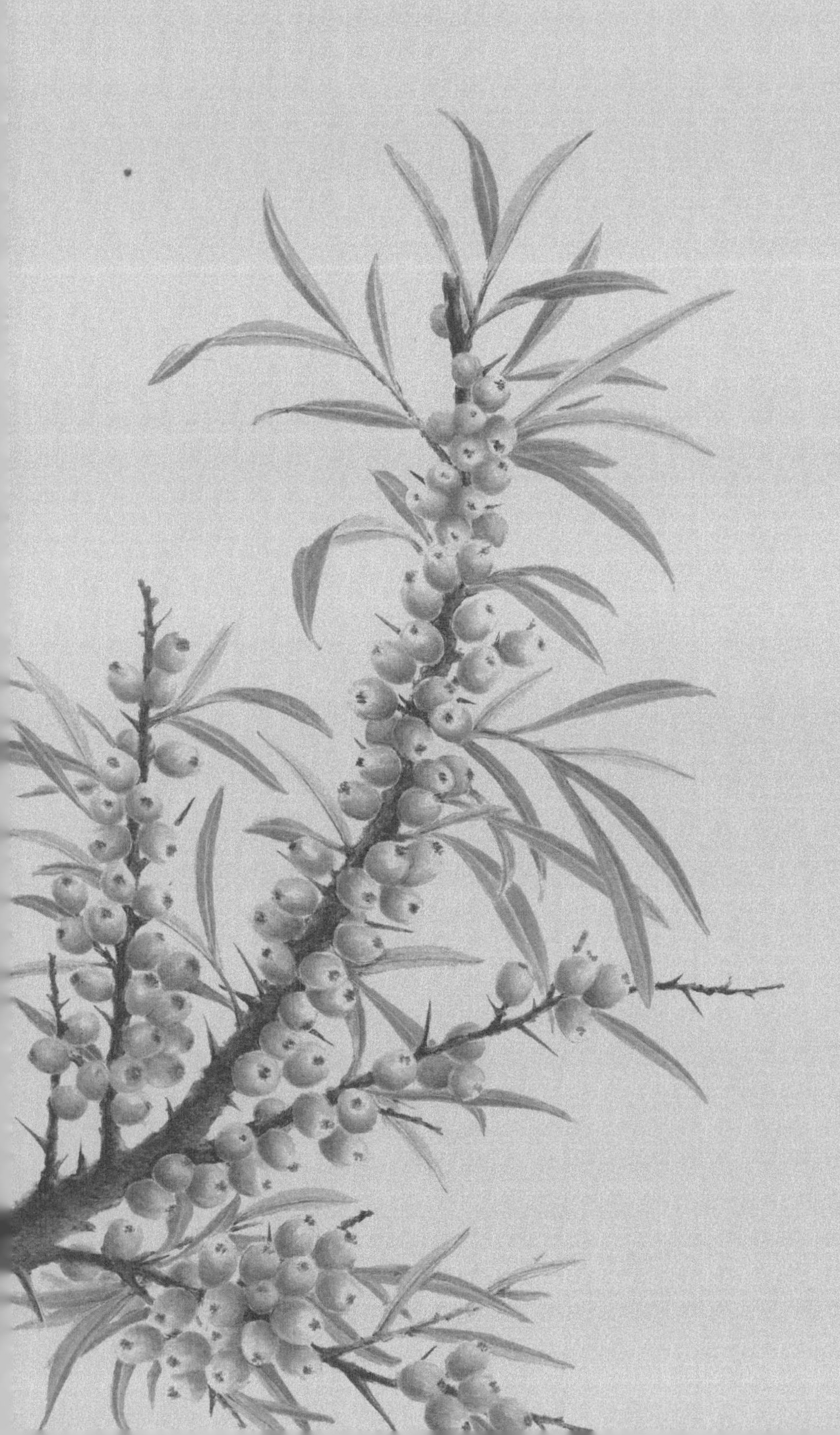

中文名索引 Chinese Index

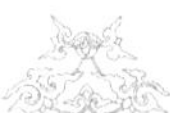

J

K

L

M

N

P

Q

R

S

拉丁学名索引
Latin Index

A

B

C

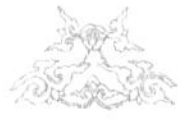

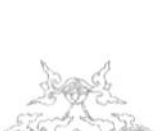

药材名索引
Medicinal Material Index

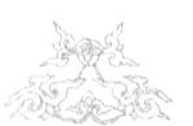

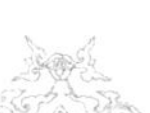

相从心生，画如其人，人如其名

《精绘中华本草》读后感

陈月明同志

参加协作纪念

《汇编》编写组赠

一九七八年六月

谢宗万教授代表《全国中草药汇编》编写组致谢月明老师

2022 年初，月明老师约我担任《精绘中华本草》一书的主审，接到此信，我心中惴惴不安，深恐难堪此重任。可当我打开书稿，一幅幅画作，映入眼帘，如诗如歌，月明老师将大自然与药用植物之美，通过自己的画笔记录，提炼，升华，让我陶醉其中、兴奋不已，我有幸成为了本书的第一个读者。

月明老师的名字，早在 1982 年，我刚到中国中医科学院中药研究所读硕士研究生时，就已经非常熟悉了。那段时间，我的导师谢宗万教授刚刚主持完成了《全国中草药汇编》，书中不少精美娴熟的墨线工笔绘图，就是出自月明老师之手。

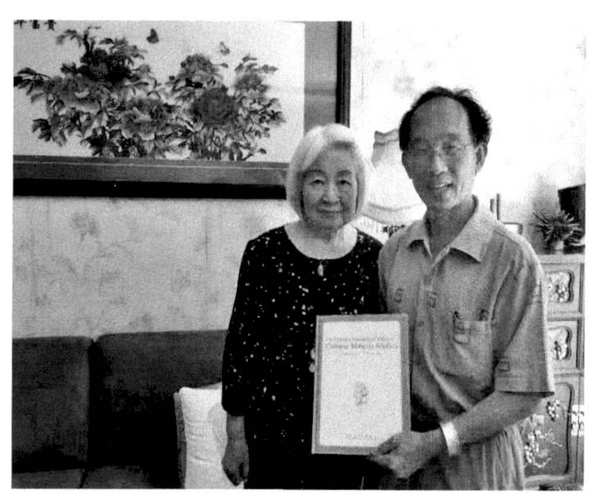

中振教授与月明老师合影

1984 年一次偶然的机会，我第一次见到月明老师，地点不是在北京，而是在中国科学院昆明植物研究所。月明老师为人真诚、和蔼可亲，全然没有艺术家的派头，但却有艺术家的气质，特别是那双清澈明亮的眼睛。

第二次与月明老师见面是在 2019

年，转瞬间，35 年过去了，月明老师依旧是那样的精神矍铄，思维敏捷、开朗健谈。

这次我是与彭勇博士一同去月明老师家共同探讨出版《精绘中华本草》的事宜。谈话之间，月明老师向我们展示了她的一幅描述植物病虫害的作品，并兴致勃勃地向我们讲起了这幅画创作背后的故事。

那是 1977 年的一天，月明老师正在植物园散步，她见到了几只小虫，正在起劲地啃着马兜铃的叶子，旁边还有两只翩翩起舞的蝴蝶相伴。强烈的求知欲与探索精神，让她停了下来，对大自然的观察，激发了她的创作灵感。她亲手用网子捕捉了蝴蝶，制成标本。并请动物学专家加以鉴定复核，以求准确无误。

月明老师把带有虫体的植物枝叶采回家，泡在水里，就像养蚕人一般，精心呵护，一只只似小蚂蚁般的幼虫逐渐长大，最后成蛹，化蝶产卵，结束了一个完整的生命周期。伴随着画作的完成，月明老师家里也俨然成了一个小的昆虫馆。有时她作画，小虫还会爬到她的手臂上相陪伴。 正是这种悉心的观察与执着，才诞生了惟妙惟肖的传神之作。

月明老师还高兴地告诉我，她的这幅作品，得到了她曾进修学习的北京师范学院（现首都师范大学）美术系工笔花鸟画教学的吴敏荣教授的高度赞许：这是一幅将中国工笔画与现代科学画结合的代表之作，也是月明老师专业日臻成熟的标志。

月明老师并没因此而满足，而是保持这种干劲、这种精神，她创作的脚步一直没有停歇，此后新作不断，艺术达到了炉火纯青的程度，这也就是今天展现在我们面前的《精绘中华本草》集锦。

月明老师人如其名，清澈如月、心地透明。她胸怀一颗永远的童心，身上永远焕发着青春的活力。年届九十的她，鹤发童颜，似从画中走来，人们常说相由心生，正所谓，腹有诗书气自华。多年的艺术熏陶、生活的感悟，历练，使得她儒雅中伴随着一股仙气。

与月明老师话别之际，她送我出门，并执意送我过马路，就像是幼儿园的阿姨在带小朋友过街一样，一边走一边叮嘱：你多年不在北京，不熟悉这里的交通秩序，别碰着呀。

致敬月明老师，我为月明老师而骄傲，而自豪。虽然现代植物科学画起源于西方，但月明老师让世界看到中国也有科学画，而且中国植物科学画的水平站在了世界级的前列。看月明老师的植物科学画，是一种专业知识的学习，是一种艺术的享受，从中能体会到艺术家笔下植物的神韵与意境。

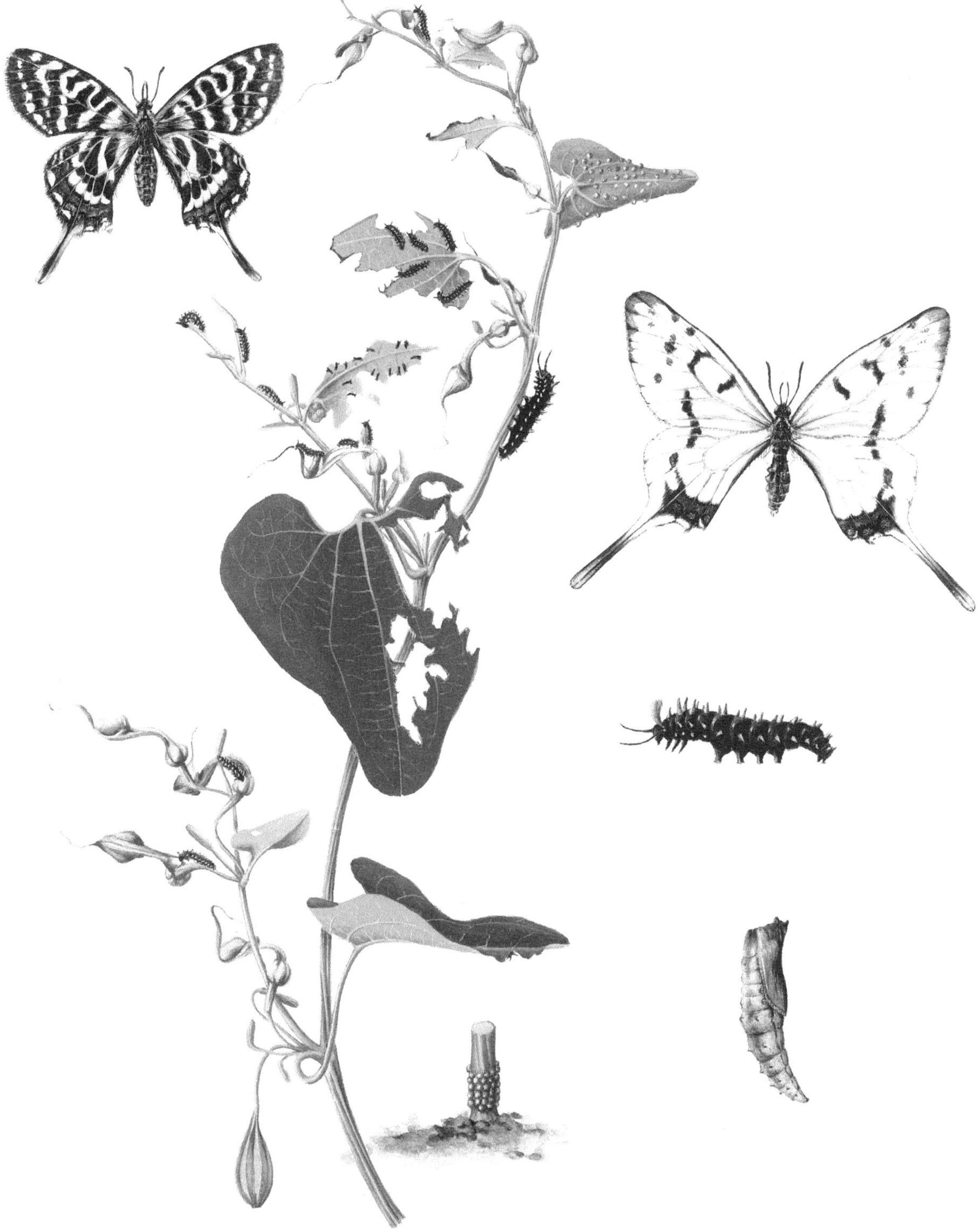

马兜铃虫害图（绘于 1977 年）

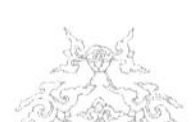

“上天给了我一双好的眼睛，我还要继续画下去。”鲐背之年还在坚持本草科学画的创作，这并不是传说，这是发生在我们身边的故事，这个传奇还在继续……

后学　中振[①]

2022 年 12 月 14 日

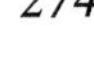

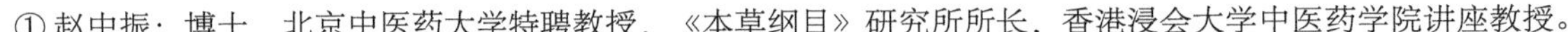

① 赵中振：博士，北京中医药大学特聘教授，《本草纲目》研究所所长，香港浸会大学中医药学院讲座教授。

Appearance reflects the heart; art reflects the person; the person reflects their name

Impressions of *Scientific Illustrations of Chinese Medicinal Plants*

In early 2022, Professor Yueming invited me to be the chief reviewer of her *Scientific Illustrations of Chinese Medicinal Plants*. When I received the letter, I was worried that I would not be able to take on this important task. However, upon opening the manuscript, the paintings captivated me like beautiful poems and songs. I was enthralled by the way that Prof. Yueming captured the beauty of nature and medicinal plants. I feel fortunate to be the first reader of this book.

Yueming's name was already very familiar to me back in 1982, when I first arrived for my postgraduate studies at the Institute of Chinese Materia Medica of the China Academy of Chinese Medical Sciences. At the time, my supervisor, Professor Xie Zongwan, had just finished the *National Compilation of Chinese Herbal Medicines* and was busy editing the *Treatise on the Varieties of Chinese Materia Medica* . Many of the exquisite, beautiful ink drawings in that book were created by Yueming.

In 1984, I met Yueming for the first time by chance, not in Beijing, but at the Kunming Institute of Botany of the Chinese Academy of Sciences. She seemed sincere and amiable; while she did not have the style of an artist, she had the distinctive quality of an artist, which was particularly evident through her clear and bright eyes.

The second time we met was in 2019. While 35 years had passed in the blink of an eye, Yueming was still energetic, sharp, cheerful and talkative.

This time I joined Dr. Peng Yong at Yueming's house to discuss the publication of *Scientific Illustrations of Chinese Medicinal Plants*. In the conversation, she showed us one of her paintings depicting plant pests and diseases, and enthusiastically told us the

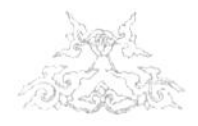

story behind the creation of the painting.

One day, while Yueming was walking in the botanical garden, she spotted several caterpillars nibbling on the leaves of an *Aristolochia* plant, accompanied by two fluttering butterflies. A strong curiosity and spirit of exploration made her stop, and the observations of nature inspired her creativity. She captured the butterflies in nets by herself and made them into specimens. She asked zoological experts to review and identify the specimens.

At the same time, Yueming collected the leaves and branches bearing caterpillars and kept them in water. Just like a silkworm breeder, she took great care of them and observed them continuously. A larva as small as an ant gradually matured and turned into a pupa, then finally transformed into a butterfly and laid eggs. As the paintings were completed, the butterfly also completed its life cycle. At times, the little black larva would even crawl on her arm as she was drawing, and her office became like a small insect museum.

Yueming happily told me that this work received high praise from Professor Wu Minrong, who taught flower-and-bird fine brushwork painting at the College of Fine Arts of Beijing Normal University (current Capital Normal University), where she previously studied. Professor Wu said: "This piece is a combination of Chinese brush painting and modern scientific painting that represents Yueming's professional maturity."

Yueming remained unsatisfied and continued with the same motivation and spirit. She has never stopped, constantly creating new pieces, and her art has reached the level of mastery. The collection *Scientific Illustrations of Chinese Medicinal Plants* presented today is an evocative work, the fruit of sixty years of her pursuit and persistence.

True to her name, Yueming is clear like the moon and bright in her heart. She has a youthful heart, and her body is glowing with vigor. At the age of ninety, she has white hair with a childlike face, as if a person stepped out of a painting. Her appearance reflects her inner heart; evoking the expression "a poetic spirit within the belly." Her years of artistic training, perception, and experience have made her an elegant with a sense of immortality.

When I left, she walked me out and insisted on taking me across the street, just like a teacher helping children cross the street. She said: "you have not been in Beijing for

many years and are not familiar with the traffic here, be careful and safe."

I am very honored to have the chance to pay my respects to Yueming. Although modern scientific botanical paintings originated in the West, Yueming showed the world that China also has world-class scientific paintings. Viewing Yueming's botanical illustrations brings together professional knowledge with the enjoyment of art, and her brushstrokes reveal the charm and spirit of the plants.

"I have been given a good set of eyes, and I will continue to paint." Even in her old age, she continues to produce scientific paintings of herbal medicines. This is not a legend, it is a story that took place around us, and it is a legend that is still continuing...

Zhongzhen

December 14, 2022

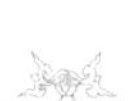